Physiology of Exercise and Healthy Aging

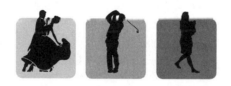

Albert W. Taylor, PhD, DSc
University of Western Ontario

Michel J. Johnson, PhD
Lakehead University, Thunder Bay, Ontario

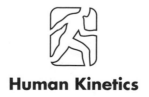

Human Kinetics

Library of Congress Cataloging-in-Publication Data

Taylor, Albert W.
  Physiology of exercise and healthy aging / Albert W. Taylor, Michel
J. Johnson.
      p. cm.
  Includes bibliographical references and index.
  ISBN-13: 978-0-7360-5838-4 (hard cover)
  ISBN-10: 0-7360-5838-9 (hard cover)
  1. Aging--Physiological aspects. 2. Exercise--Physiological aspects.
3. Exercise for older people--Physiological aspects. I. Johnson,
Michel J., 1966- II. Title.
  [DNLM: 1. Aging--physiology. 2. Exercise--physiology. WT 104 T238p
2007]
  QP86.T29 2007
  612'.044
                                                        2007019595

ISBN-10: 0-7360-5838-9
ISBN-13: 978-0-7360-5838-4

Acquisitions Editor: Judy Patterson Wright, PhD; **Developmental Editor:** Elaine H. Mustain; **Assistant Editor:** Melissa McCasky; **Copyeditor:** Joyce Sexton; **Proofreader:** Anne Rogers; **Indexer:** Sharon Duffy; **Permission Manager:** Dalene Reeder; **Graphic Designer:** Robert Reuther; **Photo Manager:** Laura Fitch; **Photo Office Assistant:** Jason Allen; **Cover Designer:** Keith Blomberg; **Photographer (cover):** Shalom Ormsby/Blend Images/Getty Images; **Photographer (interior):** © Human Kinetics, unless otherwise noted; **Art Manager:** Kelly Hendren; **Illustrator:** Mic Greenberg; **Printer:** Sheridan Books

Printed in the United States of America   10   9   8   7   6   5   4   3   2

Human Kinetics
Web site: www.HumanKinetics.com

United States: Human Kinetics, P.O. Box 5076, Champaign, IL 61825-5076
800-747-4457
e-mail: humank@hkusa.com

Canada: Human Kinetics, 475 Devonshire Road, Unit 100, Windsor, ON N8Y 2L5
800-465-7301 (in Canada only)
e-mail: info@hkcanada.com

Europe: Human Kinetics, 107 Bradford Road, Stanningley
Leeds LS28 6AT, United Kingdom
+44 (0) 113 255 5665
e-mail: hk@hkeurope.com

Australia: Human Kinetics, 57A Price Avenue, Lower Mitcham, South Australia 5062
08 8372 0999
e-mail: info@hkaustralia.com

New Zealand: Human Kinetics, Division of Sports Distributors NZ Ltd.
P.O. Box 300 226 Albany, North Shore City, Auckland
0064 9 448 1207
e-mail: info@humankinetics.co.nz

We dedicate this book to our wives, Catherine and Nicole, without whose constant love and support this book would never have reached fruition.

contents

foreword

It is a great pleasure and indeed an honor for me to commend Dr. Taylor's timely book *Physiology of Exercise and Healthy Aging*. Bert and I both remember a landmark in the Canadian history of health and fitness: the year 1961, when the federal government enacted Bill C 131, "an act to encourage fitness and amateur sport." One of the consequences of that act was a decision to establish three fitness research units to be distributed across Canada in a politically correct manner. One opened in the prairie city of Edmonton (where Dr. Bert Taylor was quickly named director), a second was opened in central Canada (which brought me to Toronto), and a third was destined for La Belle Province in Montreal. Until that point, Canadian students had lacked opportunity for doctoral studies in exercise science, but our units quickly spurred the University of Alberta and University of Toronto to remedy the deficiency.

Canadian interest in fitness quickly expanded and began to encompass not only healthy young adults but also older people and those with cardiovascular disease. Dr. Peter Rechnitzer of the University of Western Ontario initiated a multicenter, randomized controlled trial of exercise for postcoronary patients, and when this study was completed, the faculty of physical education at Western decided to apply similar tactics and techniques to a large-scale study of healthy aging. After they received their doctorates, several of my students became involved in this initiative, and Dr. Bert Taylor was tempted to move from the University of Alberta to serve as dean of an expanding faculty of physical education at the University of Western Ontario.

Bert and I have had parallel career paths for more than 40 years. I also have learned both to respect his accumulated wisdom and to admire the outstanding research conducted by the Canadian Centre for Activity and Aging (CCAA) at the University of Western Ontario. Now that Bert and I are both reaching the critical phase of our lives, I am pleased that Dr. Taylor has taken the time to refine the tremendous volume of scientific and practical knowledge accumulated by his research group and to present it in such a readable format. The integration of information on exercise, nutrition, and pharmacotherapy for very elderly people, the attention directed to female exercisers, and the careful consideration of needs in those with chronic disease are particularly valuable features of this text. In our ever-aging world,

Dr. Taylor's book should make an important contribution to the more complete instruction of students, health professionals, and allied health professionals in physical education, exercise science, and fitness and health in Canada, the United States, and beyond.

Roy J. Shephard

preface

Aging is a concept that for most of recorded history has referred to relatively few individuals, in particular those who have surpassed the age of 90. In this new millennium it appears that we will be forced to redefine what aging truly means. No longer is reaching 100 years considered an oddity or a miracle or even a rare occurrence. The fastest-growing population cohort in North America is that portion over the age of 85 years. These demographics not only demonstrate the serious population dynamics that have taken place over the past 20 or so years, but also indicate the age transition that will likely occur in the next two decades. The implications for many facets of our society are the basis for a great deal of concern in areas as diverse as geography and economics.

Society's Stake in Exercise and Aging

The rapidly aging population is a grave issue for the health care system. The decreasing birth rate in North America, when coupled with the increase in the number of senior citizens, places present health care systems in jeopardy. The increasing costs of our medical and paramedical care systems will be borne by fewer and fewer individuals and, in particular, taxpayers. A solution that is not based on increased fees and medical costs must be found in order to avoid complete collapse of the present systems. Although basic and clinical research have contributed to increased longevity, the question of reduced morbidity appears to have been responded to primarily through increased research on and the use of drug therapy. Yet the correct response must come from a combination of better living conditions, improved nutrition, and adequate physical activity.

Over the past few years, obesity has become pandemic in Canada and the United States, if not the entire industrialized world. This problem must not be permitted to become chronic. People in their teenage years are contracting type 2 diabetes and various forms of cardiovascular diseases including early onset of heart attacks. The primary causes of these maladies are poor nutrition choices and inadequate physical activity. The fact that these diseases are attacking young people does not bode well for the total population as it ages. In fact, if the present situation continues to broaden in scope, not only the health care system, but the total population, will be in serious difficulty.

Physical Activity and Health: A Report of the Surgeon General (1996) provided evidence for the beneficial effects of exercise on several diseases and maladies. Exercise is a preventive tool to reduce, or, in some instances, offset the deleterious effects of such maladies as type 2 diabetes, colon cancer in men, breast cancer in women, obesity, osteoporosis, osteoarthritis, and cardiovascular disease. Most of these medical problems are exacerbated in older individuals. In fact, it is not unusual for elderly people to suffer from a combination of several of them. Such is the not-so-wonderful world of aging. The years of life after age 65 are often referred to as "the golden years." Few people in this age-group would accept this definition if given the opportunity. Instead, a new form of discrimination has developed, called ageism, in which elderly people are looked down upon because of problems they exhibit that are, for the most part, beyond their control. However, several of the problems related to aging are controllable—or at least they can be delayed and their progress retarded. Exercise is not the elixir for healthy living, but a regular regime of physical activity has been shown to decrease morbidity and increase the quality of life enjoyed by our elderly population.

An Emerging Area of Study

Although exercise physiology has been an accepted science for more than 50 years, few papers have been written on the effects of exercise on people in older age-groups. Unfortunately, most such research has involved only males as subjects, and the majority of the papers have been about healthy individuals. However, changing demographics, which lead to the prediction that as many as 25% of the North American populace will be over 65 years of age by the year 2025, have prompted increasing investigation of the aging phenomenon and the perturbations that affect healthy aging. As well, since women, overall, lead longer lives than men in most societies, a special interest in longevity in women has arisen. It was not too many years ago that exercise was either contraindicated or thought to be inappropriate for females, especially older women. Now with the knowledge that exercise can serve as a preventive measure for a number of maladies, in particular those considered to be more prevalent in women (for example, osteoporosis), a number of research laboratories and individual researchers have taken a renewed interest in the effects of exercise on aging. The effects of aging and physical inactivity are reasonably well known for men, in relation to coronary heart disease (CHD) in particular, but preventive exercise for the elderly has seldom received adequate attention. Moreover, the renewed interest in exercise as a form of preventive medicine has resulted in the introduction of many exercise regimens that are unproven and may actually be harmful to participants.

In this book, however, we have attempted to define what healthy aging truly is and the effects that regular exercise routines have not only on longevity, but also on decreased morbidity. Too often textbooks are written with too narrow a focus. We have tried to avoid this limitation by integrating the science of exercise physiology with that of aging as an undeniable and irreversible biological phenomenon. We have attempted to show that with proper exercise prescription, this phenomenon can be retarded and also that specific diseases of aging can be delayed and their insidious effects ameliorated. We have explored the physical and cognitive processes of aging and the effects of appropriate, safe exercise on adherence and physiological improvement in seniors. We emphasize screening and assessment and the basic principles of exercise for elderly persons, as well as training programs for the complete spectrum of seniors, including frail elderly, so-called normal seniors, and masters athletes. A unique aspect of this text is that we discuss these topics in conjunction with scientific concepts of basic physiology and information on the diseases of aging.

The Focus and Substance of the Text

This text is written explicitly for students with an interest in the aging process and the effects that exercise has on the quality of life of those who are aging. It is expected that the students using this book as a course textbook or as auxiliary reading for a course will have taken at least an introductory course in human physiology. The text refers throughout to the three groups in the aging and health spectrum: the frail elderly, average aging individuals, and masters athletes.

Chapters present basic concepts of physiology as they relate to the process of aging, an exercise regimen appropriate to the topic discussed in the chapter, contraindicated exercises, and forms of physical activity that have proven to be beneficial to the aging population. Physiological responses to acute and chronic exercise perturbations are examined, including those observed in studies dealing with cardiorespiratory fitness; muscle metabolism and strength; neurophysiology and the senses; and the diseases of aging, including type 2 diabetes, osteoporosis, arthritis, and cardiovascular diseases. Questions that could serve as potential examination questions and that test the knowledge of the reader on the materials covered appear at the end of each chapter.

Additional material in the book includes information related to the process of aging, masters athletes, prevention of falls, international demographics, and theories of aging. References include Web sites where additional information can be retrieved, as well as printed sources.

Reference materials for each chapter appear in *Bibliography and References* at the back of the book. Each chapter presents tables or figures to add visual or statistical information or to reinforce the textual material.

Part I covers the physiological systems (cardiopulmonary, musculoskeletal, nervous, and sensory), age-related changes in the systems, and the effects of physical activity on these systems. Taken together, the chapters in part I review basic physiological concepts and relate these concepts to the process of aging. Chapter 1 discusses several cardiopulmonary diseases whereas chapter 2 addresses arthritis in some detail. Chapter 3 contains information on diseases of the nervous system. The perturbation effects of exercise on the systems in combination with the effects of aging are discussed as well as the effects of exercise on these diseases of aging. The senses are seldom mentioned in texts on exercise physiology, but their relative importance in the aging process makes chapter 4 highly significant.

Part II emphasizes nutritional issues in relation to aging. All aging individuals are encouraged not only to manipulate their diets to serve their daily needs, but also to realize that several diseases of aging are related to serious nutritional complications. In chapter 5 we focus on nutrition for elderly people and the effects of regular exercise on dietary control. Chapter 5 further discusses the onset of type 2 diabetes and the beneficial effects of dietary manipulation and exercise on this disease. In chapter 6 we discuss the problems associated with osteoporosis in those who are elderly, the preventive effects of early exercise, and the beneficial effects of nutrition and exercise on retardation of the disease.

Part III contains material related to physiologic adaptation to training and physical activity for older adults. Chapter 7 presents important information on screening and assessment. Because of the insidious diseases of aging, measures must be taken to protect the safety of elderly people that would not be considered for younger populations. In chapter 7 we discuss the principles of exercise for elderly persons. Although the principles may not seem to differ much from those for younger subjects, the differences are more than subtle because of the combined effects of the aging process. Chapter 8 presents material on training for aerobic and anaerobic processes, and chapter 9 is specific to training for muscular fitness by strength training. Part III also deals with the physiology of exercise for special older groups, namely the ends of the spectrum—the frail elderly and masters athletes. Although the subjects may be of the same age, their fitness levels are very different, and training techniques differ tremendously. Masters athletes are the elite among the elderly population, whereas the frail elderly must be treated with great care as they are highly susceptible to falls and are easily injured.

Additionally, part III deals with certain special and timely issues. Chapter 10 discusses exercise adherence, motivation, and safety measures. Problems specific to exercise in aging are discussed and solutions suggested. Determinants of attrition and behavior management skills and techniques are elucidated. In chapter 11 we discuss the use and abuse of drugs and supplements by elderly exercisers. This is the longest chapter in the book, but the topic is among the most important for exercising older persons and one that is consistently avoided in textbooks. Seniors differ from young individuals in many ways, and no major difference is so prevalent as the use of drugs for medical purposes, and no difference has received so little attention. In contrast to younger people, the vast majority of seniors must use drugs for everyday survival or to ameliorate the problems of aging. Incorporating legitimate drug use into the rules for athletic competitions among seniors has received little consideration from the research community. The dichotomy between abuse and survival, essentially, is nonexistent in young athletes. This question needs to be addressed immediately because of the prevalence of local, national, and international competitions for masters athletes and seniors. We have attempted to elucidate this problem and to offer some recommendations.

Thus, chapter 11 discusses several categories of drugs and relates incidents of abuse in recent world masters championships. It is difficult to comprehend that seniors are losing medals and being banned from sport competition because of drug use. The chapter is an effort to explain the differences in drug use between seniors and younger athletes. The issues of aging and the need for drug prescription for seniors creates a situation in which drug use is more than a question of ethics—it is a matter of good health or even survival.

The book also contains two appendixes that should prove to be informative and useful for students. Sources of information, usually through Web sites, are listed, and students are encouraged to locate this material, which should prove to be beneficial especially for exam purposes.

Because the authors are Canadian and because Canada has taken an international leadership role on questions of physical activity and aging, a great deal of this material has been developed in Canada, some in a collaborative effort with our American colleagues. *Canada's Physical Activity Guide to Healthy Active Living for Older Adults* is the first major attempt to establish a training regimen for the average senior. It is currently found in the office of every family physician in the country, as well as in most fitness clubs. The fact that the Canadian government, via Health Canada, financed the entire project is an excellent example of government collaborating with many private and public agencies. The American College of Sports Medicine position stand on exercise for elderly persons is also a classic example of various groups working together to formulate a most important document on exercise for the aging population.

The tests for screening and assessing elderly persons are published elsewhere, but the specific tests provided in appendix B guarantee easy access for students, in particular for those tests with limited access in the United States. These materials are excellent resource materials for students interested in the process of aging and physical activity.

It is important to note that some tests found in appendix B have been slightly modified. In some cases, we have done this so readers may photocopy the tests and use them with their clients.

We hope readers enjoy the approach taken in this book, that of combining science with practical application, to provide a unique perspective on the exercise physiology of the process of healthy aging.

acknowledgments

The authors of the book are most appreciative of the advice, assistance, and dedication to detail given to us by Dr. Judy Wright, Elaine Mustain, and Melissa McCasky of Human Kinetics. Without their continual positive attitudes and eyes for significant and useful changes, we would probably still be at the analysis stage instead of enjoying this text.

introduction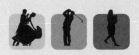

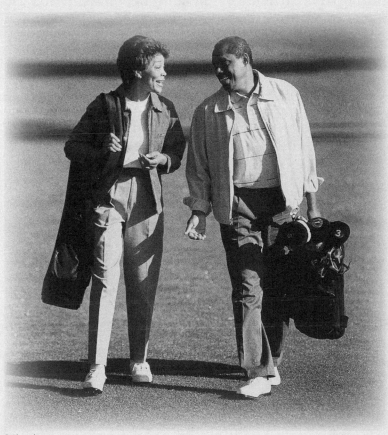
© Photodisc

Aging is a rather nebulous concept. Most of us think in chronological terms, even though we are well aware of differences in the physical appearance of individuals of similar ages. Moreover, we seldom think in terms of those physiologic functions that are not so readily apparent to the eye. The purposes of this introduction are to define the process of aging and to delineate the effects of aging and physical activity on the homeostasis of the human body, as well as to briefly review the scientific theories of aging. Aging is discussed in this book only in physiological and biochemical terms. It is recognized that the process of aging is significantly affected by sociological and psychological factors, but these concepts are beyond the framework of this text. The authors like to abide by the long-held maxim that the human body is made up of and functions through the interaction of electricity and chemicals and therefore consider that all systems are controlled by these two entities in some form.

Two types of aging must be considered: eugeric aging and pathogeric aging. Eugeric aging refers to changes in function that are not produced by disease, that is, a situation that would exist only if we lived in a perfect world or in an environmentally controlled bubble—a world in which humans and other species would reach the maximum achievable life span. Pathogeric aging refers to the aging process as it is affected by environmental perturbations, genetic mutations, and accidents of nature or the human environment.

Types of Aging

Eugeric: true aging; age-related changes that will happen to everyone, inevitably

Pathogeric: pathological aging, not a predestined part of aging

Physical and Cognitive Changes With Aging

As people age, they become aware of numerous visible physical and cognitive changes. Although many of these changes are a part of normal aging, environmental and lifestyle factors can also greatly influence the aging process. We have come to expect that with aging, hair will turn gray and thin out, the skin will lose its elasticity, body shape will change, and wrinkles will appear. Older people are weaker because of loss of muscle mass, which is generally replaced with increased fat distribution. We get shorter because of scoliosis or kyphosis or fallen arches, and older individuals tend to use more prostheses such as wigs and false teeth. Many other physiological changes are obvious with aging. The increased incidence of different stages of dementia appears to have a biochemical or physiological stimulus. Hormone imbalance occurs, the most obvious outcome being menopause, which leads to increased incidence of osteoporosis. And the onset of type 2 diabetes can be due to endocrine changes or neurophysiological changes affecting receptor site sensitivity. These topics are discussed at length in various chapters of this book.

An unanswered question about the many physiologic changes that occur with aging is, "Are these changes due to the chronological aging process or environmental factors, or a combination of the two?" The following lists include changes noted with aging that have been observed in human subjects over the last several decades (also see figure 1). These changes and functions are discussed in subsequent chapters.

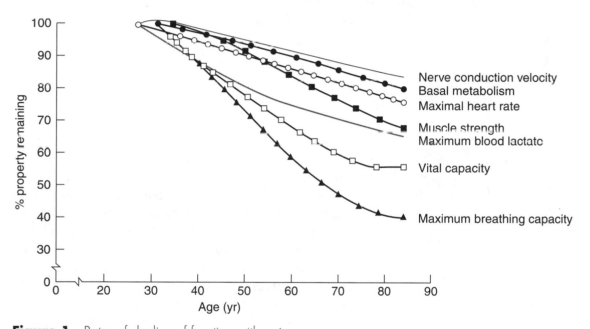

Figure 1   Rates of decline of function with aging.

Reprinted, by permission, from J.S. Skinner, 1973, Age and performance. In *Limiting factors of human performance*, edited by J. Keul (Stuttgart, Germany: Thieme), 271.

- Physiological and biochemical changes
  - Decreased renal function
  - Onset of arthritis
  - Onset of osteoporosis
  - Decreased cardiac index
  - Decreased nerve conduction velocity
  - Decreased acuity of the senses (hearing, seeing, tasting, touching, smelling)
  - Decreased iso-immunity (as measured by titers and auto-immunity titers)

- Muscle
  - Decreased strength
  - Decreased size of muscle fibers
  - Decreased number of fast-twitch fibers
  - Poorer physical fitness
- Cardiorespiratory system
  - Decreased O_2 uptake
  - Decreased maximum heart rate
  - Increased cardiovascular disease
  - Increased incidence of hypertension
- Other
  - Increased susceptibility to anxiety (which may affect decision-making abilities)
  - Increased reaction time
  - Increased movement time

The Process of Aging

But when does this process called aging really start? There are numerous religious, scientific, and even comical explanations. The complete process begins at conception and continues throughout the life span (i.e., from sperm to worm). And when does the process end?—obviously, with the death of the organism. In between these points, aging continues. As Kenny (1985) states, the physiologic hypothesis of aging and of its termination by eugeric death is that the decline of function proceeds to the point at which an internal environment compatible with the life of the cell can no longer be maintained. Aging is affected by disease and disuse. Function can include adaptability, impairment, loss in reserve of physiological capacities, and processes, eventually leading to death. Exercise as a perturbation does not usually affect primary aging if the individual is highly active, as shown in figure 2. However, exercise may affect secondary aging related to specific diseases and environmental factors.

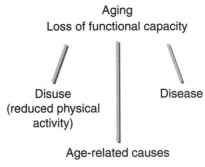

Figure 2 The process of aging as affected by disease and disuse.

Reprinted, by permission, from Canadian Centre for Activity and Aging.

Losses in function fall into four categories: (1) functions totally lost, such as reproduction and menstruation in females and high-frequency hearing; (2) structural changes—functional loss as in kidney nephrons, fast-twitch fiber numbers, and skeletal muscle diameter; (3) reduced efficiency of a unit, such as decreased conduction velocity in nerve fibers; and (4) altered control systems whereby the system, when exposed to stress, has reduced reserve; for example the female sex hormone, estrogen.

However, changes in function may affect secondary aging related to specific diseases and environmental factors. A similarity can be drawn between the death of a cell or complete organism (mortality) and a decreased quality of life because of the condition of being diseased (morbidity).

The aging process follows several stages as shown in table 1. In this text we are primarily interested in the stages of adulthood to senescence, although it must be remembered that these phases of the cycle are affected by perturbations that have occurred in earlier stages.

TABLE 1   **Stages of the Aging Process**

BIRTH TO 1 YEAR	
Neonatal	Birth to 3 weeks
Infancy	3 weeks to 1 year
CHILDHOOD	
Early	1-6 years
Middle	7 10 years
Late	Prepubertal
	9-15 years
	12-16 years
ADOLESCENCE	
Females	16-19
Males	17-19
ADULTHOOD	
Early	20-29 years
Middle	30-44 years
Late	45 64 years
SENESCENCE	
Elderly	65-74 years
Older elderly	74-84 years
Very old	85 years and above

Aging and Homeostatic Processes

Homeostasis is the maintenance of relatively stable internal physiologic conditions (body temperature, blood pH, etc.) under fluctuating environmental conditions such as physical activity. Generally, an increase in time for equilibration (i.e., increased response time) is observed with aging. These changes may be due to a number of factors, including a loss of sensitivity of receptors (temperature, pain, pressure, etc.), a compromised response of regulatory centers involved in endocrine and autonomic responses, decreased effector organ response, or a combination of these. With aging, physiological control loops no longer maintain an optimized internal environment: loops involving sensors (receptors), control (central regulation and target values), and negative feedback (reduces the deviation from the target) no longer function with the efficiency of the healthy younger body. The following are examples of changes in the homeostatic processes that occur with aging and that will be discussed throughout the text:

- An increase in time for equilibration
  - Loss of sensitivity of receptors (temperature, pain, pressure, etc.)
  - Compromised response of regulatory centers involved in endocrine and autonomic responses
  - Decreased effector organ response
- Receptors: loss of sensitivity
  - Baroreceptors, chemoreceptors
  - Loss of cutaneous receptors
- Regulatory centers
  - No major loss of neurons; only small changes in target set point
  - Loss of precision—greater deviations necessary
- Endocrine regulation (e.g., variable by organ)
  - Aldosterone for regulation of salt content markedly reduced in secretion and blood levels
  - Decreased estrogen production to complete elimination of production with menopause
- Autonomic outflow
  - Animal studies, significant age changes; transmission slowed (autonomic ganglia), but increased postganglionic sensitivity to neurotransmitter (like denervation hypersensitivity)
  - Cholinergic—reduced rate of acetylcholine synthesis
  - Adrenergic—increased neurotransmitter release, but reduced catecholamine receptors (less sensitivity and responsiveness)
- Regulatory effectors
  - Deterioration of function (e.g., heart nodal pacemaker tissue; inotropic)
  - Reduction in compliance, loss of mass, reduction in beta-receptors (e.g., sweat gland numbers reduced)

Aging Demographics

The demographics of the world are changing rapidly, but especially in North America. It has been predicted that by 2025 more than 25% of the population of the United States and Canada will be 65 years of age and older. In fact, it has been estimated that by 2050 the number of individuals 60 and older will, for the first time in history, be greater than the number of children aged 0 to 14 years. Since these changes can greatly influence both the content and delivery of physical activity interventions, a basic appreciation of the changing demographics can assist in the development of appropriate exercise regimens to meet the needs of this population. Two important demographic factors to consider are survival curves and gender differences.

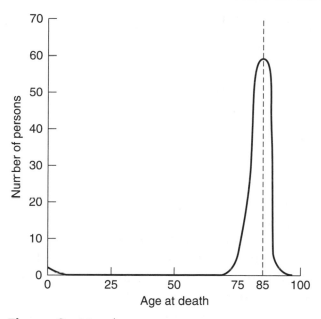

Figure 3 Mortality curve.

- **Survival curves.** The aging of a population is characterized by a survival (or mortality) curve. In figure 3, the mortality rate increases at a steady (exponential) rate. When death rates are plotted on a logarithmic scale, a straight line is obtained (Gompertz function). The slope of the Gompertz function line indicates the average rate of aging. The differences in longevity between species are the result, primarily, of differences in the rate of aging. The goal of exercise specialists is to move the curve to the right so that seniors live longer but in a healthier state.

- **Gender differences.** Over the past 100 years, more males have been born than females. However, from conception forward, females seem to have a survival advantage. That is, more spontaneous abortions, miscarriages, and stillbirths involve males. Since 1970 the gender gap has stabilized, and in fact there is some evidence to suggest that now more females are born than males. Nonetheless, as the population ages, the ratio of males to females in the United States and most industrialized nations decreases (see figure 4). Certain theories have been proposed to explain the gender differences observed. These include a genetic theory, hormonal differences, and social differences. However, to date, no theory has been proven, and the subject remains one of conjecture.

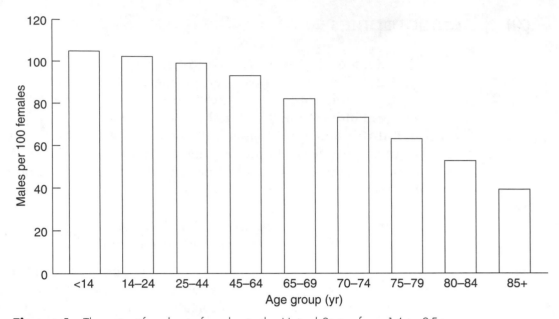

Figure 4 The ratio of males to females in the United States from 14 to 85+.

Adapted from R.C. Crandall, 1991, *Gerontology: A behavioral science approach*, 2nd ed. (New York: McGraw-Hill Companies), 49. With permission from The McGraw-Hill Companies.

Theories of Aging

Over the past century numerous theories of aging have evolved. To date, no one theory has found acceptance by the scientific community. Balcombe and Sinclair (2001) have suggested that one of the reasons for the confusion about the cause of aging is the polarization of theories, with programmed and error theories at the opposite ends of the spectrum. We suggest that, in all likelihood, aging is not caused by any single factor but is due to an aggregate of causes. All cells do not age at the same rate, and all organisms do not age at the same rate. Therefore, all humans and other mammalian species do not age at the same rate. This difference can be noted in chronological versus biological aging. Simply look at or think about how different from one another some older people look and act even if they are the same chronological age. The common denominator for all of the various groupings of aging theories is the idea that the functions of the body decline with age. Examples of different rates of decline for numerous physiological functions per decade are found in table 2. "Apex" refers to the point in time when the system or function no longer increases or plateaus but in fact begins to decline in integrity or function.

TABLE 2 **Rates of Decline of Functions With Aging per Decade After Apex**

Nerve conduction velocity	15%
Basal metabolic rate	20%
Cardiac index	30%
Vital capacity	50%
Renal blood flow	50%
Max O_2	60%-70%
Stature (height)	1 cm
Lean body mass	10%

Definitions and Aging Theory Subgroups

Biological aging refers to the slow, progressive, structural, and functional changes that take place at the cellular, tissue, and organ levels, ultimately affecting the performance of all body systems. Strehler and colleagues (1959) characterized aging by four main features:

- It is destructive, compromising functionality.
- It is progressive and irreversible.
- It is intrinsic (i.e., it is determined by internal rather than external factors).
- It is universal (i.e., all individuals of the same species display a largely uniform aging pattern, with all living beings displaying the aging phenomenon).

Esposito (1983) divided modern theoretical approaches into three distinct subgroups:

- *Causative mechanisms,* which explain aging in terms of small, sporadic, individually nonsignificant physiochemical changes that accumulate in complex organisms and lead to manifestation of the aging phenomenon
- *Systemic explanations,* which characterize aging in terms of interaction on the organ and system levels of complex organisms
- *Evolutionary explanations,* which speculate on the existence of an active genetic aging and death program for each species

As far back as the fourth century BC, Hippocrates considered the causes of aging, and numerous scientifically minded individuals have spent a great deal of time on the topic (see table 3 for a brief history up to the 1960s). None of these theories currently receives any support from the scientific community. Nonetheless, science has been concerned with the causes of aging for a long time.

TABLE 3   **Theories of Aging—Historical Figures**

Hippocrates (460-377 B.C.)	Defined aging as an irreversible and actual event dictated by the gradual loss of heat
Erasmus Darwin (grandfather of Charles)	Established one of the earliest theories of aging (1795); observed that older organisms had reduced responses to stimuli and explained this as a loss of excitability over time
Pearl (1928)	Offered a variant based on the inverse relationship between metabolic rate and life expectancy, the so-called rate of living theory of aging, which assumes a genetically determined metabolic potential that is used up at a rate determined by the actual metabolic rate of the animal
Kunze (1933)	Proposed that organ wear is caused by cosmic irradiation
Henshaw (1947)	Demonstrated that irradiation of laboratory animals at a dosage far below the dosage that would cause actual damage caused an acceleration of the aging process
Failla (1960)	Observed that the number of chromosomal aberrations increased with age, which led to the somatic mutation theory that attributes aging to accumulation of genetic errors in postmitotic cells over the life span of the cell

Categories of Modern Theories of Aging

Numerous modern theories have been proposed to explain the changes associated with aging, and these can be grouped into five broad categories: wear and tear theories, genetic theories, general imbalance theories, accumulation theories, and the dysdifferentiative hypothesis of aging and cancer (DHAC).

- **Wear and tear theories.** This group of theories is perhaps too simplistic for many, as each individual theory claims that body parts (cells, organs, etc.) wear out with continued use and stop functioning. Damage may result from internal or external causes, leading to an accumulation of incompletely repaired insults. Cells lose the ability to regenerate, which leads to mechanical or chemical exhaustion. Causes may include chemical micro insults found in the air, in food, in smoke, or internally in basic cellular metabolism. Viruses, trauma, free radicals, cross-linking, environmental radiation, and high body temperature are examples.

- **Genetic theories.** These theories hold that genes program aging from birth to death; that is, cells have a biological clock or are programmed for death (apoptosis). This is seen, for example, in puberty and menopause. It has been suggested that there may be one or more positively acting genes for longevity. Genes dictate cellular aging within the nucleus of the cell, or are expressed or repressed with normal development. Gene mutation and cellular error are other examples of genetic complications that accelerate aging.

- **General imbalance theories.** These theories suggest that the brain, endocrine glands, or immune system (or a combination of these) gradually fail to function appropriately. The rate of failure varies in different systems. The central nervous system (CNS) and neuroendocrine systems are important regulators and integrators of cell function and organ systems, and the failure of the immune system leads to susceptibility to disease.

- **Accumulation theories.** These theories suggest that functional decline associated with aging is the result of the accumulation of certain elements (some foreign and others the result of natural cell metabolism). Examples include lipofuscin in the cell, free radical accumulation, and excess membrane permeability to potassium.

- **Dysdifferentiative hypothesis of aging and cancer.** Joseph and Cutler (1994) postulated that underlying most of the vast complexities of aging is a primary aging process: the drifting away of cells from their proper state of differentiation (a process whereby unspecialized cells acquire specialized structures and functions). This is thought to be due to regulatory changes of highly differentiated cells. Dysdifferentiated cells, in important regulatory systems, initiate a cascade of changes throughout the organism. The summation of these changes is the aging process. It is important to understand several issues about the DHAC, including its uniqueness among current theories of aging and the supporting arguments.

- The DHAC differs from other genetic-based models in three key ways. (1) The model is not dependent upon gross changes in genes themselves, thus lacking the gross impairment of vital functions brought about by gross changes in genes; (2) regulatory changes, not gene mutation, lead to dysdifferentiation (the majority of DNA in a cell is involved with gene regulation and therefore has a greater probability of getting hit by a mutagen); and (3) very small changes occur in the genetic apparatus that are insufficient to alter genes responsible for housekeeping functions, but are sufficient to alter specialized genes in highly differentiated cells.

- The DHAC theory postulates special stabilizing mechanisms for maintenance of a differentiated state of cells. Such mechanisms are considered more effective in longer-lived species and similar in mammalian species. Species differences are likely quantitative rather than qualitative. However, there may be a relationship with antioxidant capability. In humans, the pituitary, hypothalamus, and other regulatory regions of the brain have highly differentiated characteristics. Therefore, small changes would result in massive functional changes (defects) in an organism dependent upon them. The DHAC suggests a common mechanism behind aging and cancer: cell dysdifferentiation. Properties consistent with a dysdifferentiated state include synthesis of foreign proteins, loss in sensitivity to normal controlling elements in cell division, altered isozyme patterns, and shifts in membrane properties. In fact, aging does show altered membrane, protein, and immune responses, as well as metaplastic cells (cell types of one tissue that are found in other cells).

- Arguments in favor of the DHAC include the facts that older cells do show a greater tendency toward dysdifferentiation with age; metaplastic cells have been observed (e.g., intestinal cells have been found in the lining of the stomach); membrane composition and properties become altered and the appearance of abnormal proteins has been observed; and age-dependent increases in autoimmune phenomena have been detected.

Recently an old hypothesis, the caloric restriction hypothesis, has been revisited and seems to be gaining momentum. Once this hypothesis is supported by an adequate amount of strong scientific evidence, it too might become a theory. It has been observed in laboratory animals, and alluded to via anecdotal material for humans, that caloric restriction (approximately 60% of the subject's normal diet) results in an extended life span. The mechanism or mechanisms responsible for this result have yet to be elucidated, and we await further clarification and scientific scrutiny before offering acceptance of this hypothesis.

Physical Activity and Aging

As we age, we become more dependent on the health care system. Although seniors make up about 12% of the population in North America, almost 30% of total health care expenditures go toward their needs. For example, injuries following falls alone can cost several billion dollars per year. More than a quarter of those aged 65 and over are limited in their activities due to long-term health problems, and approximately four out of five seniors living at home suffer from at least one chronic health condition (see figure 5). The vast majority (84%) of seniors use at least one medication regularly. Not surprisingly, emphasis in gerontology research has shifted from lengthening life to increasing years of health, thus compressing morbidity.

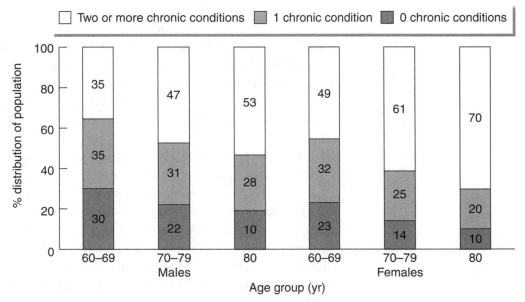

Figure 5 Percent distribution of population 60 years and older by number of chronic conditions, according to age-group and sex in the United States, 1984.
U.S. government

Cardiovascular and muscular fitness can greatly contribute to continued or improved quality of life in seniors, and numerous organizations now promote the benefits of physical activity for health and wellness for all ages. In middle age (see table 4 for definitions used almost universally by gerontologists in North America) and in the young old, fitness helps maintain peak performance and postpone premature aging. In the old, fitness will enhance quality of life (beyond just activities of daily living). In the oldest old, fitness will help with maintaining independence. Numerous groups have tried to ascertain the level of inactivity in older adults, and it has proven useful to use a questionnaire to estimate physical activity levels based upon self-reported types, frequency, and intensity of exercise.

TABLE 4	**Age Categories for Seniors**
Middle age	45-64
Young old	65-74
Old	75-84
Old old	85-99
Oldest old	100+

Canada's Physical Activity Guide to Healthy Active Living for Older Adults suggests that about 60% of older adults are inactive and thus unable to enjoy the health benefits of regular exercise. Certain groups of seniors seem particularly inactive, including those with low incomes or low education levels; the oldest seniors; those living in institutions; seniors with illness, disabilities, or chronic diseases; senior women; and isolated individuals. According to data collected by the Canadian Fitness and Lifestyle Research Institute, the proportion of seniors not active enough fell from 81% in 1981 to 70% in 1988, and increased again to 79% in 1998. In Canada, the most popular physical activities reported by adults 60 years of age and older are walking (69%), gardening and yard work (48%), home exercise (29%), swimming (24%), and bicycling (24%). Though the specifics vary from country to country, these statistics are not dissimilar to those from other developed nations, especially those from the United States.

Programming Recommendations

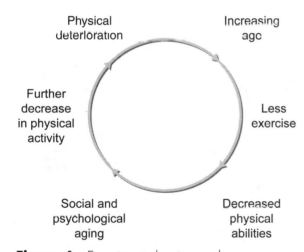

Figure 6 Exercise and aging cycle.

Adapted, by permission, from Canadian Centre for Activity and Aging, 2000, *Canada's Physical Activity Guide to Healthy Active Living for Older Adults.*

Although figures may vary depending on the population and methods used, there is general agreement that greater participation in physical activity must be promoted in seniors worldwide (Health Canada Division of Aging and Seniors, 2002b). The primary goal of exercise is to shift the physiological and biochemical curves to the right (i.e., to decrease the incidence of disease and increase the quality of life during aging). The exercise and aging cycle (figure 6) is an insidious cycle with start and end points throughout. All individuals working in the fields of gerontology or geriatrics should memorize this cycle, as it is applicable to nearly all seniors whether they exercise regularly or not.

Summary

Aging is associated with a variety of physiologic and cognitive changes. Although certain changes are undoubtedly a normal part of aging, lifestyle and environment also play a considerable role in the process. Increasingly, physical activity is widely supported as a means to enhance quality of life in the elderly.

The changes in our population will contribute to an increasing prevalence of functional impairment and chronic disease. Among those over the age of 65, 80% will have at least one chronic health problem, 42% will suffer some functional limitations, and 10% will require long-term institutionalization.

In addition, about 33% of those over the age of 85 will have some degree of dementia. Increased longevity results in an increase in degenerative diseases and a decrease in the quality of life, and the average 65-year-old will spend 7.5 years of the remaining 17 years living with functional disability.

The aging process has been under investigation for more than a thousand years, and numerous theories have been devised. It is now well known that chronological aging and biological aging are dissimilar for most cells, tissues, and whole animals within the mammalian kingdom. However, this has not deterred the emergence of numerous theories of aging. The common denominator for the aging process is the decline in function and structure that has been observed.

Questions to Consider

1. Do automobile exhaust fumes affect the aging process?

2. Are the commonly recognized secondary aging signs, such as graying of the hair, due simply to aging or decreased function of homeostatic processes or enviornmental factors?

3. Why would the population demographics differ between Canada and the United States? Points to consider in the response could include ethnic differences, climatic differences, dietary differences, work ethic, leisure time, and economics.

4. Describe the changes observed in, for example, the lens of the eye with aging (or any other selected functional or structural change). Apply two theories of aging and describe how they are applicable and how they support the changes described. Would more than two theories be applicable?

5. Select one theory of aging and demonstrate how it can explain the onset of type 2 diabetes (after you have studied chapter 5). Does only one of the theories fit this model?

6. What is the "usual" rate of decline (i.e., percentage loss per year) of several physiological functions?

7. Should the DHAC be a theory or a hypothesis, and why?

8. Dolly, the world's most famous sheep, lived to be only about 6 years of age, whereas the average sheep attains about 12 to 14 years. When Dolly's telomeres were measured, they were found to be much shorter than would have been suspected. She appeared to have inherited all the wear and tear of replication from her mother, a 6-year-old sheep at the time of the cloning. With this example in mind, what effect do you suspect cloning could have on longevity, and thus the aging process, in humans?

part I

Physiological Systems, Age-Related Changes, and the Role of Physical Activity

I t is the hope of the authors that students of exercise physiology already have a firm grasp of the effects of exercise on the physiologic systems of the body. The primary purposes of this text are to outline the effects of the aging process and the ways in which these deleterious effects (and there are none to the best of our knowledge that are not deleterious) can be positively affected by exercise.

The first section of the book groups together chapters 1 through 4 for very specific reasons. In these chapters we describe four of the primary physiologic systems of the human body: the cardiopulmonary system (chapter 1), the musculoskeletal system (chapter 2), the nervous system (chapter 3), and the sensory systems (chapter 4). It is important for readers to have a rather brief review of these systems as a framework for the succeeding sections of the book, parts II and III. Furthermore, in these chapters we describe the effects of aging on the four physiologic systems, and then demonstrate the effects of physical exercise and training on these systems and on the consequences of the aging process. Each chapter also includes programming recommendations, a summary, and a list of questions readers can consider in order to better understand the contents of the chapter and prepare for tests and examinations.

In contrast to other exercise physiology texts, the chapters in this part of the book present detail on age-related changes to the physiologic systems, as well as the various diseases or pathologies of the aging process. Chapter 1, for example, emphasizes the effects of aging on cardiovascular disease, providing details about atherosclerosis and arteriosclerosis and vascular remodeling. In chapter 2, we discuss the musculoskeletal diseases of aging, including sarcopenia and several types of arthritis. In chapter 3, we emphasize dementia and Alzheimer's disease. Chapter 4 describes the effects of aging on the sensory system. This material is unique to the book as an exercise physiology text, as little research has addressed the effects of exercise on the various components of the sensory system (hearing, sight, taste, feel, and smell). The chapter describes the structure and functions of the senses and offers recommendations for problems related to sensory impairment. The effects of aging on the sensory system are of particular importance to our aging population.

chapter 1

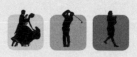
Cardiopulmonary System

Dr. Kevin Shoemaker

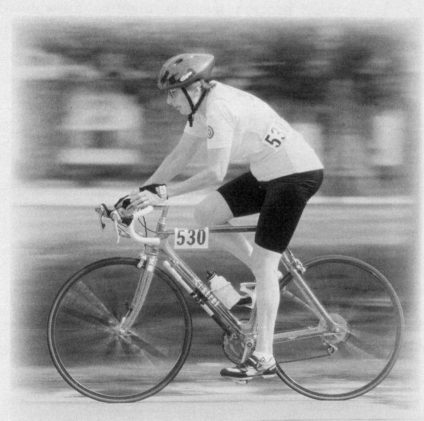

chapter outline

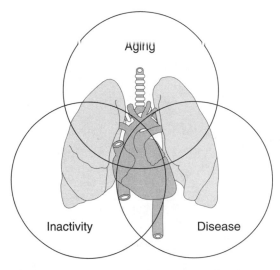

Figure 1.1 Aging, disease, and inactivity interact in the cardiopulmonary system.

Activities of daily living as well as leisure pursuits rely on the heart, lungs, and vasculature to adequately eliminate waste and deliver oxygen and other nutrients to active skeletal muscle. In addition to the normal process of aging, inactivity and disease can change the structural and functional features of the cardiopulmonary system (see figure 1.1). In this chapter, we will review some of the changes observed in the structure and function of the heart, the pulmonary system, and the vasculature with aging. The impact of these changes on exercise capacity, as well as some current recommendations for endurance training in elderly persons, will also be reviewed.

Structure and Function

The heart, the pulmonary system, and the vascular system make up the cardiopulmonary system. The heart is a muscle that is a reservoir for and pumps blood to all areas of the body. The pulmonary system ensures that tissues receive oxygen and eliminate carbon dioxide. The vascular system is composed of arteries that are essential to the function of the entire cardiopulmonary system. The next sections describe the structures and functions of these systems and how they work together to form the cardiopulmonary system.

The Heart

The heart is a muscular organ (myocardium) weighing between 250 and 350 g (0.8 lb) in healthy adults and enclosed in a fibrous sac called the pericardium. It comprises four hollow chambers (atria and ventricles) separated by walls (septa) lined by the endocardium, which is continuous with lining of blood vessels. The heart serves both as a reservoir (atria) and as a pump (ventricles) for blood. Deoxygenated blood enters the right atrium through the superior and inferior vena cava and passes to the right ventricle through the tricuspid valve. Blood is then pumped through the pulmonary semilunar valve into the pulmonary arteries to the lungs, where it is oxygenated (pulmonary circulation). It returns to the left atrium via the pulmonary veins and passes through the bicuspid (mitral) valve on its way to the left ventricle, where it is then pumped through the aortic semilunar valve into the aorta and systemic circulation.

Myocardial muscle cells (myocytes) are made to contract and relax via a specialized conduction system. The initial depolarization usually arises from the sinoatrial node (SA) or pacemaker (±100 beats per minute). The action potential then spreads out through the atria and then into the ventricles (sinoatrial node → atrioventricular node (slight delay) → bundle of His → left and right bundle branches → Purkinje fibers). A cardiac cycle consists of the full sequence of contraction (systole) and relaxation (diastole) of the heart (see figure 1.2). The volume of blood at the end of ventricular filling is termed end-diastolic volume (EDV), and the amount of blood ejected from each ventricle during systole is the stroke volume (SV). The amount of blood remaining in the ventricles after the end of contraction is the end-systolic volume (ESV).

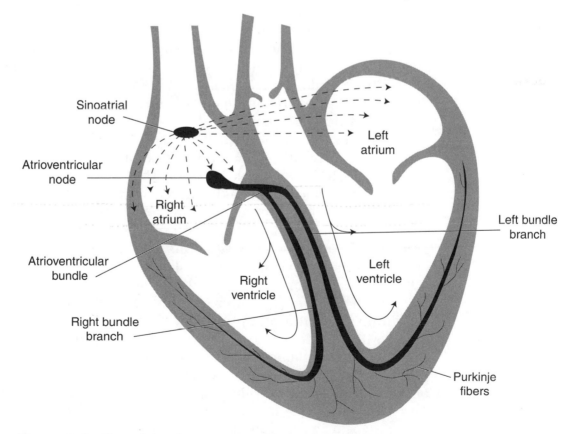

Figure 1.2   Flow of depolarization across the cardiac tissue.

Reprinted, by permission, from P.J. Maud and C. Foster, 2005, *Physiological assessment of human fitness*, 2nd ed. (Champaign, IL: Human Kinetics), 40.

Determinants of Stroke Volume

Preload: atrial filling pressure and its effect on the stretch of the ventricles prior to contraction

Afterload: resistance that must be overcome by the left ventricle

Contractility: strength of left ventricular contraction

The percentage of the EDV pumped from the ventricles is the ejection fraction (EF). The volume of blood pumped by each ventricle per minute (stroke volume × heart rate) is termed the cardiac output (CO).

The endocrine and autonomic nervous systems greatly influence myocardium contraction strength (inotropic effect) and rate (chronotropic effect). Sympathetic neurons (excitatory) innervate the SA and AV nodes and the myocardium of the atria and ventricles. Sympathetic activity can increase cardiac output more than 100%. Parasympathetic neurons (inhibitory) innervate the SA and AV nodes and mostly the myocardium of the atria. In certain situations, parasympathetic activity (vagal) can stop the heart from beating for a few seconds. In addition, circulating hormones such as norepinephrine (NE) and epinephrine (Epi) also stimulate increases in heart rate and contractility. Owing to these combined influences, in humans the resting heart rate (RHR) is normally between 60 and 100 beats per minute.

Until the 1970s, based mostly upon autopsy data, it was commonly believed that the heart decreased in size with age. Although this can be true in certain pathologies, the advancement of new technologies (echocardiography, radionuclide imaging, etc.) and longitudinal studies suggest that the heart might in fact increase in mass with age. It has been observed that a thickening of the left ventricle occurs with senescence in healthy populations, due primarily to the hypertrophy of myocytes. It is reasonable to believe that this is an adaptation to the heightened workload due to the increased vessel stiffness observed in aging (increased peripheral vascular resistance). Systolic blood pressure at rest and during moderate exercise is as much as 40 mmHg greater in older versus young adults. A slight increase in the volume of the left atrium may occur as well.

The myocardium in older adults is slower to relax following contraction due to the (1) slower calcium reuptake by the sarcoplasmic reticulum's calcium pump protein, (2) changes in the myosin heavy chain (MHC) composition of myocytes, and (3) prolonged action potential. Although the longer time for contraction may be advantageous in pumping blood into stiffer vessels, it may also lead to a greater incidence of arrhythmias and fibrillation. Increased fat and collagen deposits may also contribute to increased stiffness and decreased compliance of the myocardium. Changes in the conduction system in aged hearts

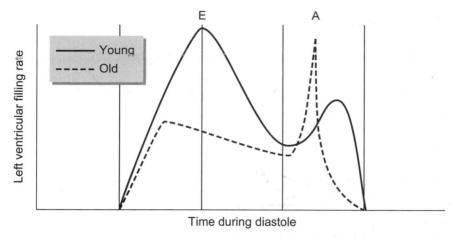

Figure 1.3   Effects of age on filling rate of the left ventricle during diastole.

also occur. In particular, a decreased number of sinus node pacemaker cells along with decreased cells in the AV node, bundle of His, and Purkinje network have been observed.

Cardiac output is an important indicator of the cardiovascular system's ability to adequately meet the circulatory needs of the body, and is greatly influenced by metabolism, activity level, age, and body size. Cardiac output is the product of heart rate and stroke volume. In turn, the primary factors that determine stroke volume include preload, afterload, and contractility. In order to compare cardiac output between individuals, it is often adjusted for differences in body surface area: cardiac index (L/min/m^2). Although the cardiac index at rest is maintained with aging, the structural changes observed do influence the functional mechanisms involved. The slower myocardium relaxation time leads to a smaller early diastolic volume (50% reduction by age 80; see figure 1.3); however, the late diastolic filling is greater due to an increased blood volume contained in the enlarged atria. In addition, studies suggest that aging in populations screened for cardiovascular disease does not greatly influence heart rate or stroke volume at rest. However, during sampling in the general population (not screened), cardiac output and stroke volume are observed to decrease with age (see table 1.1). In these cases, starting in early adulthood, cardiac output decreases about 1% per year, and stroke volume may decrease by as much as 30% before the age of 85.

TABLE 1.1   **Approximate Resting Values for Healthy Cardiac Function**

Variable	Young	Older
Cardiac index (L/min/m^2)	3	3
End-diastolic volume (mL/m^2)	75	85
End-systolic volume (mL/m^2)	25	30
Stroke volume (mL/m^2)	42	50
Ejection fraction (%)	66	66
Heart rate (beats/min)	70	60

The Pulmonary System

The pulmonary system consists of the nose, pharynx (throat), larynx (voice box), trachea (windpipe), bronchi, and lungs. The primary role of the pulmonary system is to provide oxygen to and eliminate carbon dioxide from tissue. Other functions include the regulation of blood pH, the production of vasoactive substances, speech, and defense against microbes.

With aging, the number of alveoli and corresponding capillaries gradually decreases. There is a noticeable increase in the size of the surviving alveoli as their elastic properties are compromised due to changes in collagen and elastin. A thickening of the larger pulmonary arteries is also observed. Calcification of rib cartilage along with a weakening of respiratory muscles is also present. Taken together, the decreased elasticity of the lungs, increased stiffness of the chest walls, and reduction in respiratory muscle strength result in a reduced compliance of the thorax. This causes an approximately 20% increase in the work of respiratory muscles. As we age, increased ventilation becomes more dependent on increasing respiratory rate rather than increased depth of breathing. Pulmonary ventilation is the process by which ambient air is brought in (inspiration) and out (expiration) of the lungs.

Inspiration is an active process, achieved by the contraction of inspiratory muscles (diaphragm and external intercostal muscles) that causes an increase in intrathoracic volume so that air flows into the lungs. Expiration is a passive process by which recoil of stretched lung tissue and relaxation of inspiratory muscles move air out of the lung. Pulmonary ventilation is controlled by the depth and frequency of breathing, and this is most often expressed in terms of volume per minute, or minute ventilation.

Minute ventilation is the product of the frequency of breathing and the tidal volume (air inspired or expired with each normal breath). Lung volumes are important tools for evaluating the state of the pulmonary system, and can be measured readily at rest or during exercise with the aid of spirometers.

Definitions

Tidal volume: air inspired or expired with each normal breath

Vital capacity: maximal tidal volume

Inspiratory reserve volume: extra volume of air that can be inspired over and above the normal tidal volume

Expiratory reserve volume: extra air that can be expired by forceful expiration after the end of a normal tidal expiration

Residual volume: volume of air remaining in lungs after a forceful expiration

With aging, it has been observed that residual volume can increase by as much as 30% to 50%. By the age of 70, vital capacity may decrease by as much 40% to 50%.

Pulmonary circulation is the movement of blood from the heart, to the lungs, and back to the heart again. Pulmonary circulation supplies mixed venous blood to pulmonary capillaries at the rate required for delivery of CO_2 and uptake of O_2 in the gas-exchanging regions of the lungs. In the ideal lung, inspired air reaches all the alveoli, and all the alveoli have the same blood supply. However, neither alveolar ventilation nor pulmonary capillary blood flow is really uniform, and the supply of air and blood is never perfectly matched even in healthy individuals. Ventilation and perfusion are not matched as well in the lungs of elderly people as they are in lungs of younger people (ventilation–perfusion distribution), and a decreased blood flow to lower regions of the lung is observed.

Although improvements in ventilation with training are reported, pulmonary function does not seem to be a limiting factor for exercise in healthy elderly persons. In fact, during moderate exercise, pulmonary ventilation and mechanical efficiency are similar in the old and the young. During intense exercise, ventilation is also adequate for the task. However, increased shortness of breath is often observed in elderly people due not only to increased respiratory muscle work, but also to changes in the perception of exertion.

The Vascular System

Blood pressure is the product of cardiac output and peripheral vascular resistance. Thus, an understanding of age-related cardiovascular diseases such as hypertension, atherosclerosis, stroke, and peripheral vascular disease must take into account age-related changes to cardiac output and the vasculature. Issues associated with cardiac output were discussed earlier. Within the arterial system, it is the small arterioles that exert the primary muscular influence over vascular resistance, and it is in these vessels that the majority of control over the amount of blood flow to the organ (muscle) occurs. The role of these arteries is to conduct oxygenated blood to metabolically active tissues. Adequate delivery of blood to any organ depends on the pressure driving the blood and the state of the resistance in the arteries and arterioles in the organ.

A complete explanation of blood flow control is beyond the scope of this chapter. Rather, we will examine the structural aspects of arteries (i.e., endothelium, vascular smooth muscle, and connective tissue) and how changes in these are fundamental to cardiovascular disease.

Figure 1.4 provides structural details of a muscular conduit vessel, such as the brachial or femoral arteries. The smaller resistance vessels (arterioles) that penetrate the organ have similar anatomical components but with progressive reductions in diameter and smooth muscle

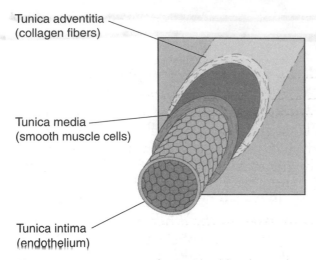

Tunica adventitia
(collagen fibers)

Tunica media
(smooth muscle cells)

Tunica intima
(endothelium)

Figure 1.4 Structure of a conduit blood vessel.

layer thickness. Nonetheless, the proportion of smooth muscle to arteriole luminal area increases in the arteriolar branching so that these smaller vessels just before the capillaries provide the bulk of resistance to blood flow and, therefore, form a major contributor to blood pressure regulation.

• **Endothelium.** A crucial determinant of tone in vascular smooth muscle cells and blood pressure is the endothelial layer that lines the lumen of cardiovascular tissues. This endothelium consists of simple squamous epithelium cells. This layer of cells covers the luminal (inside) surface of all cardiovascular structures including the heart, arteries, arterioles, and veins. The endothelial cells are the sole tissues composing the capillary networks. These cells are in close contact and form a slippery layer that prevents blood cells from contacting the vessel wall. The endothelium plays a critical role in the mechanics of blood flow, the regulation of blood clotting, leukocyte adhesion, and vascular wall growth and stiffness; it also serves as a barrier to the movement of liquids and solutes between the blood and the organ interstitial space. Thus, this dynamic tissue performs many active functions to maintain organ perfusion and blood vessel health.

• **Vascular smooth muscle (tunica media).** As indicated previously, peripheral vascular resistance and cardiac output are the determinants of blood pressure. In turn, vascular resistance (or its inverse variable of conductance) is determined by vascular smooth muscle cells that make up the muscular resistance vessels. Vascular smooth muscle is a contractile tissue that can acutely change the lumen size of an arteriole so that conductance of flow through that region is controlled. The contractile state of vascular smooth muscle is affected by many influences from multiple sources. For example, the endothelial layer produces compounds that affect the size of the arteriole lumen by changing the contractile tone of the smooth muscle layer (see later). The major endothelial compounds that dilate blood vessels are nitric oxide and prostaglandins. These dilatory factors are released by several stimuli, including the friction (shear) stress caused by blood as it rubs the endothelial cells. There are also endothelial products that cause constriction of blood vessels, namely endothelin-1 and some varieties of prostaglandins. Local sympathetic neurons also influence the contractile status of the arteriolar size by releasing vasoconstrictor neurotransmitters that affect postjunctional receptors on the outside (abluminal) side of the vessel. In addition, circulating catecholamines and other hormones can affect vascular resistance (tone) either directly, by acting on the smooth muscle, or indirectly, by acting on endothelial cells to produce their vasoactive factors. Thus, at any point in time, the current state of a blood vessel's tone is the balance between competing dilatory and constrictor influences.

- **Connective tissue (tunica media and adventitia).** The media of a blood vessel, being reduced in thickness from the largest to the smallest arterial vessels, is composed of collagen and elastin, with other basement membrane materials, fibroblasts, and so on. The collagen fibers are relatively stiff compared to elastin fibers. Therefore, the stiffness of a blood vessel is determined by the ratio of collagen to elastin tissue. For example, the aorta is a highly elastic tissue with high compliance compared to the smaller and stiffer brachial or femoral arteries. This means that there is a larger change in cross-sectional area of the aorta for any given change in pressure than in the other peripheral conduit arteries. Thus, the aorta has a high balance of elastin versus collagen. This ratio changes with age such that all vessels become stiffer as the content of collagen increases relative to elastin. This stiffening of aging vessels is discussed in greater detail later.

Age-Related Changes

Changes to exercise capacity and blood flow to limbs occur as individuals age. In sedentary older people, exercise capacity and blood flow decreases. Sedentary adults can benefit from increases in maximum oxygen consumption and vasodilation, as described in the following two sections.

Exercise Capacity

Maximum oxygen consumption ($\dot{V}O_2$ max) is a widely used index of cardiopulmonary fitness. It is calculated using the Fick equation, which describes the relationships among cardiac output, oxygen consumption, and arterial-venous oxygen difference:

$$\dot{V}O_2 \text{ max} = \text{cardiac output} \times \text{arterial-venous (a-}\bar{v}O_2) \text{ difference}$$

A linear loss from age 30 to 65 years has been described for various measures, and in sedentary individuals it is often suggested that maximal oxygen uptake declines at a rate of about 10% per decade after the age of 25. The decline observed in maximal oxygen consumption has been attributed to a decreased cardiac output, a decreased arterial-venous (a-vO_2) difference, and a loss in muscle mass. Cardiac output during maximum exercise decreases by about 30% between the ages of 20 and 80, and the myocardium's increased relaxation time and decreased sensitivity to catecholamines can decrease maximum heart rate by as much as 30% to 50% between the ages of 25 and 85 years. Nonetheless, the central cardiovascular capacity, despite some suggested age effects, would appear to be adequate to support the decreased muscle mass observed with aging. Thus, despite the losses in absolute exercise capacity with age, the ability to sustain a relatively high intensity of aerobic exercise appears to be preserved.

In those who are elderly, the improvement in maximum oxygen uptake following training is explained by an increased cardiac output along with enhanced muscle oxygen extraction. However, the greatest gains are observed in cardiac output. Since maximum heart rate generally remains unchanged after training, it is stroke volume that is the critically modified variable. It is thought that an increased sensitivity to circulating catecholamines, along with a decreased peripheral resistance, contributes to the observed increase in stroke volume. With moderate-intensity exercise, elderly people can expect gains of 20% to 30% in maximum oxygen uptake (see figure 1.5). This is comparable to the increases observed in younger subjects. This is especially important since exercise capacity remains a strong predictor of mortality in both healthy elderly people and those with cardiovascular disease. In fact, once data were adjusted for age, peak exercise capacity was shown to be a stronger predictor of increased risk of death than hypertension, smoking, and diabetes.

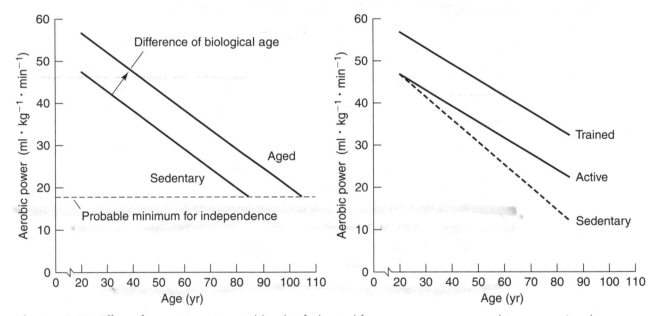

Figure 1.5 Effect of increasing age and levels of physical fitness or activity on aerobic power. Aerobic power declines with age; but at any given age, physical activity can maintain a higher level of fitness.

Blood Flow in Aging Limbs

As already discussed, exercise cardiac output is decreased with age. Similarly, the majority of evidence suggests that limb blood flow to aged skeletal muscle is reduced at rest compared with that in young controls (Seals and Dinenno, 2004). However, debate continues about whether aging per se affects blood flow during exercise. Possible contributions to alterations in exercise blood flow, when they are observed, could include diminished ability to dilate blood vessels in skeletal muscle, or a reduction in number of blood vessels available due to the inactivity associated with advancing age, or both. Thus, researchers have investigated the ability of blood vessels to dilate in aging individuals. A common test for vasodilation is the peak reactive hyperemia test. This test involves measuring the blood flow response to muscle after a period (e.g., 3 to 10 minutes) of ischemia. The conclusion from this line of research is that peak reactive hyperemia to a short period of forearm ischemia is reduced in elderly individuals (Proctor et al., 2005), but not necessarily because of age. Rather, the decrease is due to reductions in activity levels. Thus, the ability of the vascular tree to adapt to the ongoing chronic levels of oxygen demand is not affected by age.

Cardiovascular Disease and Age

Aging is associated with many chronic disorders. Within the cardiovascular system there are several separate conditions, including coronary artery disease, cerebrovascular disease, peripheral vascular disease, and congestive heart failure. As indicated in table 1.2, heart disease, stroke, and hypertension may be grouped under a larger condition called cardiovascular disease (CVD). Cardiovascular disease accounts for more deaths than any other disease. As many as 25% of North Americans have some form of heart disease or disease of the blood vessels or are at risk for stroke. In general, the risk of developing CVD is greater for males compared to females. However, with increasing age, females also have a high incidence of CVD. Age is an independent risk factor and is also implicated in the development of hypertension and hypercholesterolemia. Epidemiological studies have determined several risk factors that are associated with the development of CVD, as outlined by the World Health Organization (2002):

TABLE 1.2 **The Eight Major Modifiable Risk Factors for Cardiovascular Diseases and Other Leading Noncommunicable Diseases**

Risk factor	Cardiovascular diseases*	Diabetes	Cancer	Chronic obstructive pulmonary disease
Smoking	X	X	X	X
Alcohol	X		X	
Physical activity	X	X	X	
Nutrition	X	X	X	
Obesity	X	X	X	X
Raised blood pressure	X	X		
Dietary fat/lipids	X	XX	XX	
Blood glucose	X			

*Includes heart disease, stroke, and hypertension.
Source: World Health Organization.

The Physiology of CVD and Aging

While each disease has its separate features with respect to etiology, the organ affected, the symptoms generated, and ultimate pathology, it may be argued that there are fundamental aspects of cardiovascular structure and function that change with age, leading to the development of these diseases. There are independent effects of age on cardiovascular form and function—effects that in some cases are influenced by one's level of physical activity.

The current determination is that several factors interact in the development of CVD. A proposed model of this complex interaction is shown in figure 1.6. In this model, advancing age has three primary effects on the cardiovascular system. First, there is a change in the structure of blood vessel walls that reduces their compliance, that is, makes them stiffer. This occurs primarily in the large conduit vessels such as the aorta and carotid arteries. Concurrently, there is an age-related increase in sympathetic nerve activity. This heightened sympathetic level is affected by stress, body mass (obesity), and perhaps some genetic aspects. Third, the endothelial lining of blood vessels becomes less "functional."

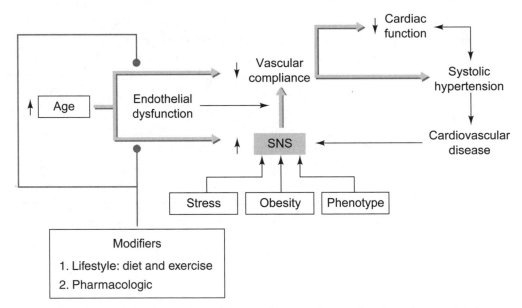

Figure 1.6 Model outlining the multifactorial nature of age-related cardiovascular disease and how it is modified by lifestyle. Lines with blunt ends indicate factors that likely diminish the detrimental effects of age on processes that contribute to cardiovascular pathology. See text for explanation.

The effects of heightened sympathetic nervous system and endothelial function augment the independent effect of age on vascular compliance. In turn, stiffer blood vessels place additional stress on cardiac function (as mentioned earlier) through elevations in systolic pressure, ultimately leading to systolic hypertension and, finally, diseased cardiovascular tissues. A common finding in chronic CVD is that sympathetic outflow and endothelial function are further changed, causing the adverse cycle to continue. It is also clear that a positive lifestyle including appropriate diet and exercise can minimize the adverse effects of age as outlined.

Thus, what may be determined as critical elements of this model are the following: (1) vascular stiffening, (2) endothelial function, (3) elevated sympathetic nervous system, (4) vascular remodeling, and (5) exercise interventions. Each of these is discussed separately in the following sections.

Vascular Stiffening

With aging, the major conduit arteries such as the aorta get stiffer and longer. Current evidence indicates that these large vessels become stiffer due to two factors: a thickening of the structural materials that make up the vessel wall and an increase in sympathetic tone of the smooth muscle. These vessels grow thicker because of a disorganization of endothelial and connective tissue cells, as well as through an increased amount of connective tissue. It is noteworthy that this growth of the blood vessel is considered to be independent of plaque deposition along the arterial wall. Thus, this wall thickening is an independent effect of age and not an effect of diseases associated with age. From this perspective it may be helpful to define some terms before we consider the independent effects of age on vascular stiffening.

It is also important to recognize that the age-related remodeling of conduit blood vessels is not the same type of remodeling associated with onset of elevated blood pressure, as happens with essential hypertension occurring earlier in life. In the latter case, the arterial wall gets thicker, but the lumen size is reduced (inward remodeling). This response protects the blood vessel by high circumferential tension stress. In age-related vascular remodeling, the lumen of the vessel is often increased while the vessel wall gets thicker and stiffer. This thickening and stiffening process is not accounted for by an atherosclerotic process but is related to changes in the material structure of the wall, resulting in a higher balance of collagen with respect to elastin fibers.

Endothelial Function and Aging

In patients, the risk of arteriosclerosis is associated with impaired endothelium-dependent vasodilation in the coronary arteries, a response that is correlated with diminished endothelial control in the forearm (Anderson et al., 1995; Celermajer et al., 1994). Consequently, the magnitude of change in brachial artery diameter during the first minute or so following a brief period of forearm ischemia is used as

Definitions

Arteriosclerosis: a group of diseases characterized by thickening and loss of elasticity of arterial walls; includes atherosclerosis, arteriolosclerosis, and Mockenberg's arteriosclerosis

Atherosclerosis: a common form of arteriosclerosis in which deposits of yellowish plaques containing cholesterol, lipoid material, and lipophages are formed within the intima and inner media of large and medium-sized arteries

the index of endothelial function in the coronary vessels. Endothelial dysfunction represents one of the earliest signs of developing CVD.

There is a strong coherence between age and reductions of endothelial function, particularly after the age of 45 years and in the presence of other cardiovascular risk factors (Walther et al., 2004). Thus, it is tempting to think that age has a direct and negative impact on endothelial function, leading to risk of CVD. However, some studies strongly suggest that age-related endothelial dysfunction is a highly reversible situation, caused by a sedentary lifestyle, rather than an independent effect of age. The dependency of endothelial function on a healthy lifestyle is consistent with accumulating knowledge that the relative risk of death due to hypertension, chronic obstructive pulmonary disease, diabetes, smoking, obesity, or elevated cholesterol is greatly reduced in active individuals compared with sedentary people (Laughlin, 2004). Even extremely obese children are characterized by diminished forearm endothelial function that is reversible by exercise training (Watts et al., 2004).

Elevated Sympathetic Nervous System Activity

The autonomic nervous system is critical in the normal function of heart rate, cardiac output, blood pressure, and vascular structure. Inadequate sympathetic responses to simple maneuvers such as standing upright result in lower blood pressure and fainting. On the other hand, levels of sympathetic nerve activity (SNA) that are too high result in increased peripheral vascular resistance, remodeling of cardiovascular tissue, and, ultimately, hypertension if these persist over a long period of time. Levels of baseline plasma NE concentrations (Palmer et al., 1978; Sowers et al., 1983) and SNA (Iwase et al., 1991; Sundlöf and Wallin, 1978) are increased with advancing age, with apparently greater effects in females (Matsukawa et al., 1998). Thus, elevated SNA has been identified as an important risk factor for age-related CVD possibly through deleterious effects on vascular (Pauletto et al., 1991) and cardiac (Cechetto, 1993; Du et al., 1999; Kaye et al., 1995) function. Indeed, among other disorders (Benarroch, 1993), elevated baseline SNA is believed to contribute to vascular (Izzo and Taylor, 1999) and cardiac (Hachinski et al., 1986; Hachinski et al., 1992; Pauletto et al., 1991; Stoney et al., 1987) damage as well as many types of chronic hypertension (Grassi et al., 2000; Pauletto et al., 1991); these are major risk factors for CVD (Doyle and Donnan, 1990; Hachinski et al., 1992).

Alterations in parasympathetic nervous system outflow also occur with age and are equally important in the overall health of the cardio-vascular system, particularly the heart. This system is particularly important for normal rhythms of the heartbeat. There is also evidence that the intrinsic ability of the heart myocytes to control their rhythm is altered with age as well.

The reason or reasons for the elevated sympathetic nerve outflow and decreased parasympathetic outflow are not known. There are receptors located within the heart, aorta, and carotid blood vessels that inhibit SNA and heart rate if pressure rises. Thus, some have investigated whether alterations in this baroreflex-control feature is affected by age, accounting for the elevated sympathetic and dimin-ished parasympathetic levels in senescence. However, age-dependent reductions in baroreflex function do not occur (Seals and Esler, 2000) and cannot explain age-related alterations in the autonomic nervous system. Therefore, augmented sympathetic drive by the central nervous system has been proposed (Seals and Esler, 2000); but there have been no direct tests of this hypothesis, and specifics regarding focal control centers have not been addressed.

It has been noted that dysregulation of both SNA and ventilation (i.e., dyspnea in heart failure patients) is present in patients with CVD (Grassi et al., 1995; Middlekauff, 1997; Narkiewicz et al., 1999). Thus, an emerging hypothesis is that altered chemosensitivity is mechanisti-cally involved in the chronic elevations in sympathetic outflow in CVD. In addition, others are examining the role of centers within the brain that respond to angiotensin II and nitric oxide to control chronic levels of sympathetic and parasympathetic outflow, and perhaps the balance between these two systems (Zucker et al., 2001).

Vascular Remodeling and Systolic Hypertension

The thickening and stiffening of aging conduit vessels have remarkable consequences for blood pressure. Normally, the large conduit blood vessels have some degree of elasticity (due to the elastin component) so that they absorb some of the energy associated with the heart ejecting a volume of blood into the blood vessel system. Because of absorption of some of this energy, the systolic blood pressure will not be as high as it might otherwise be. Similarly, absorbing energy during the sys-tolic phase of the cardiac cycle allows the energy to dissipate during diastole so that diastolic pressure is kept high enough to push the blood down through the capillaries through the cardiac cycle. This is a normal function. However, with stiff vessels, the ability to absorb some of the energy during systole is reduced. This causes systolic pressure to increase to above-normal levels. Concurrently, diastolic pressure falls below normal because there is less "recoil" of the elastic conduit vessels during diastole. The functional ability of conduit blood vessels to store energy during systole, and to recoil to release that energy during diastole, is called the Windkessel effect. This is not the only explanation for higher systolic pressure in elderly individuals, but it provides a conceptual framework within which to envision how these vessels change over time.

This scenario of elevated systolic pressure and lower diastolic pressure leads to a widening of the pulse pressure (systolic pressure – diastolic pressure). This widened pulse pressure with high systolic pressure is called systolic hypertension. Systolic hypertension is a major risk factor for CVD and is highly associated with death rate.

The stiffness of blood vessels is also accomplished by the neurotransmitters emitted from sympathetic neurons that innervate the smooth muscle of arteries. The primary neurotransmitters from the sympathetic neurons in skeletal muscle are adenosine triphosphate (ATP), NE, and neuropeptide Y (NPY). As already noted, SNA increases with age. Consequently, the reduction in muscle blood flow with age has been directly linked with the elevated SNA (Seals and Dinenno, 2004).

While elevated sympathetic outflow may directly affect the acute status of arterial tone, it may also influence the structural changes that occur in conduit blood vessels with age. Recent evidence has shown that NE and NPY released from sympathetic neurons can act as growth factors, causing these blood vessels to get thicker. However, it appears that two conditions must coexist. First, there must be a chronic elevation in release of the transmitter. Second, this must occur while the endothelial layer is damaged or dysfunctional (Zhang and Faber, 2001a; 2001b). As outlined earlier, both of these scenarios do develop with age.

Exercise and Vascular Health in Aging

The beneficial aspects of an active lifestyle on cardiovascular health are undisputed. Booth has commented, "Physical inactivity is part of the disease process for a large number of important chronic disease states" (Booth et al., 2000, p 774). The challenge is that the number of individuals participating in regular leisure-time rigorous physical activity declines from 30% to 45% at age ~20 years to 15% to 25% at age 75 (Bassuk and Manson, 2003). Regular physical activity of moderate intensity can abolish the age-related decline in endothelial function outlined here (Laughlin, 2004; Walther et al., 2004) and enhance vascular compliance. However, it is not yet clear how regular physical activity affects levels of sympathetic outflow.

It is undisputed that aerobic training has positive impacts on both maximal and submaximal exercise performance in elderly people. During maximal exercise, increased ventilation, oxygen consumption, cardiac output, and a-vO$_2$ difference have all been observed following training. Aerobic training also helps to decrease ventilation, heart rate, stroke volume, and blood pressure during submaximal exercise. These changes can significantly benefit activities of daily living.

Programming Recommendations

Kinesiologists are increasingly asked to provide guidance in a variety of settings (home, hospitals, gyms, etc.). Regardless of the venue, exercise programs for elderly people can be beneficial in many ways. They can

- improve self-care capabilities and general well-being;
- improve cardiovascular condition and general endurance;
- increase muscular strength and endurance;
- maintain or improve flexibility, coordination, and balance;
- maximize social contact and enjoyment of life;
- improve weight control and nutrition;
- aid digestion and reduce constipation;
- promote relaxation;
- relieve anxiety, insomnia, and depression; and
- sustain sexual vigor.

Exercise Management

Some simple management guidelines can help create a successful environment for elderly participants. Above all, try to make the experience as fun as possible for everyone involved. Be open and seek out participant feedback. Be enthusiastic and get to know your group! Here are a few suggestions to help better manage exercise programming with elderly persons.

- Explanations
  - Give slow, clear instructions; repeat.
  - Speak loudly.
  - Use simple language.
  - Use demonstrations.
  - Don't talk down to participants.
- Environment
  - Encourage social interaction.
  - Provide background music when appropriate.
  - Minimize distractions.

- – Do not encourage undue competition.
- – Encourage self-paced work.
- Safety
  - – Insist on proper footwear.
  - – Choose appropriate activities (according to fitness level, disease, etc.).
  - – Allow freedom to opt out.
  - – Assess the difficulty of getting down to and up from mats or floor.
  - – Be ready for emergencies (CPR, first aid, 911, etc.).
  - – Practice emergency response.

Endurance Exercise Training

A number of organizations now recognize the protective effect of regular exercise against heart disease, and habitual physical activity is recommended for both young and old. In addition, the Canadian Society for Exercise Physiology (CSEP) and the American College of Sports Medicine (ACSM) have presented detailed, specific exercise prescription guidelines for endurance training in elderly people.

- **Canadian Society for Exercise Physiology.** In 1999, CSEP and Health Canada produced *Canada's Physical Activity Guide to Healthy Active Living for Older Adults.* The guide recommends that older adults participate in endurance activities four to seven days per week (examples: walking, swimming, dancing, skating, cross-country skiing, cycling, hiking). Participants should work up to doing at least 10 min of continuous activity at a time and try to accumulate 30 to 60 min per day. Important safety considerations include beginning with activities that can be done comfortably, progressing gradually to more demanding activity, using comfortable footwear and clothing, and choosing boots that will grip on ice and snow for winter activities.

- **American College of Sports Medicine.** In addition to the CSEP norms just listed, the ACSM indicates that the training intensity should be >55% of one's maximal oxygen uptake level, or >40% of one's heart rate reserve (the difference between maximal heart rate and resting heart rate). The lower intensity values are most applicable to individuals who are quite unfit.

Summary

Advancing age has profound effects on the cardiac, vascular, and pulmonary systems. These changes lead to a significant reduction in exercise capacity and increasing risk of various CVDs. It is noteworthy, however, that many of the deleterious cardiovascular consequences of age either are attributable to the effects of reduced physical activity, such as a decline in endothelial function, or can be delayed or minimized through an active lifestyle.

Questions to Consider

1. Describe the mechanical and neural control of heart rate and stroke volume.

2. Describe the changes in heart structure and function that occur with age.

3. How does age affect resting heart rate and stroke volume?

4. List the effects of age on lung characteristics. How do these changes affect breathing patterns in senescence?

5. Describe cardiac factors that contribute to the decline in exercise capacity with advancing age.

6. Outline the anatomy of conduit blood vessels and how these change with age, physical training, or both.

7. What is the consequence of age-related blood vessel stiffening on blood pressure?

8. List the risk factors for cardiovascular disease.

9. Describe why, or how, age-related increases in sympathetic nervous system activation are believed to be a risk factor for cardiovascular disease.

chapter 2

Musculoskeletal System

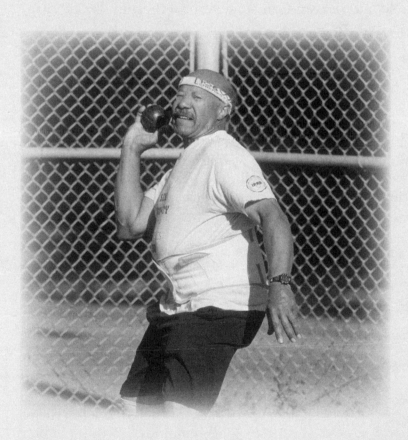

This chapter discusses basic skeletal muscle physiology, elementary muscle biochemistry related to energy pathways, and activity and aging. We consider in some detail the primary disease related to movement and joint-muscle stiffness—arthritis. The chapter also outlines acceptable and proven forms of exercise therapy and contraindicated exercise therapy.

Muscle Morphology

Mammalian skeletal muscle is composed of more than one fiber type. Most mammals have at least three fiber types (Abernethy et al., 1994; Noble et al., 2004); but human skeletal muscle (see figure 2.1) is known to possess only two distinct fiber types (Lexell et al., 1983, 1988), fast twitch (FT) and slow twitch (ST), although there are various subtypes of each (Noble et al., 2004). Animal fibers are most often blocks of fibers, whereas human fibers form a mosaic pattern. Under normal conditions, the cross-sectional area (CSA) of FT and ST fibers in humans is rather similar (for an example see figure 2.1 and Larsson and Ansved, 1985). However, it is well known that specific types of training can produce hypertrophy in either of these fiber types. For example, strength training can produce growth primarily in FT fibers (McDonagh and Davies, 1984), and extended endurance training can result in a slight hypertrophy of the ST fibers (Taylor et al., 1978). The remainder of this chapter concerns only human skeletal muscle.

With aging, CSA decreases (see figure 2.2). This phenomenon is caused by the gradual disuse of muscle fibers as elderly people become much less active than before. The preferential loss in area is principally seen in the FT fibers. The rationale for this loss is due to a lack of explosive movements as the

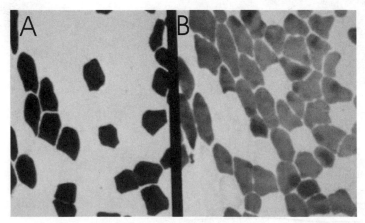

Figure 2.1 Note the mosaic pattern of this cross section of a human vastus lateralis muscle. In this myosin ATPase reaction, the left picture shows the FT fibers stained darkly at ph 10.2. The right section is the reverse stain at ph 4.6 and the ST fibers are stained more darkly.

Adapted with permission from A.W. Taylor et al.,1978, "Effects of endurance training on fiber area and enzyme activities of skeletal muscle of French Canadians," *Third International Symposium in Biochemistry of Exercise.* (Miami, FL: Symposium Specialists Inc.), pp. 267-278.

individual ages. A second factor that results in a greater proportion of ST fibers appears to be the selective loss of fast motoneurons (Doherty et al., 1993) to the atrophying FT fibers, some of which are thought to be reinnervated by slow motor units (collateral sprouting) (see figure 2.3). Despite the relatively greater proportion of ST fibers available for force generation, fatigue resistance of aging muscle is not enhanced. The reason for this is unknown; but it may be that due to a lack of training, the capacity of aged muscle is not optimized (Grimby et al., 1992; Taylor et al., 1992).

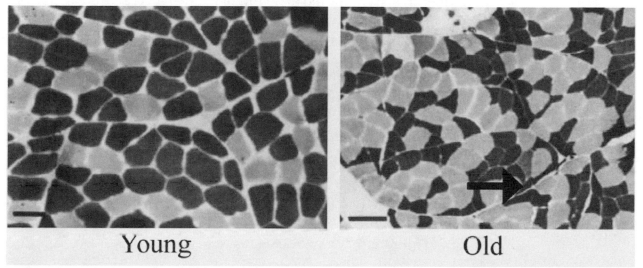

Figure 2.2 A myosin ATPase (pH 10.2) stain of a cross section of a human vastus lateralis biopsy sample. Note the differences in fiber size from *(left)* a young subject and *(right)* an older subject. Fiber size decreases as aging occurs.

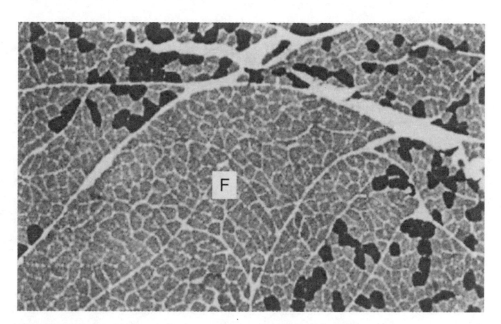

Figure 2.3 Adductor pollicic muscle of the hand (autopsy sample, transverse section) from an elderly woman with no clinical neurological signs. F, fascicle containing only type 1 fibers indicating reinnervation. (ATPase pH 9.4, type 2 fibers stain dark.)

Body Composition

As aging continues and the muscle becomes less active, areas previously designated as muscle are replaced by fat and connective tissue (Rice et al., 1989, 1990). Note in figure 2.4 the cross sections of human arms, the photograph on the right from a healthy young man and that on the left from an inactive older person. The area that was once muscle tissue is atrophied, and muscle has been replaced with connective tissue, fat, and vacuous space (the dark areas).

In figure 2.5 are computed axial tomography (CAT) scans taken from the leg of an older subject (82 years of age) before (left) and after (right) an intensive six-month endurance exercise regimen.

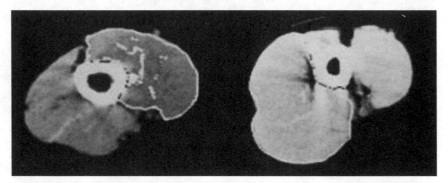

Figure 2.4 Cross section of human arms with humerus in middle showing fat (black), muscle (gray), and bone (white). *(Right)* healthy young muscle. *(Left)* inactive old muscle filled with connective tissue and fat. The outlined area on the left image shows the elbow flexor compartment including biceps and brachialis. Triceps compartment is on the bottom slightly to the left of the humerus on both panels.

Reprinted from Rice et al., 1989, "Arm and leg composition determined by computed tomography in young and elderly men," *Clinical Physiology* 9: 207-222.

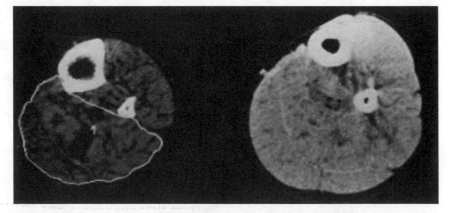

Figure 2.5 Cross section of a human leg showing tibia (larger bone) and fibula. Fat appears as black areas and muscle as gray areas. The left image shows the old and inactive leg and the right image is the same leg after 6 months of endurance training. Note the return to a healthy condition for this 82-year-old subject's muscle. The outlined compartment on the left panel is the plantar flexor compartment and includes soleus, gastrocs, and other deeper plantar flexors.

Reprinted from Rice et al., 1989, "Arm and leg composition determined by computed tomography in young and elderly men," *Clinical Physiology* 9: 207-222.

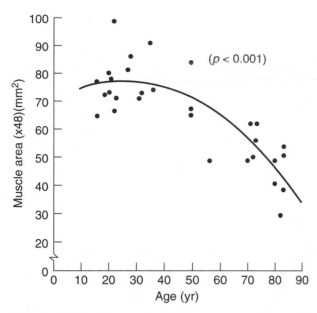

(p < 0.001)

Figure 2.6 Relationship between age and muscle area.

Reprinted, by permission, from J. Lexell, C. C. Taylor, and M. Sjostrom, 1988, "What is the cause of the ageing atrophy? total number, size and proportion of different fiber types studied in whole vastus lateralis muscles from 15- to 83-year-old men," *Journal of Neurological Science* 84: 275-294.

Note that the muscle has hypertrophied and that the infused fat and connective tissue have been replaced with skeletal muscle. These CAT scans demonstrate that the rate of decline in fiber area can be decreased with exercise. In fact, regular exercise appears to reverse most of the atrophy.

Lexell and colleagues (1988) noted, when working with human autopsy samples, that by the age of 50, muscle had suffered a 10% loss in mass; by 80 years of age, a 50% loss was prevalent. Similar findings have been obtained by other researchers around the world using other techniques such as ultrasound scanning (Young et al., 1984) and computed tomography (Rice et al., 1988). Figure 2.6 demonstrates the relationship between age and muscle area.

Fiber Size

In nonactive persons, fiber size decreases with age after reaching a maximum at about 20 years of age. Individuals who exercise regularly maintain a very high proportion of fiber size until approximately 60 years of age. It must be emphasized that the only muscles that maintain size are those that undergo regular exercise. Therefore, as one ages and loses whole-muscle mass, the decrease is due to two factors: a decrease in fiber number (mainly FT fibers) and a decrease in size of individual fibers (once again, this loss is seen mainly in the FT fibers of locomotory muscles). It is reported in the scientific literature that the major decrements in size occur between the ages of 60 and 80. The underlying mechanisms appear to be twofold: (1) inactivity and immobilization and (2) changes in functional demands for force, velocity, and duration.

Figure 2.7 demonstrates the relationship between ST and FT fiber areas and age, verifying the effect of the loss of FT fibers on the decrease in muscle size with age. However, it is now well accepted that even nonagenarians can increase fiber size with weight training (Fiatarone et al., 1990). It appears that progressive exercise has the same effects on the skeletal muscle of nonagenarians as it does on 25-year-olds (see table 2.1).

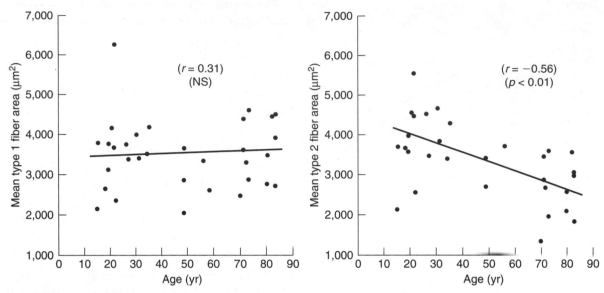

Figure 2.7 The relationship between age and mean slow-twitch and fast-twitch muscle fiber cross-sectional areas.

Reprinted, by permission, from J. Lexell, C.C. Taylor, and M. Sjostrom, 1988, "What is the cause of the ageing atrophy? total number, size and proportion of different fiber types studied in whole vastus lateralis muscles from 15-83 year old men," *Journal of Neurological Science* 84: 275-294.

TABLE 2.1 **Effects of Aging and Progressive Exercise on Muscle Mass**

Age	Sex	Training program	Aging effect	Training effects
25	M	Progressive resistance exercises at high load and low repetitions	↓	↑
25	F		↓	↑
60	M		↓	↑
60	F		↓	↑
90+	M		↓	↑
90+	F		↓	↑

Note: ↑ = increase; ↓ = decrease.

Fiber Number

As noted earlier, the number of fibers decreases with age. This loss is closely related to the marked loss of alpha motor units (MU) (see chapter 3 for more information on the nervous system). A loss of alpha motor neurons (spinal cord) and degeneration of their muscle fibers continue progressively until the seventh decade, with rapid acceleration thereafter. Tomlinson and Irving (1977), using postmortem materials, found no change in motor unit counts (L1-L3) up to the age of 60.

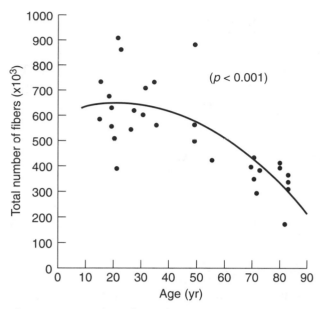

Figure 2.8 The relationship between age and the total number of fibers.

Reprinted by permission, from J. Lexell, C.C. Taylor, and M. Sjostrom, 1988, "What is the cause of the ageing atrophy? total number, size and proportion of different fiber types studied in whole vastus lateralis muscles from 15-83 year old men," *Journal of Neurological Science* 84: 275-294.

Thereafter, motor unit counts started to decrease. However, Lexell and colleagues (1988) observed a loss of muscle fibers from the age of 25, with an accelerated loss after 60 years of age (see figure 2.8). A question that remains is whether muscle degeneration is of neurological or intrinsic origin. For more advanced reading on this controversial and intriguing topic, students are referred to the works of Doherty and Brown (1993), Klitgaard and colleagues (1990), and Noble and colleagues (2004). To date, no scientific evidence exists that shows a reversal of the loss of fibers that occurs with aging. However, the rate of loss is attenuated, especially that of the FT fibers, with strength training (MacDougall et al., 1984).

Capillaries

Limited research has been carried out on the effects of aging and exercise on skeletal muscle capillarization. Since without regular exercise fiber size decreases, and the number of fibers also decreases, one would expect the number of capillaries carrying blood and its nutrients to the muscle to decrease also. And this is apparently what occurs. Table 2.2 contains data, collected by Coggan and colleagues (1992), demonstrating the expected decreases in capillary density, capillary-to-fiber ratio, and the number of capillaries in contact with each muscle fiber.

TABLE 2.2 **Skeletal Muscle Capillarization in Men and Women With Aging**

	Young men	Old men	Young women	Old women	Age effect	Gender effect
Capillary density (cap/mm²)	308 ± 16	228 ± 13	328 ± 19	248 ± 12	$p < .001$	Nonsignificant
Capillary/ fiber ratio	1.72 ± 0.14	1.39 ± 0.13	1.56 ± 0.15	0.94 + 0.07	$p < .001$	$p < .01$
Capillaries in contact with each muscle fiber	4.39 ± 0.28	3.55 ± 0.30	3.96 ± 0.35	2.67 ± 0.16	$p < .001$	$p < .05$

Reprinted, by permission, from A.R. Coggan et al., 1992, "Skeletal muscle adaptations to endurance training in 60-to 70-yr-old men and women," *Journal of Applied Physiology* 75: 1780-1786.

One other interesting aspect of the question of the effects of exercise and aging on capillarization of skeletal muscle fibers was addressed by Chilibeck and colleagues (1997), who found that capillary density (that is, the number of capillaries per cross-sectional area [CSA]) did not change with regular exercise. Once again, a beneficial aspect of regular endurance exercise has been pointed out.

Age-Related Changes in Biochemical Properties

One of the more prominent age-related changes in biochemical properties is a change in metabolic enzyme activities. Metabolic energy follows several pathways that depend on enzymes to generate energy. As discussed in the following section, results do show a decrease in the regulatory or marker enzymes as people age. Three other enzymes, hexokinase, lactic dehydrogenase, and adenosine triphosphatase, are also used to measure enzyme changes.

Metabolic Enzyme Activities

Metabolic energy potential in skeletal muscle is represented by the concentration of substrates and the concentration and activity levels of enzymes in the biochemical energy-producing pathways. These pathways include the glycogen cycle, glycolysis, the Krebs cycle, the free fatty acid (FFA) oxidation pathway, the electron transport chain, and in certain instances the transamination pathways for the utilization of protein as a substrate. These pathways generate usable energy through a variety of reactions, which are dependent on various enzymes. In the literature, the commonly used marker enzymes (indicative of the rate of a pathway) or regulatory enzymes (enzymes that control the rate of a pathway) are glycogen phosphorylase (a), phosphofructokinase (PFK), succinate dehydrogenase (SDH) or citrate synthase (CS), and beta-hydroxyacyldehydrogenase (BHAD) in the glycogen cycle, glycolytic, Krebs, and FFA oxidation pathways, respectively. Concentrations of these enzymes have been shown to change with aging; these findings offer a further explanation for reduced skeletal muscle function in elderly people.

Three other important enzymes are measured to indicate metabolic changes in pathways associated with energy production or as direct measures of energy production. These are (1) hexokinase, which is an indirect measure of the transport of glucose into the muscle cell from the circulation; (2) lactic dehydrogenase (LDH), which converts lactic acid to pyruvic acid; and (3) calcium-activated (found on the actin-myosin complex) adenosine triphosphatase (ATPase), which breaks off the phosphates from ATP to generate energy. Generally, the concentrations or activity levels (or both) of these enzymes are indicative of any changes in the metabolic rate of the given pathway.

With aging, the activity levels of all of these enzymes have been demonstrated to decrease. With exercise training, though, the concentrations or activity levels (or both) of most of them increase. This is important because the activity levels of these enzymes determine the rate, and probably the total amount, of energy available to the older person. In this context one must not forget that systems in the body seldom work in isolation. Substrates must be delivered to the working muscle, and the waste products must be carried away, or eliminated, or converted to useful products. For example, with prolonged exercise, the duration of the activity is highly correlated with the activity of the enzymes of the relevant metabolic pathways *and* the ability of the cardiovascular system (see chapter 1) to deliver oxygen to the working muscle, as well as the muscle's ability to utilize the oxygen substrate. One should also note that enzyme activities are somewhat specific and highly correlated with the type of training and the roles of the enzymes; that is, anaerobic training primarily affects the anaerobic enzymes, and aerobic training mainly affects the aerobic enzymes. Table 2.3 summarizes the effects of aging and endurance training on the activities of the skeletal muscle metabolic enzymes we have been considering.

It is interesting to note the effects of chronological aging and exercise on two of the most often studied enzymes from the Krebs cycle and the glycolytic pathway, namely SDH and PFK, respectively. In figure 2.9, note that for SDH, exercise endurance training shifts the curve to the right, which is indicative of a training effect, but in the long run the

TABLE 2.3 **Effects of Aging and Training on Skeletal Muscle Enzyme Activities**

Enzyme	Age	Sex	Training program	Aging effects	Training effects
Ca²⁺ ATPase	60-79	M	Endurance	↓	↓ or →
Hexokinase	60-79	M	Endurance	↓	→
PFK	60-79	M & F	Endurance	↑→↓	→
LDH	60-79	M & F	Endurance	↓	↑→↓
SDH	60-79	M & F	Endurance	↓	↑
CS	60-79	M & F	Endurance	↓	→
CPK	60-79	M & F	Endurance	↓	→ or ↑

Note: ↑ = increase; ↓ = decrease; → = no change.

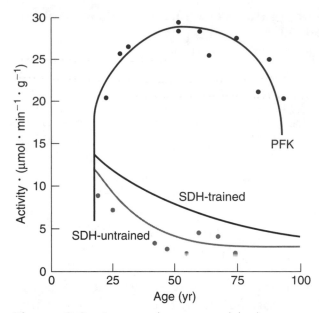

Figure 2.9 Aging and succinate dehydrogenase and phosphofructokinase activities with endurance training.

effects of aging prevail. For PFK, however, endurance exercise has little impact on the effects of aging.

Other Biochemical Parameters

Other biochemical parameters are equally important to the skeletal muscles of older people as to those of a younger population. These parameters include substrates for energy production such as glycogen, FFAs, and protein. Metabolites, electrolytes, special consequences (remember the infiltration of fat into muscle), and free phosphate concentration all play roles in the production of energy of the muscle. Table 2.4 summarizes the effects of aging and various types of exercise on selected biochemical parameters. Note that for many of these factors, relatively little research on aging and training effects has been carried out.

TABLE 2.4 **Effects of Aging and Training on Physiological and Biochemical Parameters Related to Skeletal Muscle**

Parameters	Age	Sex	Training program	Aging effects	Training effects
Fatty acids	65+	M	N/A	N/A	N/A
Cholesterol	65+	M	N/A	→	N/A
Glycogen	65+	M	Endurance	N/A	N/A
PCr/Pi	65+	M	Endurance	↓	→
Na/K pump	65+	M	Endurance	N/A	N/A
Fatty infiltration	65+	M	Endurance	↑	↓
Fiber area	65+	M	Endurance	N/A	→↓
Fiber area	65+	M	Strength	↓	↑
Protein breakdown	58+	M	Strength	N/A	N/A

Note: ↑ = increase; ↓ = decrease; → = no change

Skeletal Muscle, Aging, and Training

While the North American life expectancy continues to increase due to advances in medicine, the quality of life in individuals in their later years appears to decline. Loss of the ability to perform essential daily tasks is a direct cause of this decline and is most often associated with reduced muscular strength. Recent studies demonstrating an ability of elderly persons to increase muscular strength offer seniors the hope of maintaining independence for many years.

The observable decline in muscular strength with aging is often associated with both a decrease in activity and a decline in various skeletal muscle functions. These physiological changes in muscle include reduced contractility, muscle atrophy (accompanied by a reduced hypertrophic capacity), enzymatic changes (influencing muscle function and performance), and an increased prevalence of various neuromuscular diseases. The consequences of such changes in muscle function are reduced flexibility and muscular strength. However, resistance training provides an excellent means of combating the debilitating effects of aging on muscle function. Proper exercise prescription can allow for considerable changes in strength and ultimately the quality of life of elderly people.

Muscle Contractility

Skeletal muscle is composed of many individual muscle fibers made up of many myofibrils, which are in turn made up of many actin and myosin filaments (sarcomeres) (see cross section of skeletal muscle in any anatomy text). When a muscle contracts, myosin heads bind to actin, and ATP breaks the bond. Myosin then bonds to an adjacent binding site (actin) and the sarcomere shortens. As already discussed, age brings about a decrease in muscle cross-sectional (contractile tissue) area and an increase in nonmuscle tissue (fat and connective tissue). The result is reduced strength caused by reduced muscle size and contractility. A number of other noticeable changes occur to the muscle fiber with aging:

- Decrease in ATPase activity
- Decrease in motor neuron number
- Increase in length of contraction
- Lower muscle excitation threshold
- Increase in twitch tension
- New axonal nerve branches
- Decrease in nerve conduction

Hypertrophic Response and Atrophy in Skeletal Muscle

Muscle growth occurs mainly as a response to mechanical stress (e.g., exercise). This stress can induce muscle injury, primarily with eccentric exercise; and repair is often a function of the type, intensity, and duration of the stimulus. Muscle regeneration ultimately induces increases in strength through neural and hypertrophic mechanisms. It has been hypothesized that increases in muscle CSA also occur as a result of an increase in muscle fiber number (hyperplasia). However, this hypothesis remains controversial, as it is assumed that fiber number is determined at, or shortly after, birth. Increases in strength are thought to occur mainly by increased fiber diameter.

The pathway appears to be as follows:

exercise (stimulus) → muscle damage → disruption of intracellular homeostasis → proteolysis of various muscle proteins → gene expression (protein phenotype dependent on stimulus) → protein synthesis → satellite cell proliferation → hypertrophy → "ceiling size?" → fiber splitting (hyperplasia?)

Muscle atrophy or decreased CSA is caused by a loss of fibers, a decrease in fiber area, or a combination of both of these factors operating simultaneously. It is well known that fiber atrophy occurs with a decline in muscle activity, with a loss in protein, and as a result of several dystrophic diseases. Atrophy is a well-known phenomenon accompanying aging. However, it is also well documented that the rate of decline in muscle size can be slowed with regular exercise, in particular resistance training.

Sarcopenia

Sarcopenia is the age-associated loss of skeletal muscle mass, strength, and quality of contractile function. Although the cause per se of sarcopenia has yet to be identified, the main groups of factors that could be responsible are neurogenic (i.e., an age-related motor unit remodeling) (see chapter 3) and myogenic (i.e., caused by contraction-induced injury, selective primary muscle fiber atrophy, changes in contractile protein hormonal influences, or alterations in muscle fiber signal transduction), or a combination of neurogenic and myogenic factors.

Myogenic Factors

Contraction-induced injury causes morphological damage to small focal groups of sarcomeres as a result of mechanical disruption of thick and thin filaments, or Z-disc attachments (eccentric contractions). Further, injury presents as an inflammatory response that could be caused by free radical damage (delayed-onset muscle soreness, DOMS). Muscle from older subjects shows greater susceptibility to injury and delayed recovery compared with muscle from young subjects. This leads to atrophy and degeneration and may have the potential to induce age-related remodeling.

It is difficult to attribute muscle atrophy solely to aging. In all likelihood the atrophy is due to reduced activity and weight-bearing activities. Because of the observed great decrease in specific tension (F/CSA) of the muscle fibers of older people (~20%), there must be something more than selective loss and hypotrophy of fibers to explain the muscle weakness associated with aging. These factors could include changes in the myosin heavy chain (MyHC) isoforms, which are related to speed of contractile shortening (Larsson et al., 1997), or reductions in muscle protein synthesis rates, which also affect myosin ATPase activity.

Another consideration could be anabolic hormone levels, as shown in table 2.5, which may affect protein turnover rates. Hormonal influence on muscle growth is substantial at various stages of growth. In those who are elderly, a decline in hormones known to exert an anabolic effect (testosterone, insulin-like growth factor-1, insulin, etc.) may provide some insight into a reduced hypertrophic capacity and a general decline in strength. Reduced satellite cell proliferation may also be a key limiting factor to work-induced muscle growth. However, the most obvious determinant of muscular strength is muscular activity (tension), and the reduction in physical activity with aging is often the most important determinant of muscle fiber atrophy and reduced muscular strength.

Another myogenic factor to be considered is age-associated alterations in excitation contraction coupling (ECC)—the events that link the propagation of an electrical nerve impulse to muscle contraction. In particular, ECC changes related to mechanisms of sarcoplasmic reticulum (SR) Ca^{++} release and uptake are thought to be modified. The number or quality of the Ca^{++} receptor-controlled channels that govern the release of Ca^{++} from the SR is modified with age. For each wave of depolarization, the amount of Ca^{++} released in muscle from aged individuals to

TABLE 2.5 **Hormone Changes With Aging**

Hormone	Relative change
Insulin levels	↑ (→)
Insulin sensitivity*	↓
IGF-1	↓↓
Growth hormone	↓↓
Testosterone (biologically active)	↓
DHEA-S	↓↓

*May relate to fat distribution.

Note: ↑ = increase; ↓ = decrease; → = no change. IGF, insulin-like growth factor; DHEA, dehydroepiandrosterone.

trigger contraction is less than that found in younger individuals. Thus, contractile force is reduced. The evidence is not as strong for impairment of Ca^{++} uptake after contraction has been triggered. Any of the myogenic factors mentioned here may inhibit feedback and promote denervation of the fibers. Unfortunately, the effects of exercise training on these factors have yet to be studied.

Neurogenic Factors

Neurogenic factors are discussed in more detail in chapter 3. It is most difficult to separate the neuromuscular system into two distinct parts, so contractile properties are discussed briefly in this section. Whole-muscle contractile properties can be studied invasively or indirectly using electrical stimulation techniques. Most laboratories, in the past, have utilized the latter method because of the complications associated with invasive techniques. Rice's research team (Rice, 2000; Rice et al., 1988, 1989, 1990; Klein et al., 2001) found that aging has a severe effect on skeletal muscle contractile properties: time to peak tension (TPT); peak tension (Pt); tension at 10, 20, and 50 ms (Po10, Po20, Po50); and maximal contractile velocity (MCV). Table 2.6 shows the

TABLE 2.6 **Effects of Aging and Training on Contractile Properties**

Contractile property	Age	Sex	Results	Muscle	Aging effects	Training effects
TPT	25	M	105 ms	TS		
TPT	63-76	M	127 ms	TS	↑	↓
TPT	80-100	M	133 ms	LG	↑	→
TPT	80-100	F	145 ms	LG	↑	→
Pt	25	M	87 N	TS		
Pt	69	M	92 N	TS	→	→
Po10	25	M	493 N	TS		
Po10	63-76	M	388 N	TS	↓	↑
Po20	25	M	832 N	TS		
Po20	63-76	M	618 N	TS	↓	↑
Po50	25	M	1027 N	TS		
Po50	63-76	M	760 N	TS	↓	↑
MCV	25	M	1579 N	TS		
MCV	63-76	M	1248 N	TS	↓	↑

Note: ↑ = increase; ↓ = decrease; → = no change; TPT = time to peak increase; Pk = peak tension; Po10 = tension at 10 s; Po20 = tension at 20 s; Po50 = tension at 50 s; MCV = maximal contractile velocity.

effects of aging and training on these contractile properties in several skeletal muscles. It is noteworthy that regular exercise training is able to at least delay some of the debilitating effects of the aging process. Although differences exist between males and females, the trend is the same both for the aging process and for the training response.

Age-Related Diseases Limiting Exercise

Numerous diseases of the elderly population are attributed directly to the aging process. Many of these affect or are affected by the musculoskeletal and neuromuscular systems. It is important that exercise leaders be aware of the maladies as well as the symptoms of these diseases (see chapters 1, 3, 5, and 6 for additional information). The following are movement diseases and disorders of elderly persons, along with telltale signs:

- Diseases and telltale signs that directly affect the ability to exercise include the following:
    - *Parkinson's disease:* dopamine deprivation to the brain; leads to stiff muscles and joints, tremor, bradykinesia
    - *Ophthalmoplegic muscular dystrophy:* becomes manifest in adulthood; affects the extraocular muscles and those used for swallowing; facial appearance is altered
    - *Essential tremor (ET):* similar to Parkinson tremor; affects hands, legs, neck, facial, and phonatory muscles
    - *Huntington's disease:* characterized by a movement disorder, dementia, and personality change
    - *Dystonia:* involuntary movement that is twisting, repetitive, and continuous; affects neck and arms
    - *Myoclonus:* sudden involuntary contraction of muscle or group of muscles; may be a sign of other pathological conditions
- Diseases and telltale signs that indirectly affect the ability to exercise include these:
    - *Osteoarthritis:* disease in which joint structure weakens and begins to break down; gout is a form of arthritis
    - *Osteoporosis:* reduction in bone mass; weakens the body's capacity to support weight (see chapter 6)
    - *Dementia:* loss in two areas of complex behaviors such that it interferes with a person's daily activities (see chapter 3)

Of these diseases and disorders, arthritis is the most common. In fact, arthritis is the leading cause of long-term disability in North America, affecting one in seven individuals. The number of people with arthritis in North America is expected to increase by approximately 10 million per decade. The greatest increase in incidence is expected to be in the over-45 age-group. Today, it is surmised that arthritis and the complications from the disease cost North Americans approximately $200 billion a year in lost wages and health care. There are several types of arthritis, but only a few (the most prevalent) are considered here.

Ankylosing Spondylitis

Few are aware of the term ankylosing spondylitis (AS), but many are aware of the symptoms of the disease. Ankylosing means fusing together, and spondylitis is the inflammation of the vertebrae. This is a painful, progressive type of rheumatic disease that affects the spinal area as the joints and bones fuse together. It usually strikes men in their late teens and early 20s. The symptoms are as follows:

- Slow or gradual onset of back pain and stiffness over weeks or months rather than hours or days
- Possible persistence of pain down to the buttocks and thighs
- Early-morning stiffness and pain, wearing off or decreasing during the day with exercise
- Pain persistence for more than three months

The causes of AS are uncertain at this time. All AS patients seem to have a specific gene called human leukocyte antigen B27 (HLA-B27). Having this gene does not guarantee that one will contract AS, but chances are increased (about 20%). There is no conclusive evidence, but it seems that the gene must interact with certain unknown proteins in the body and that the combination alters the human immune system and causes AS.

There is no known cure for AS, but maintenance of proper posture, nonsteroidal anti-inflammatory drugs (NSAIDS), and physical activity are known to alleviate the symptoms. In order for people to feel better after exercise, maintaining little excess weight is important to alleviate stress on the affected joints. Therefore it is important that AS be diagnosed early to provide certainty that it is not a case of simple back pain, as the AS could be exacerbated by an inappropriate exercise program. The onset of the disease is usually before the age of 40, and the first sign is morning stiffness of the spine. Obviously, exercises that rotate or forcefully bend the spine are contraindicated. There appears to be improvement in pain relief with regular movement that does not overtax the spinal column.

Fibromyalgia

Fibromyalgia is estimated to affect between 2% and 6% of the population. The symptoms include widespread pain for at least three months and tenderness in 11 of 18 active tender points, as well as signs of fatigue and disturbed sleep, stiffness and numbness, joint or soft tissue swelling, and dry eyes. People with fibromyalgia have an intolerance to cold; sensitivity to foods, allergens, and medications; feeling of weakness; poor memory or concentration, which may also be accompanied by depression, tension, or migraine headaches; irritable bowel and bladder; chronic fatigue syndrome; and temporomandibular joint dysfunction. The causes of fibromyalgia are unknown, but possible factors include the following, singly or in combination:

- Mechanical problems in the neck and lower back
- Motor vehicle accidents
- Work-related injuries
- Viral illnesses
- Surgery
- Infections
- Emotional trauma
- Physical or emotional stress

The treatments for this debilitating disease include medication, physical therapy, and a lifestyle management program. Regular endurance activity at a slow walking pace has shown some signs of mild success in alleviating the symptoms.

Rheumatoid Arthritis

Rheumatoid arthritis (RA) is a chronic, progressive, systemic disorder that is classified as an inflammatory disease. Women appear to be affected more than men (3:1); but as age increases, the difference tends to decrease. The onset of the disease is generally between the ages of 20 and 50 years. The disease occurs bilaterally and is severely debilitating. The extent of the debilitation is such that many individuals with the disease experience the psychological disorders of depression, anxiety, and learned helplessness. The signs and symptoms are as follows:

- Pain and swelling of joints
- Morning stiffness of joints and muscles
- General weakness and fatigue
- Fever and weight loss
- Tenderness, deformity, and limited motion
- Wrists, ankles, and toes commonly affected
- Elbows, shoulders, feet, ankle, knees, and hips also generally affected

Although the mechanism behind the cause is unknown, RA is caused by a failure of the body's immune system. An inflammatory response prevents the white blood cells (WBC) from removing foreign products from the joints, and the congregation of blood cells leads to further inflammation. There appear to be a defect in the inflammatory process, which persists and which exacerbates the swelling from edemic fluid in the joint (infiltration of leukocytes), and a proliferation of synoviocytes, blood vessels, and lymphatics. Synoviocytes grow and divide abnormally, causing the synovial membrane to become thicker, tender, and more swollen. Two types of white blood cells (lymphocytes and leukocytes) are the primary infection-fighting units in the body. The lymphocytes are divided into two subtypes (T-cells and B-cells). T-cells mistake the body's own collagen as a foreign antigen and therefore attempt, with good success, to destroy it. This process stimulates the B-cells to produce antibodies that attack the antigen (the body's own cells). The ensuing cascade of events leads to a vicious cycle by which collagen is destroyed; this in turn leads to the deterioration of the articular collagen, necrosis, and thus contracture. The bottom line is a crippling effect that is irreversible.

The treatment for RA is heat to decrease pain, ice to decrease inflammation, and stretching and strengthening exercises to help slow the progress of the disease. Apparently the exercise also alleviates some of the psychological problems. NSAIDS, disease-modifying antirheumatic drugs (DMARDS), and corticosteroids are sometimes of assistance; and surgery is the last resort.

Osteoarthritis

Osteoarthritis (OA) is a functional disorder of the joints, characterized by altered joint anatomy, especially the loss of articular cartilage. There are three types of OA: primary, secondary, and generalized primary. Osteoarthritis increases in prevalence parallel with age; by age 70, about 85% of the populace will have some degree of OA. Racial patterns, varying occupations, and lifestyles have been noted, and about 10% of North Americans are affected. The signs and symptoms include the following:

- Persistent joint pain and stiffness
- Common effects on weight-bearing joints such as the knees, hip, spine, and feet
- Effects also on the finger joints and base of the thumb
- Altered joint anatomy, not cartilage, as the source of pain
- Inflammation, usually mild if present
- A possible grating sound when roughened cartilage rubs together

The risk factors for this disease are well known as excess weight, heredity, injury, and age. The clinical symptoms are well defined by changes in joint anatomy that can be seen by simple X-ray. There is a gradual narrowing of the joint spaces due to loss of cartilage, thickening of bone endings, development of fluid-filled cysts deep in the bone, and growth of bony spurs (osteophytes) at the edges of the bone joints. Other changes occur that cannot be seen on the X-ray. Cartilage becomes pitted and cracked with tiny fissures; the lining of the joint is thickened and may be inflamed; the joint capsule becomes thickened; and synovial fluid increases in volume and water content.

The resultant pain is caused by tendons, ligaments, and muscles contracting in spasm to protect the joint from movement. Inflammation occurs when eroded cartilage floats in synovial fluid and irritates the synovial membrane. When cartilage is weak or damaged, the nerve endings on bone sense pain from weight-bearing forces, which causes increased blood flow (hyperemia), which leads to further pain. Due to the erosion of cartilage, bones rub against one another, again increasing the pain. It should be recognized that OA is not an inflammatory disease, although it shows some similar symptoms. Nor is it a simple disease in terms of finding the causal mechanism. Once again, a very complex cascade of events describes the pathology of OA, including the structural breakdown of cartilage and the proliferation of new bone. When reparative processes fail to keep pace with degenerative changes, OA ensues. Some 20% to 30% of the populace over 65 have OA of the knee, and women are twice as likely as men to develop OA in this joint. The spine is the other joint most often affected by OA.

Osteoarthritis can be treated with medication, heat or cold application, weight control, viscosupplementation, exercise, and finally, surgery. Before one begins exercise therapy, one should consult a registered physiotherapist or kinesiologist. The primary aims of the exercise programs are to reduce pain, improve range of motion, increase strength, normalize gait, and permit the individual to perform activities of daily living. The overall goals of the exercise are to reduce joint stress, improve shock attenuation, maintain active joint motion and alignment, and prevent disability and improve overall health. The exercise program must include aerobic conditioning as well as flexibility, strength, and neuromuscular exercises. If joint pain is already prevalent, then non-weight-bearing training should be initiated, with a gradual buildup to weight bearing, if possible. Remember, encouragement by the exercise leader or health care provider is very important with respect to initiation and maintenance of an exercise program.

Programming Recommendations

ACSM Weight-Training Exercise Guidelines for Individuals over 50 (American College of Sports Medicine, 1998) recommend the following parameters for basic training for older individuals:

- Perform one set of 10 to 15 reps, 8 to 10 exercises, two to three days per week.
- Use minimal resistance for the first eight weeks.

- Maintain a normal breathing pattern during all exercises.
- Increase repetitions; then increase the amount of weight being lifted.
- Never use a weight so heavy that you can't perform at least eight reps.
- Perform all exercises in a controlled manner. Take 2 sec to lift the weight and 4 sec to lower it.
- Perform all the exercises within a "pain-free arc." Never "lock out" the joint when attempting to straighten your arms or legs.
- If you have arthritis, do not participate in any exercise session during a period of pain or inflammation.
- Do not overtrain.
- Do a minimum of two strength training sessions per week to produce positive results.
- Do not do the same exercises two times in a row within the same session.
- Engage in a year-round resistance training program on a regular basis.
- If you have to take time off from this program, gently ease back into your routine.
- When returning from a layoff, start with resistances no greater than 50% of the intensity at which you had been previously training; then gradually increase the resistance.

Summary

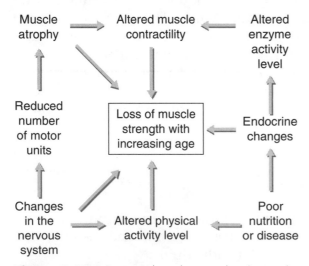

Figure 2.10 Proposed mechanisms leading to the loss of muscle strength with increasing age.

Reprinted by permission, from M.M. Porter, A.A. Vandervoort, and J. Lexell, 1995, "Aging of human muscle: Structure, function and adaptability," *Scandinavian Journal of Medicine and Science in Sports* 5: 138.

In the first part of this chapter we reviewed the basic physiology of human skeletal muscle and explored the effects of aging and physical exercise on muscle physiology. Fiber types were discussed in terms of size, total number, CSA, and capillarization. Enzymes of the several metabolic pathways, which lead to the generation of energy, were discussed with particular reference to endurance exercise and aging. Sarcopenia was defined; and the causative factors, both myogenic and neurogenic, that are thought to lead to muscular atrophy were discussed. In particular, contractile properties as they affect muscle and are affected by the aging process and exercise were emphasized. Much of the material in this chapter is consistent with a mechanism proposed by Porter and colleagues (1995) for the loss of strength with aging and the effects of exercise (see figure 2.10). Limitations to exercise because of several disease states were introduced, and arthritis was emphasized in detail. The weight training guidelines for elderly persons as outlined by the American College of Sports Medicine were listed.

Questions to Consider

1. What fiber types are found in human skeletal muscle? Do they differ from those of other mammals? What are the effects of aging on these fiber types?

2. Are capillary beds affected by aging? By exercise?

3. Which are the primary enzymes controlling the metabolic pathways for energy production? Are the same pathways found in all mammals?

4. Does skeletal muscle of older people respond the same to exercise as that of young subjects?

5. How is muscle force produced?

6. What is sarcopenia?

7. Can the muscle of older people adapt with weight training? If so, how? If not, what are the mechanisms preventing the changes?

8. How are muscle fiber size and mass affected by aging and by exercise? Remember to consider different types of exercise.

9. Is there an aging–muscle area curve? If so, how does it differ from a fiber–age curve? If not, what are the reasons a curve would not be appropriate?

10. Is there a linear relationship between any of the marker or regulatory enzymes in the energy pathways and aging?

11. How specific is exercise training to the regulatory enzyme activities? To their concentrations?

12. Why does skeletal muscle of females react differently to exercise and aging than muscle of males? And how does it do this?

13. Which type of arthritis can be cured by exercise?

14. Can arthritis be induced by exercise? If so, how? If not, why not?

15. Why is flexibility so important for older people?

chapter 3

Nervous System

Michel J. Johnson, PhD, and Anthony A. Vandervoort, PhD

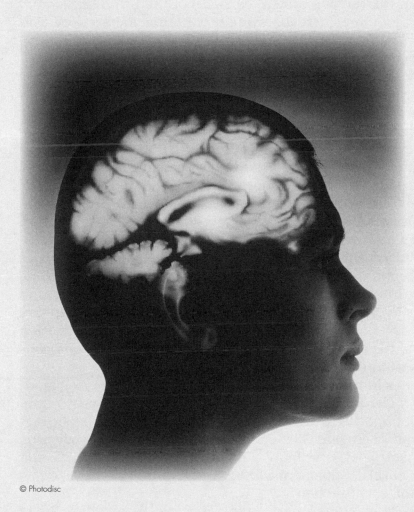

© Photodisc

In elderly people, alterations in nervous system function can be observed, including changes in functional capacity and cognitive ability. Changes associated solely with the aging process are difficult to identify since disease and lifestyle, for example, and prolonged inactivity and nutrition can also influence the function of the nervous system.

Overview of the Nervous System

The nervous system consists of both a central and a peripheral component. The central nervous system consists of the brain and spinal cord, and the peripheral nervous system contains the sensory and motor neurons that relay information from the periphery to the central nervous system and vice versa.

We find two types of neural tissue within the nervous system, neurons and neuroglia. Neurons generate and transmit electrical impulses, and they are the functional unit of the nervous system. Neurons typically consist of a soma (cell body), an axon, dendrites, and axon terminals (figure 3.1). Dendrites convey signals from other nerve cells to the soma. The soma contains the nucleus and organelles of the cell, and integrates information from the dendrites. Nervous impulses are conducted along the length of the axon to the axon terminals that contact other nerve cells or effectors such as muscles or glands. The axons are surrounded by a myelin sheath with regular gaps called nodes of Ranvier. Nerve impulses can leap from node of Ranvier to node of Ranvier (saltatory conduction) leading to faster conduction speeds. Neurons can be divided into three functional classes: afferent, efferent, and interneurons. Afferent neurons transmit information from the periphery to the central nervous system. Efferent neurons transmit information from the central nervous system to the periphery. Interneurons connect neurons within the central nervous system.

Most of the cells in the nervous system are made up of neuroglia, or glial cells. Neuroglia provide neurons with nourishment, protection, and structural support. The three types of neuroglia are oligodendroglia, astroglia, and microglia. Oligodendroglia form the myelin covering around axons. Astroglia serve many functions, including metabolism, signaling, and neural development within the nervous system. Microglia contribute to immune function.

As the numbers of human nerve and muscle cells are thought to become fixed in a postmitotic state before or shortly after birth, their decline in later life is representative of important principles of the aging process: It is intrinsic, progressive, deleterious, and irreversible.

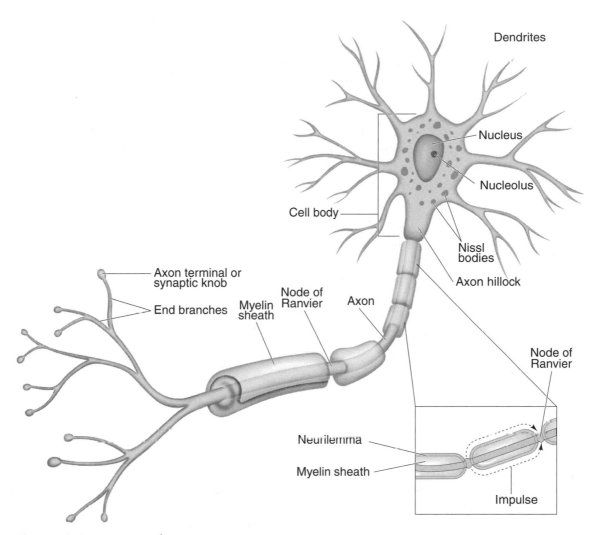

Figure 3.1 Structure of a neuron.

Reprinted, by permission, from J. Wilmore and D. Costill, 2003, *Physiology of sport and exercise*, 3rd ed. (Champaign, IL: Human Kinetics), 62.

However, as Fries and Crapo (1981) noted in their influential book, it is important to remember that normal aging is often confounded with the effects of a sedentary lifestyle. In one sense, the remarkable longevity of a human neuron or muscle fiber must be admired. Some people will live for over a century, and some of their cells will have been generating action potentials and manufacturing a wide array of proteins throughout that time. However, other excitable cells that were present at maturation will have disappeared, leaving a reduced reserve. This loss of neurons has been demonstrated throughout the nervous system, although there are regional variations in the extent to which this occurs.

The existence of neuronal loss may be subtle and generally well compensated for, in even the oldest individuals; but excessive localized degeneration and cell loss are found in clinical conditions such as Parkinsonism (basal ganglia), senile dementia of the Alzheimer's type (neocortex and hippocampus), or Friedreich's ataxia (cerebellum). It should also be noted that motor cells may be present on anatomical observation yet still be dysfunctional because of biochemical changes within (MacIntosh et al., 2006). Nerve cells communicate via neurotransmitters; hence it has been of considerable interest to investigate the effect of aging on these chemical messengers. Such research is complicated because of the complex nature of signaling—synthesis, release, diffusion, reception, postreceptor action, and degradation of a given neurotransmitter—and the ever-growing variety of neurotransmitter chemicals found in the nervous system (e.g., acetylcholine, dopamine, norepinephrine, serotonin, gamma-aminobutryic acid [GABA], and many peptides including endorphins). However, for the ubiquitous neurotransmitters such as acetylcholine and dopamine, differences between young and aged nervous systems have been noted for each aspect of signaling (Magnoni et al., 1991). Finally, nerve cells also show a loss of dendritic and synaptic connections in aged nervous systems, along with microscopic changes such as accumulation of lipofuscin and neurofibrillary triangles. However, the remarkable redundancy of the nervous system also becomes apparent when it is realized that despite these changes, mental function of most aged people remains adequate for an independent lifestyle.

Central Nervous System

The central nervous system (CNS) is made up of the brain and spinal cord. The CNS is critical in initiating and regulating motor, cognitive, autonomic, and sensory mechanisms. A brief review of its structure and function will help readers better appreciate the potential impact of CNS changes associated with aging.

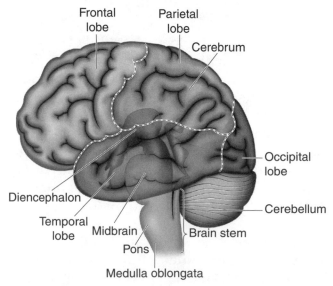

Figure 3.2 Anatomical divisions of the brain.

Reprinted, by permission, from J. Wilmore and D. Costill, 2003, *Physiology of sport and exercise*, 3rd ed. (Champaign, IL: Human Kinetics), 69.

The Brain

The anatomical subdivisions of the brain are the cerebrum, diencephalon, brainstem, and cerebellum (figure 3.2).

• **Cerebrum.** The cerebrum is divided by a deep longitudinal fissure into left and right cerebral hemispheres. The two cerebral hemispheres are connected by the corpus callosum. Each cerebral hemisphere consists of a cerebral cortex, underlying nuclei, and myelinated fiber tracts forming the white matter.

  – *Cerebral cortex.* The cortex of each hemisphere is divided into four lobes: the fontal lobe, the parietal lobe, the occipital lobe, and the temporal lobe. Certain areas of the cerebral cortex are dedicated to the processing of sensory or motor information. These areas are called primary, secondary, or tertiary depending on the level of processing. Association areas surround the primary, secondary, and tertiary areas and also help integrate information.

– **Subcortical nuclei.** Deep within the cerebrum lie a number of subcortical nuclei. The basal ganglia, made up of the caudate nucleus, putamen, globus pallidus, subthalamic nucleus, and substantia nigra, are subcortical nuclei that participate in the control of movement, posture, and behavior.

– **White matter.** The white matter represents dense collections of myelinated axons. Myelin is a protein with a high lipid content that serves to insulate the axon. This insulation facilitates transmission of electrical impulses down the axon to the synapse.

• **Diencephalon.** The diencephalon is centrally located and is nearly surrounded by the cerebral hemispheres. It includes the thalamus, hypothalamus, and epithalamus. The thalamus serves as a relay station for sensory impulses. The hypothalamus plays a key role in maintaining homeostasis, regulating heartbeat, body temperature, and fluid balance. The functions of the epithalamus include the secretion of melatonin and the regulation of hunger and thirst.

• **Brainstem.** The brainstem is composed of the midbrain, the pons, and the medulla oblongata. The midbrain helps regulate hearing and vision reflexes. The medulla is involved in breathing, swallowing, blood circulation, and muscle tone. The pons is involved in the control of movement, sleep, and arousal.

• **Cerebellum.** The cerebellum is located below the occipital lobes of the cerebrum. The cerebellum plays an important role in the coordination and learning of movements and the control of posture and balance. The cerebellum receives information from the muscles, joints, skin, eyes, ears, viscera, and other parts of the brain involved in movement.

The Spinal Cord

The spinal cord extends from the foramen magnum at the base of the skull to the level of the first lumbar vertebra. The spinal cord has two main functions. It serves as a conduction pathway for impulses going to and from the brain and acts as a reflex center. Many reflexes are mediated in the spinal cord without going to the higher brain centers.

Age-Related Changes to the CNS

Tissue loss in the brain begins as early as the third decade, and brain weight can decrease by about 10% between the ages of 30 and 90. Average tissue losses are estimated to be 14% in the cerebral cortex, 35%

in the hippocampus, and 26% in the cerebral white matter (Jernigan et al., 2001). Particularly high losses are reported in the frontal, parietal, and temporal cortices. Decreases in certain enzymes, receptors, and neurotransmitters in the brain are also observed with aging. The number of cells in the spinal cord decreases with age as well.

It is suggested that aerobic exercise may, in addition to providing cardiovascular fitness benefits, slow down the progress of age-related changes. Diminished tissue loss in the frontal, parietal, and temporal cortices in older adults has been linked to aerobic fitness in older adults (Colcombe et al., 2003). Cardiovascular fitness may affect the cortical structures, blood flow, or neurotransmitter activity in the brain (Colcombe et al., 2004).

Peripheral Nervous System

The peripheral nervous system (PNS) contains 43 pairs of nerves: 12 pairs of cranial nerves and 31 pairs of spinal nerves (8 cervical, 12 thoracic, 5 lumbar, 5 sacral, 1 coccygeal) that carry efferent and afferent information. The PNS can thus be divided into afferent and efferent divisions. The efferent division consists of the autonomic nervous system (ANS) and the somatic nervous system (SNS). In general, the ANS (involuntary) neurons innervate smooth muscle, cardiac muscle, and glands while the SNS (voluntary) neurons (motor neurons) innervate skeletal muscle.

Structure

Neurons use chemical messengers called neurotransmitters to communicate with each other or with other target cells. Hundreds of substances have been identified as possible neurotransmitters. The major classes of neurotransmitters are (1) the biogenic amines, which are synthesized from amino acids and contain an amino group (acetylcholine, catecholamines, serotonin, histamine); (2) amino acids (glutamate, aspartate, gamma-aminobutyric acid, glycine); (3) neuropeptides, which are two or more linked amino acids (beta-endorphin, enkephalins, dynorphins, substance P, somatostatin, etc.); (4) gases (nitric oxide, carbon monoxide); and (5) purines (adenosine, adenosine triphosphate).

The cell bodies of motor neurons are located in the cerebral cortex and brainstem. The axon of each motor neuron reaches all the way from its origin in the CNS to its target muscle fibers. Nerve impulses sent along the motor neurons trigger the release of the neurotransmitter acetylocholine (Ach) at the neuromuscular junction. In contrast to the single neuron organization of the motor system, the descending pathways of the ANS use a two-neuron chain to reach target organs. The cell body of the first neurons (preganglionic) are located in the CNS while their axons synapse in autonomic gangli located in the peripheral nervous system. From the autonomic ganglion, a second neuron (postganglionic) reaches the target organs (smooth muscle, cardiac muscle, glands) where neurotransmitters are released. The ANS is divided into sympathetic and parasympathetic components. Nerve fibers from these two components leave the CNS at different levels. Those from the sympathetic division (thoracolumbar division) leave the CNS from the thoracic and lumbar regions of the spinal cord, while those from the parasympathetic division (craniosacral division) exit from the brain and sacral portions of the spinal cord. Acetylcholine is released between postganglionic fibers and the target tissue in the parasympathetic system, while norepinephrine (NE) is the major neurotransmitter released between the postganglionic fiber and the target tissue in the sympathetic division. However, some sympathetic postganglionic fibers release acetylcholine, and one or more cotransmitters can also be released (adenosine triphosphate, dopamine, etc.). Certain sympathetic preganglionic neurons reach the adrenal medulla where they initiate the release of epinephrine (80%) and a little norepinephrine (20%) into the bloodstream.

The two major types of cholinergic (acetylcholine) receptors are muscarinic (respond to muscarine, a poison from mushrooms) and nicotinic (respond to the drug nicotine). They interact with G proteins that in turn affect different enzymes and ion channels. There are also two major types of adrenergic (norepinephrine) receptors: the alpha- and beta-receptors. The adrenergic receptors are divided into alpha-1 and alpha-2 and beta-1 and beta-2 receptors (identified on the basis of reaction to certain drugs).

Age-Related Changes to the PNS

Nerve conduction time decreases with age through demyelinization; nonetheless, this does not result in a significant change in peripheral nerve function. Reinnervation of damaged nerves is slower in elderly than in younger people. Physical activity may not only retard age-related changes, but may also facilitate recovery following injury in those who are elderly (Vaynman and Gomez-Pinilla, 2005).

The CNS puts movement plans into action by activating motor units (MUs), each consisting of a single motoneuron and its family of innervated muscle cells. Considerable flexibility is built into the peripheral motor pathways due to the variability in contractile properties between these MUs. With use of the electrophysiological technique of MU estimation, a striking decline in the number of excitable MUs present in skeletal muscles has been demonstrated beginning in the seventh decade (see Doherty et al., 1993; McComas, 1996). The functional implications of this loss of muscle mass are widespread; hence the atrophy is of much interest from both a biological and a rehabilitation perspective.

Modern radiological techniques allow accurate measurements of muscle cross-sectional areas in healthy people of different ages. The thigh muscles show significant reductions (25-35%) in size for older adults versus young, yet muscles of the upper limb do not always atrophy to the same extent (Lexell and Vandervoort, 2002; Doherty, 2003). This regional difference suggests that the leg muscles studied were demonstrating a form of disuse atrophy (i.e., older adults had stopped exercising them as much). While this is an attractive hypothesis when one is trying to promote increased weight-bearing activity, gerontologists are also studying other factors such as changes in trophic supply from motoneurons and systemic levels of circulating hormones. It is also important to remember that simple anthropometric measurements may be misleading in estimating muscle mass in older groups. The overall shape and exterior girth of older people's limbs can appear to be unchanged if fat and connective tissue have replaced the disappearing muscle.

Among a number of skeletal muscles investigated, the vastus lateralis, of the quadriceps group, has received particular attention from gerontologists (Lexell and Vandervoort, 2002). In one study of cadavers, the total number of muscle fibers observed decreased substantially with increasing age, such that an 80-year-old had about 50% fewer fibers than a young adult. There was also evidence of fiber atrophy, but this was specific to the type II fast-twitch fibers and not observed in the type I slow-twitch fibers. It is not known why the type II fibers would be more susceptible to age-related deterioration, yet one encouraging finding is that those that remain appear to be capable of hypertrophy during a weightlifting program (Porter, 2001; Lexell and Vandervoort, 2002).

The preferential atrophy of type II fibers, and some evidence of fiber type grouping as well, have been interpreted as evidence of an ongoing denervation and reinnervation process that may favor the preservation of type I fibers in older muscles. It is also postulated that some of the type I motoneurons actually enlarge their own MU territory by capturing neighboring fibers "orphaned" by their deteriorating original axon. In support of this theory, the decline in the number of functional MUs is coupled with the appearance of some very large electromyographic potentials in the profile of an older muscle (McComas, 1996). It is suggested that frail elderly persons manifest this physiological change more than those who are healthy.

The changes in fibers and MUs contribute to slower muscle contraction. Slowing of contraction has a disadvantage because it gives older muscle a reduced capacity for rapid production of force in protective reflexes (i.e., when ballistic, phasic reactions are required). This slowness factor combines with other changes in the neuromuscular system to magnify the functional deficit (Vandervoort, 1999). For example, if an older person steps on an obstacle, the kinesthetic and pain sensations are less intense and nerve impulses slower to travel around the reflex loop to the muscle. After the signal arrives at the muscle, the actual generation of restorative torque is slower as well and may not occur in time to prevent a loss of balance. Also, the muscle response must act against increased passive resistance of the connective tissue structures of the antagonistic muscles, a factor that hinders rapid stretch and therefore rotation of aged joints, particularly in very old women.

There is clear evidence for deterioration throughout the postural control system in association with the aging process. Although at some point these degenerative changes may seem to be small and insignificant, the summation of deficits will increase the risk of incorrect or inefficient responses and a subsequent loss of coordination, particularly when one is attempting a taxing functional activity (e.g., going down stairs while carrying a load, moving sideways quickly to avoid a collision). Slower postural reflexes alone will not always be the cause of a fall, but, combined with other biological changes such as delay in the detection of imbalance and disorganization of central processing, put the older individual at increased risk.

Age-Related Diseases

A large number of diseases can affect central and peripheral nervous system function, and a discussion of each is far beyond the scope of this text. Therefore, we chose to explore dementia because this syndrome is associated with a number of illnesses, and its impact extends to both those individuals with dementia and their caregivers.

Types and Demographics of Dementia

The term dementia is used to describe the group of symptoms associated with changes in the brain that cause cognitive problems. Some of the most common symptoms include confusion, memory loss, difficulty performing familiar tasks, problems with language, and changes in mood or behavior. For our purposes, we will distinguish between three types of dementia in elderly people: Alzheimer's disease, vascular dementia, and Lewy body dementia. Alzheimer's disease is the most common type of dementia, accounting for approximately two-thirds of all dementia cases. It is characterized by a gradual onset and a continuing decline of memory and is not explained by other disorders. Vascular dementia is associated with problems in the circulation of blood to the brain (cerebrovascular disease). Vascular dementia usually results from damage to brain function from single or multiple strokes (multi-infarct dementia) and accounts for approximately 20% of all cases of dementia in Canada. In 1991, 1.5% of the population 65+ had some form of vascular dementia. Lewy body dementia is associated with abnormal protein deposits called Lewy bodies found in neurons. Dr. Frederick Lewy first described them in the early 20th century. Some of the common presentations include progressive cognitive decline, fluctuating symptoms, recurrent visual hallucinations, movement difficulties, hypersensitivity to neuroleptics (antipsychotic drugs), and repeated falls.

Although dementia can strike at any age, it is mostly a disease of elderly people, affecting more than 15% of persons over the age of 65 and as many as 40% of persons over the age of 80. In 1991 (National Advisory Council on Aging, 1996), 8% of Canadians (±250,000) over the age of 65 suffered from dementia, and the economic cost of dementia was estimated to be over $3.9 billion annually (±5.8% of total health care costs). In 1991, women accounted for 68% of dementia cases. The greater number of women with dementia mainly reflects the greater number of women in older age-groups in which the likelihood of dementia is even higher. It is expected that the number of cases will triple by 2031, and costs will rise to upward of $12 billion per year. Approximately 50% of seniors with dementia live in the community while the rest reside in an institutional setting. The net economic cost of caring for a dementia patient in the community is $10,100, compared with $19,100 in an institution. As many as 10,000 deaths per year can be attributed directly to dementia (1985 data).

Alzheimer's Disease

Alzheimer's disease (AD) is the leading type of dementia, and the number of people who have this disease is expected to triple over the next 20 years as the population ages. It is estimated that by 2025, as many as 22 million people around the world may suffer from AD. This disease was not recognized as a unique form of dementia until the 1960s, although the German neurologist Alois Alzheimer characterized the syndrome at a meeting in Munich in 1906. During this meeting, he described the symptoms observed in a 51-year-old female patient (Auguste D) who died after years of progressive dementia. The symptoms described included progressive memory impairment; altered cognitive function; changed behavior including paranoia, delusions, and loss of social appropriateness; and a progressive decline in language function. During an autopsy, Alzheimer also observed that the patient's brain tissue had abnormal clumps and irregular knots of brain cells. These signs remain the hallmark of the disease even today.

It is estimated that 8.5% of the world population 65+ and 28% of the world population 85+ suffer from AD. In 1991, it was estimated that 5.1% of the Canadian population 65+ had AD (±161,000). This accounted for approximately two-thirds of all dementia cases.

Risk Factors and Diagnosis

Although no definite cause of AD has been identified, a number of factors have been associated with a greater risk of developing the disease:

- History of head trauma
- Heredity
- Slow-acting virus
- Environmental toxins
- Mitochondrial genetic defect
- Decreased blood flow to the brain (inadequate oxygen and glucose delivery)

In the early stages of AD, some of the changes may be very subtle, and we often do not recognize the problems immediately. There is no single diagnostic test that can detect if a person has AD. Standard clinical methods combine physical and neuropsychological testing with caregiver input and the physician's judgment. A large part of the diagnosis remains the exclusion of other illnesses that may cause intellectual impairment (brain tumors, thyroid problems, etc.) whereby the evaluator has come to the conclusion that symptoms are most likely the result of AD: probable diagnosis. Current clinical diagnostic tools can accurately diagnose AD in about 90% of cases. Alzheimer's disease is associated with changes in neurotransmitters (i.e., loss of acetylcholine and serotonin) and structural changes within the brain. A definite diagnosis of AD can be made only through an autopsy at the time of death. During the autopsy, three distinct structural abnormalities are observed in AD: (1) loss of neurons, (2) amyloid plaques, and (3) neurofibrillary tangles.

Treatment

The progression of AD is variable (2-20 years), and can be influenced by such factors as age of onset, environment, and concomitant pathologies (stroke, Parkinson's, etc.). Although there is presently no known cure, proper management may slow down the progression of the disease. Proper management strategies include the following:

- Control of medication
- Maintenance of normal wake/sleep cycles
- Ensured adequate nutrition
- Optimization of physical health
- Minimization of social isolation

Drug therapy in AD seeks to improve memory (cholinergic drugs) and slow the progression (nerve growth factor, calcium channel blockers) of the disease. Some of the more common medications include these:

- **Tacrine (Cognex).** Tacrine can improve mental abilities in about 30% of people with mild to moderate AD by slowing the breakdown of neurotransmitters in the brain. However, the drug has been linked to liver complications.
- **Donepezil (Aricept).** This medication also decreases mild to moderate symptoms of Alzheimer's by improving levels of neurotransmitters

in the brain. Its side effects, which include nausea, diarrhea, and fatigue, are usually mild and do not last long.

- **Rivastigamine (Exelon).** Like tacrine and donepezil, rivastigamine blocks the breakdown of neurotransmitters in the brain, lessening symptoms. Side effects may include nausea and vomiting.

- **Other.** Medications aimed at improving behavioral symptoms that often accompany Alzheimer's are also often prescribed. These symptoms include sleeplessness, wandering, anxiety, agitation, and depression.

Programming Recommendations

Exercise is an important part of the management plan for seniors with dementia because daily routine will help people retain a sense of self-esteem and keep disruptive behaviors in check. There is also evidence of a positive relationship between fitness and cognition. Moreover, exercise will enable the person to remain functionally mobile, active, and healthy.

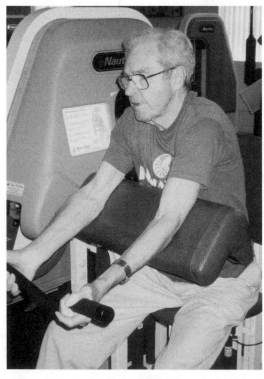

This gentleman (89 years old at the time of this photo) engaged in a fitness program that included a daily walk of at least 1.6K as well as a Nautilus 15-exercise strength training circuit 3 times a week. He had experienced Alzheimer's onset at age 87, but maintained a high quality of life for more than a decade, aided by a fitness level achieved through the exercise program he continued until well into his 97th year.

Courtesy of Wayne A. Westcott.

Guidelines

Here are guidelines that should be followed for exercise programs for seniors with dementia:

- What type of exercise is best?
  - Aerobic activity (walking) is highly recommended, as it will increase cerebral blood flow.
  - Modified games, dancing, and intergenerational activities are recommended.
  - Repetitive and familiar movements such as household tasks should be encouraged.
  - Consider physical abilities, perceptual processes, and cognitive functions.
  - Plan activities that will create opportunities for success.
  - Organize activities at the most appropriate time of day.
  - Monitor participants' functional ability (increase or decrease level of difficulty of exercises accordingly).
  - When planning activities, keep them familiar, simple, repetitive, structured, flexible, successful, and fun.
- FITT principle
  - Frequency: Participants should exercise a minimum of three times per week at an intensity to elicit improvement in functional capacity.

- – Intensity: The intensity should be sufficient to challenge the individual without being perceived as unduly difficult.
- – Time: A structured exercise program of 20 to 30 min in length is recommended.
- – Type: The activity should be specific to the desired goal.
- Walking programs
  - – Have participants walk in noncrowded areas.
  - – Participants will walk more securely when provided with a visual target.
  - – Break up a long walk into shorter legs.
  - – Warn of obstacles and irregularities in the terrain.
  - – Establish a walking rhythm; you can help by setting a somewhat exaggerated rhythm.
  - – If a participant is having difficulty, use single-word commands.

Leadership Implications

Seniors with dementia require a unique style of leadership.

- Presentation of activity
  - – Inform participant of the goals of activity.
  - – Break down exercise into logical and simple steps.
  - – Use concise statements (e.g., "Stand up").
  - – Limit distractions (i.e., clutter, noise, interruptions).
  - – Ensure that all equipment is present.
  - – Encourage routines within the exercise group so that the process becomes familiar to participants.
- Guidance during exercise
  - – Provide only as much guidance as required.
  - – Start with a verbal cue (e.g., "Throw ball") and then try gesturing (i.e., pretend to throw ball); next, demonstrate (i.e., throw ball while person observes); finally, try hands-on direction (i.e., put ball in person's hand with your hands over top, demonstrate throw).
  - – Fade out guidance as soon as participant is on track.
- Verbal instructions
  - – Give only one-step instructions.
  - – Support verbal instructions with visual clues.
  - – It helps to say the participant's name to get his or her attention before making a statement.
  - – Keep phrases short and consistent.
  - – Reassure when needed, but avoid distracting the participant.

- Hands-on direction
    - If you are out of sight of a participant, warn the person that you are going to provide guidance.
    - Let your hand rest on the participant for a second before you start directing a movement.
    - Never persist in moving a totally passive or resistant limb.
    - Provide as little manual guidance as is necessary.

Summary

Important changes occur in the nervous system with age. Many of these changes have very little functional impact, while others greatly influence quality of life. With an aging population, the role of physical activity in the management of dementia and AD is of great interest to researchers and practitioners. Special care must also be taken when one is assessing the role and responsibilities of caregivers.

Questions to Consider

1. How might exercise be adapted for the different stages of AD progression?

2. Discuss the similarities and differences between theories of AD and those relating to general aging.

3. How might regular physical activity counteract potential risk factors for AD?

chapter 4

Sensory Systems

Michel J. Johnson, PhD, and Anthony A. Vandervoort, PhD

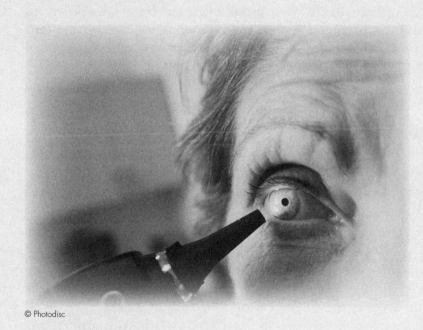

© Photodisc

> *We don't stop playing because we grow old; we grow old because we stop playing.*
>
> George Bernard Shaw

A decline in function of the body's various sensory systems can easily be observed in the frail elderly. One of the most prevalent changes is the loss of visual acuity; and sometimes the first sign of this change occurs in middle age, when there is new need for reading glasses. Other visual changes relevant to movement include decreased spatial discrimination, restriction in upward gaze, and reduced ability to track objects.

Another well-known sign of aging is hearing loss, which usually appears later in life than visual changes. Both the acoustic apparatus and related nerve pathways appear to undergo functional decline, which may produce communication problems in older people. As well, morphological changes appear in the vestibular organs; these contribute to decline in the ability to detect orientation in space. The olfactory system and taste receptors are also affected, and the losses in these senses may lead to reduced appetite and poor nutritional status.

Hearing

Hearing difficulties can range from an inability to understand certain words or sounds to total deafness. Changes in auditory abilities with age can greatly influence the individual's social interactions in difficult listening conditions.

Structure and Function

The ear is made up of three areas, the outer, middle, and inner ear (figure 4.1). The structures of the outer and middle ear are involved in hearing, while the inner ear is involved in both hearing and balance.

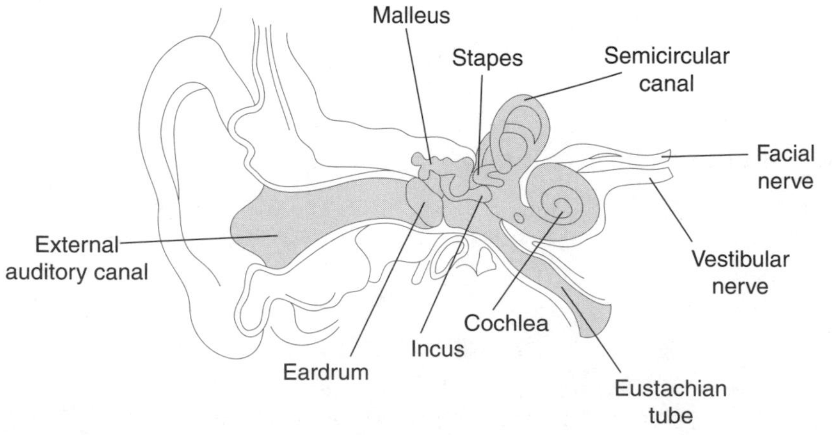

Figure 4.1 Structure of the ear.

The outer ear is made up of the auricle and external auditory canal. The auricle, the outermost part of the ear, is connected to an opening called the auditory canal. At the end of the auditory canal is the tympanic membrane, or eardrum, which serves as a boundary between the outer and middle ear. Sound waves go through the auditory canal and make the eardrum vibrate, which in turn causes small bones (ossicles) that span the middle ear to vibrate. The malleus is connected to the center of the eardrum, on the inner side. When the eardrum vibrates, it moves the malleus from side to side like a lever. The other end of the malleus is connected to the incus, which is attached to the stapes. The stapes fits into the oval window between the middle and inner ear. When the oval window vibrates, fluid in the inner ear transmits the vibrations into the hearing organ of the inner ear, the cochlea. Inside the cochlea is the organ of Corti, which contains thousands of hair cells that are the actual vibration receptors. The cilia (the hair) of the hair cells make contact with another membrane called the tectorial membrane. When the hair cells are excited by vibration, a nerve impulse is generated in the auditory nerve. These impulses are then sent to the brain.

Hearing Loss

With hearing loss, an individual loses the ability to distinguish and discriminate between sounds. Hearing loss affects 30% of adults aged 65 to 74 years and 50% of those aged 75 to 80 (Wallhagen et al., 2006). Hearing impairment causes a decline in the ability to communicate efficiently and may lead to withdrawal and depression. Such physiological states can have a negative effect on exercise adherence. Balance is also something to consider when one is designing programs. Individuals with such a deficit will require unique adaptations or provisions in an institutional program setting to achieve their potential. The two most common types of hearing loss are presbycusis and loss caused by occupational or lifestyle factors.

- **Presbycusis (sensorineural impairment).** Presbycusis involves changes in the delicate inner ear. Older people are more often affected by presbycusis than by heart disease, blindness, and arthritis. Although the direct development is unknown, the best correlation has to do with age-related sound sensing of the auditory nerve. A progressive loss of high tones occurs, making it difficult for the person to understand speech and tolerate loud noises. At first only those high tones outside of the speech range may be affected, but the lower range may be eventually inhibited, reducing voice comprehension. Since the inner ear also functions in the maintenance of balance, this sensory loss contributes to a higher incidence of falling. It is not curable or correctable.

- **Occupational or lifestyle hearing loss.** Hearing loss may also be due to controllable factors such as lifelong exposure to environmental noise rather than physiological degeneration (table 4.1). Prolonged exposure to high levels of sound is one of the leading factors in permanent hearing loss. It is not uncommon for individuals to report a mild hearing loss of up to 25 decibels. However, those who expose themselves to excessively high intensities, frequencies, and tones may experience a profound loss greater than 99 decibels. Many workplaces

TABLE 4.1   **Sound Levels and Human Response**

Common sounds	Noise level decibels (dB)	Effect
Jet engine (near)	140	Pain and damage
Shotgun firing, jet takeoff (100-200 ft)	130	Threshold of pain (about 125 dB)
Thunderclap (near), discotheque	120	Threshold of sensation
Power saw, pneumatic drill, rock music band	110	Regular exposure of more than 1 min risks permanent hearing loss
Garbage truck	100	No more than 1 min unprotected exposure recommended
Subway, motorcycle, lawnmower	90	Very annoying
Electric razor, many industrial workplaces	85	Level at which hearing damage begins after 8 hr or more of exposure
Average city traffic noise	80	Annoying; interferes with conversation
Vacuum cleaner, hair dryer, inside car	70	Intrusive; interferes with telephone conversation
Normal conversation	60	

have implemented programs like the Workplace Hazardous Materials Information System (WHMIS) to stress the importance of taking protective measures toward delaying the onset of hearing loss.

Vision

The eye is the organ of vision. It is a complex light-gathering structure that focuses light onto nerves that become stimulated and send messages to the brain.

Structure and Function

The eye is made up of an outer, middle, and inner layer (figure 4.2). The outer layer consists of the sclera, a tough fibrous tissue that composes the white outer wall of the eye, and the cornea, a strong clear bulge located at the front of the eye that permits light to enter. The middle layer consists of the choroid, ciliary body, and iris. The choroid absorbs light in order to minimize internal reflection in the eye and contains blood vessels to supply nutrients and eliminate waste. The ciliary body contains the ciliary muscles that attach to the lens, a clear and flexible structure located behind the iris and the pupil. Together,

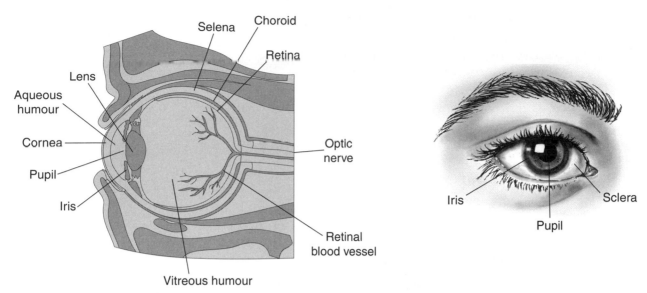

Figure 4.2 Structure of the eye.

the lens and the ciliary muscles help control the focusing of light as it passes through the eye. The iris has two sets of muscles that work together to regulate the size of the pupil in order to manage the entry of light into the eye.

The inner layer consists of the retina, which contains the photoreceptors—rods and cones. Rods are responsible for vision in low light, and cones are responsible for color vision and detail. In the back of the eye is the macula. The macula is made up mostly of cone cells and is responsible for central vision. In the center of the macula is an area called the fovea that contains only cones and is responsible for seeing fine detail. Nerve fibers in the retina carry information to the brain through the optic nerve. The point of departure of the optic nerve through the retina does not have any rods or cones and thus produces a "blind spot." The lens and ciliary body separate the eye into two fluid-filled chambers. The anterior cavity is filled with a clear watery fluid called aqueous humor that supplies nutrients to the cornea and lens. The vitreous chamber lies behind the lens and ciliary body and is filled with a firm jellylike material called vitreous humor, which helps maintain the structure of the eye.

Age-Related Changes and Eye Disease

Certain changes in the eye begin in our 30s, and by our 50s most of us will probably need glasses at least part of the time. Vision impairment can significantly affect quality of life, leading to loss of basic skills, loss of ease of communication, loss of confidence, and a lack of the sense of belonging within our community. Significant changes in the structures of the eye are observed as we age. The cornea changes shape from kidney-like to a more flat surface, and a greater scattering of light rays causes a blurring effect on our vision. In the iris, muscles weaken and the pupil becomes smaller, reacts more slowly to light, and dilates more slowly in the dark. This contributes to greater difficulty in seeing when we are moving from darker to lighter areas, or lighter to darker areas. The lens thickens and takes on a yellowish tinge, and less light can reach the photoreceptors.

In most cases vision loss can be attributed to one of four age-related pathologies. These are cataracts, glaucoma, macular degeneration, and diabetic retinopathy (Whiteside et al., 2006).

• **Cataracts** occur when the lens interior becomes cloudy and opaque as a result of chemical changes in the lens itself. Almost half of the population 65+ have some degree of clouding. The most common treatments are these:

– *Cataract surgery*—restores sight in over 95% of all cases

– *Eyeglasses*—increase object size by 25%

– *Contact lenses*—increase object size by 6%

– *Bifocal glasses*—increase image size by 1%, correct central and peripheral vision

• **Glaucoma** causes a disturbance to the optic nerve fibers with an increase of pressure on the eye due to a buildup of fluid. Symptoms include difficulty adjusting eyes to a darkened room, foggy vision, and focus that fluctuates. Glaucoma is treated medically with eyedrops.

• **Macular degeneration.** The macula is a small spot near the center of the retina. It contains an extremely high concentration of cone cells, and is the primary source of central vision. Macular degeneration results in the loss of central visual field and contrast sensitivity. There are two types of macular degeneration: wet and dry. The dry type is the most common, accounting for 90% of cases. The wet type accounts for approximately 10% of cases of macular degeneration. In this type, damaged blood vessels beneath the macula leak fluid and cause the retina to become distorted. Treatment with laser photocoagulation can be used to seal the damaged blood vessels. However, the treatment is often not effective and recurrences are common.

• **Diabetic retinopathy** is caused by changes in the blood vessels of the retina, and it is an important cause of blindness. The more advanced and severe form of the disease is called proliferative retinopathy. During proliferative retinopathy new blood vessels appear within the eye. These newer blood vessels are fragile and can bleed, causing vision loss and retinal scarring. All people with diabetes are at risk for the development of diabetic retinopathy. Treatment includes strategies to control blood sugar, blood pressure, and cholesterol.

Touch

The somatosensory system contains various receptors located in the skin that provide information on touch (mechanoreceptors), temperature (thermoreceptors), and pain (nociceptors). The somatosensory pathways bring sensory information from the peripheral receptors to the brain (figure 4.3). The dorsal column–medial lemniscal pathway carries information about touch and vibration from the skin, as well as proprioceptive information from the limbs. The spinothalamic pathway carries information about pain and temperature.

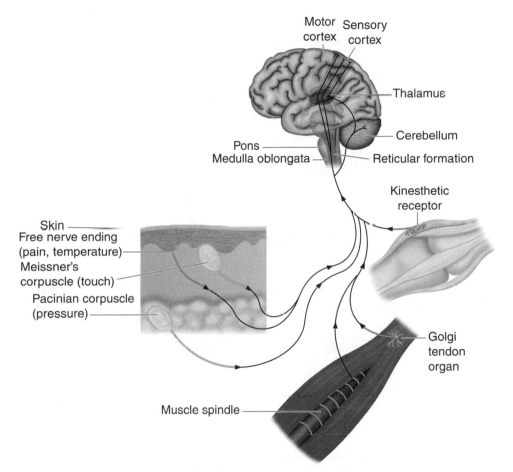

Figure 4.3 Somatosensory pathways.

Reprinted, by permission, from J. Wilmore and D. Costill, 2003, *Physiology of sport and exercise*, 3rd ed. (Champaign, IL: Human Kinetics), 75.

Mechanoreceptors respond to pressure. There are two forms of mechanoreceptors—rapidly adapting and slowly adapting. Both types of receptors respond to pressure; however, the rate at which the receptor terminates firing is different. Pacinian corpuscles and Meissner's corpuscles are rapidly adapting mechanoreceptors. Pacinian corpuscles are highly sensitive pressure receptors deep within the skin, while Meissner's corpuscles are fine-touch receptors that are abundant in the fingertips. Merkel's discs and Ruffini endings are slowly adapting mechanoreceptors. Merkel's discs are touch receptors that respond best to gradual skin indentation. Ruffini endings respond to gradual tension and stretch in the skin. Free nerve endings throughout skin, muscle, bone, and connective tissue perceive changes in temperature and pain. Reduced or changed sensations of pain, vibration, cold, heat, pressure, and touch have been reported with aging; however, it remains unclear whether these changes are due to the process of aging or the impact of disease.

Smell and Taste

Smell and taste receptors are chemoreceptors, and the brain needs information about both smell and taste to distinguish most flavors. Taste receptors are stimulated by food dissolved in saliva, while smell receptors detect airborne chemicals dissolved in fluids coating the nasal membranes.

Structure and Function

The area of the mucous membrane that lines the roof of the nasal cavity, the olfactory epithelium, contains neurons called olfactory receptor cells. Cilia from the olfactory receptor cells extend into the mucosa of the olfactory epithelium. Airborne molecules (odorant) enter the nasal cavity, dissolve in the mucosa, and bind to receptors in the cilia. Signals are transmitted from the cilia through nerve fibers that extend through the roof of the nasal cavity (cribriform plate) and connect to the olfactory bulbs that form the olfactory nerves traveling toward the brain (figure 4.4).

Food stimulates taste receptors that detect sweet, sour, salty, and bitter qualities. The tip of the tongue is most sensitive to sweet and salty tastes, the sides to sour, and the back to bitter. The taste receptors, located in taste buds, are found mostly on the tongue in taste papillae, tiny bumps that cover the upper surface and sides of the tongue. Taste buds are also found in the palate, pharynx, and upper portion of

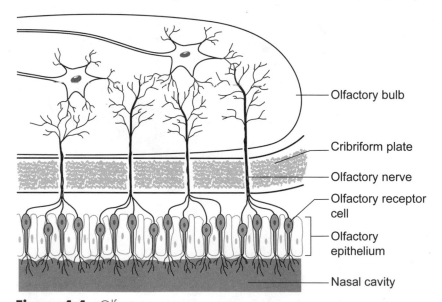

Figure 4.4   Olfactory sense.

Labels: Olfactory bulb; Cribriform plate; Olfactory nerve; Olfactory receptor cell; Olfactory epithelium; Nasal cavity

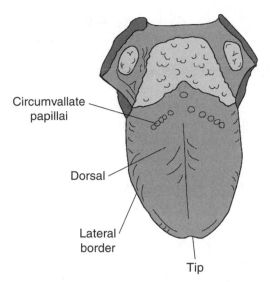

Circumvallate papillai

Dorsal

Lateral border

Tip

Figure 4.5 The fungiform papillae, where the taste buds at the back of the tongue are located, are clearly visible.

the esophagus. Most taste buds are found in the round circumvallate papillae at the back of the tongue and in the mushroom-shaped fungiform papillae abundant in the tip and sides (figure 4.5). Taste buds have specialized receptors, gustatory cilia (gustatory hairs), that extend through a taste pore to the surface of the tongue where they are bathed by saliva. Food molecules stimulate the cilia, triggering a nerve impulse in associated nerve fibers that are connected to the cranial nerves of taste (the facial and glossopharyngeal nerves). The impulse travels along these cranial nerves to the brain, which interprets the impulse as a distinct taste.

Age-Related Changes in Smell and Taste

Smell and taste are chemical senses that are already very sharp at birth; however, beginning in our 40s, our senses of smell and taste begin to diminish. By our 60s, our decreased senses may make food taste bland, and appetite can diminish greatly. Over 77% of older people have a substantial loss in taste and smell sensitivity. The loss becomes noticeable in the average person between the ages of 70 and 80. More than 2 million Americans have taste and smell disorders, with men suffering more than women, and the sick more than the healthy. Chronic disorders of taste and smell have been largely neglected because they are seldom fatal and, unlike deficiencies in sight and hearing, are not considered a serious handicap; they are more "nagging problems" affecting the quality of life (Boyce and Shone, 2006). Exercise helps to increase appetite, slow the aging process, and lessen the effects of sensory loss; but there are no special adjustments that need to be made for deficits of smell and taste.

Programming Recommendations

Even very minor modifications to the environment can make physical activity both safer and more enjoyable for seniors with sensory loss. Although more significant changes may sometimes be required, a well thought out, commonsense approach is often sufficient.

It is important to obtain a baseline medical report of deficits and recommendations before getting a senior with sensory impairment involved in an exercise protocol. When adapting an exercise program it is important both to promote physical fitness and well-being and to avoid disappointing and risky situations. One must take into account that there may be people of varying hearing and physical activity levels in the group.

For Individuals With Hearing Impairment

Follow these guidelines for exercise programs for individuals with hearing impairment:

- Place seniors with hearing impairment at the front of the class and speak directly to them. Don't turn your back while instructing. Facing participants allows people to lip-read or at least see that you are speaking.
- Provide physical cues and sight cues. Eliminate loud sounds. Use arm signals and physical gestures.
- Proper acoustic treatment of walls, floors, and ceilings keeps sounds from echoing.
- Speak distinctly, slowly, and in lower tone frequencies.
- Reduce background noise such as the sound of fans, other groups talking, and music playing while instructions are being given. Avoid the use of sudden loud noises, which could be damaging to hearing aid users.
- If people must wear hearing aids, care should be taken to avoid blows to the ear or quick movements (which may dislodge a hearing aid). It can also be confusing for people to get two noise inputs at the same time.
- Avoid the use of sudden loud noises or whistles; these may be damaging to a participant with a hearing aid.
- Take precautions to ensure that seniors are not put in situations in which they may lose their balance.

For Individuals With Visual Impairment

These are special considerations you should incorporate into any exercise program involving seniors with visual impairment:

- Speak to people in a normal tone, address them by name, and give them accurate directions.
- Do not assume that someone needs help. Ask first, assist by touching the arm, and always describe the surroundings.
- Facilities should have bright lights and matte surfaces to reduce glare, and use contrasting background colors.
- Consider choice of color for equipment, keeping in mind people who are color-blind, as well as safety of equipment (e.g., balls should be soft; equipment should have no sharp edges). All lettering should be enlarged.

For Individuals With Tactile Impairment

Appropriate adaptations to exercise are

- affixing tape to bats, stick handles, rackets;
- using balls with pebbly surfaces; and
- including a partner or mirror.

Heat and pain sensitivity are major concerns among elderly people (air conditioning, bathing water, needle pricks, frostbite). To prevent injury, watch for

- shoes that are too tight;
- temperature of pools, heating pads, and bathwater; and
- appropriate dress.

Summary

Sensory loss affects people to varying degrees and at different ages. Genetics, environment, and lifestyle are all factors that lead to a decline in sensory capabilities. Sensory changes can have tremendous impact on an individual. These changes may make it hard for a person to communicate, enjoy certain activities, and interact with others. This can lead to feelings of isolation and loneliness. Adaptations to exercise programs can greatly enhance the experience of older adults with sensory loss. Many simple modifications can be made to the exercise environment so that individuals of all ages can participate together.

It is important to consider the function of the somatosensory system in older people. Anatomical studies have demonstrated changes in the number and structure of specialized nerve ending receptors in the skin such as Meissner's and Pacinian corpuscles (Katzman and Terry, 1983). Older groups have been shown to be less sensitive to vibration, touch pressure, cutaneous pain, and temperature. Age-related reductions also occur in the ability to tolerate and adapt to cold and hot ambient temperatures in the environment (Wilmore and Costill, 2004). Factors such as deterioration in hypothalamic control of body homeostasis, in combination with altered autonomic nervous system function and temperature sensation, lead to reduced ability to regulate body temperature. Hence extra precaution should be taken in situations such as strenuous exercise or in hot or humid climates.

Questions to Consider

1. In general, what changes are observed in the senses as we age?

2. Describe the structure and function of the outer, middle, and inner ear.

3. What is presbycusis?

4. Describe the structure and function of the eye.

5. List and describe the most common causes of vision loss in aging.

6. Describe the mechanoreceptors.

7. Describe the processes of taste and smell.

8. How can we change exercise environments to accommodate the changes in sensory ability that are associated with aging?

9. How would an exercise leader lead a class composed of nonimpaired and impaired individuals? What strategies would benefit both groups?

10. What activities could be used to help younger fitness professionals appreciate age-related sensory losses?

part II

Nutrition, Common Diseases, and the Role of Physical Activity

Part II of the book comprises chapters 5 and 6, which deal with nutritional aspects of aging. In chapter 5 we discuss healthy food choices and important nutrients. All components of healthy nutrition are important. However, specific nutrients are more important for older adults than for younger people because of the complicating effects of the aging process. The most insidious disease of aging is type 2 diabetes. It is well known that the onset of this disease occurs around the age of 55 in most individuals of Caucasian descent. However, the onset has been shown to occur 5 to 10 years earlier in African Americans and in those of Hispanic or Aboriginal descent. Most importantly, the age of onset is declining rapidly, so that the disease is now being identified in teenagers. There is a direct correlation and cause-and-effect relationship between type 2 diabetes and obesity. The disconcerting fact is that type 2 diabetes can be controlled rather simply by a combination of good dietary selection and daily physical activity. In chapter 5 we outline the contents of a healthy diet and define the benefits of a functional exercise program for the elderly.

Chapter 5 also contains information about the types of diabetes, the control of glucose transport, the symptoms of the disease, the major risk factors, and the various methods of diagnosis currently being used. Furthermore, we explain the effects of proper nutrition and the effects of a good exercise program on the disease itself, as well as the signs of hyper- and hypoglycemia. Most importantly, we delineate the complications of diabetes and the ways in which nutrition and exercise can offset these complications and lead to a healthier quality of life.

In chapter 6 we discuss bone nutrition and the effects that good nutrition and exercise can have on osteoporosis. It was long thought that osteoporosis was found primarily in postmenopausal women. Today we are well aware that the onset of the disease occurs at approximately 30 years of age and that osteoporosis attacks also men and premenopausal women. The causes, risk factors, and methods of diagnosis are delineated. Much of this chapter deals with the treatment of osteoporosis, from pharmacologic, nutritional, and physical activity points of view.

It has not been shown that osteoporosis can be completely controlled. However, it is well known that good nutrition and impact types of physical activity can delay perhaps the onset, but certainly the progress, of the disease. We offer a lengthy section on the exercises thought to best combat the progress of osteoporosis, as well as other ways and means to lessen the effects of the disease, including the influence of good posture.

chapter 5

Nutrition and Diabetes

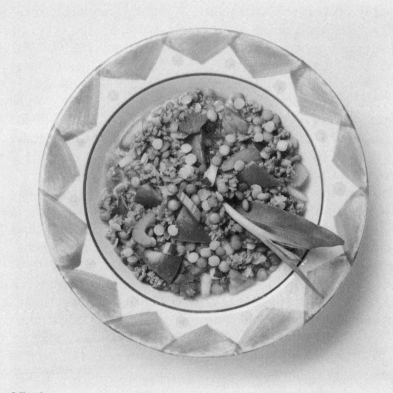

© Photodisc

> " *Regular physical activity and healthy eating are each known to contribute to overall well-being. Physical activity not only reduces the risk factor for developing certain chronic diseases but also leads to favorable changes in body composition, fitness level and functional capacity. Similarly, healthy eating has been shown to influence the onset and management of various chronic conditions, as well as body composition and functional capacity.* "*

Shanthi Johnson, PhD, PDt (2004, ALCOA *Research Update*, p. 1 #7, March)

In this chapter we discuss a healthy diet for those who are elderly. Such topics as healthy food choices, important nutrients, and recommended doses of specific nutrients are covered. Nutritional needs change throughout the life cycle, but a balanced, varied, nutritionally sound diet is vital to good health at all stages of our lives.

Proper nutrition and regular activity are two of the most effective tools in the prevention of heart disease, diabetes, osteoporosis, and other conditions commonly associated with aging. Keeping oneself healthy will help reduce the likelihood of becoming sick.

Exercise plays a very important role in achieving body fat (weight) loss for many reasons. Dieting alone often results in the loss of lean tissue, which will slow the metabolic rate and impair progress, along with significantly decreasing strength. In addition to improving body composition, exercise has positive effects on blood pressure, serum cholesterol levels, and cardiorespiratory function. Therefore for optimal health benefits it is wise to combine a healthy eating pattern with a regular program of physical activity.

This chapter also contains information related to the effects of nutrition, aging, and exercise on the onset and control of diabetes, in particular, type 2 diabetes, one of the prime diseases of aging. The physiological changes that accompany aging include factors that affect the pancreas, hence insulin secretion and the insulin-sensitive sites on skeletal muscle. Therefore, exercise can and does have direct consequences for insulin secretion and for the transport of glucose into skeletal muscle. Risk factors, symptoms, diagnostic techniques, common medications, glucose transport, and the effects of hypoglycemia and hyperglycemia are outlined. The primary roles played by exercise and nutrition in the control of this disease are discussed. Furthermore, the complications that derive from uncontrolled type 2 diabetes are outlined.

Nutrition for Older Adults

As adults age, many factors may influence their food choices, including economic factors, social variables such as the loss of a loved one, loneliness, lack of appetite, and boredom. In addition, insufficient resources, lack of financial and personal support, and the inconvenience of meal planning and preparation may interfere with proper dietary intake patterns. Ultimately, this may lead to changes in health and nutritional status. Some of the physiological changes that are commonly associated with aging and are directly implicated with nutrition include the following:

- A decrease in lean body tissue with a concomitant increase in body fat
- A decreasing resting metabolic rate and reduced energy needs
- A decreased exercise capacity (decreased $\dot{V}O_2$max, decreased number of red blood cells, diminished sense of balance)
- A loss of bone mass, increasing the risk of osteoporosis
- A decline in immune function, which increases the risk of infection
- A reduced sense of taste and smell, which contributes to a lack of appetite
- Tooth loss and dry mouth, compromising food intake
- Declines in kidney function and the thirst mechanism, which increase the risk of dehydration
- Changes in gastrointestinal function, contributing to constipation and impaired nutrient absorption

Healthy Food Choices

While aging is inevitable, it is highly variable across individuals. Eating well and living well can make successful aging a reality. Healthy food choices for older adults should focus on and include the following:

- Nutrient-dense foods to meet vitamin and mineral needs within reduced energy requirements
- Milk products, which are excellent sources of calcium and vitamin D, to maintain bone health
- Foods rich in protein and vitamins A, B_6, C, D, and E, as well as zinc, for a healthy immune system
- Colorful and tasty foods to stimulate appetite
- Texture-modified foods to facilitate chewing and swallowing
- Increased fluid and fiber intakes to minimize dehydration and digestive disturbances, respectively

Some common nutritional deficiencies in the elderly population are fiber, protein, calcium, zinc, iron, and certain vitamins. Each of these important nutrients is discussed in the following section.

Important Nutrients

All known nutrients are important for humans to consume. However, the basic metabolism of the older adult is confounded by the aging process, and as a result, certain constituents become more important than others as people age. Here we outline these constituents and explain why they are essential for older adults.

Fiber

Fiber, a complex carbohydrate, is generally defined as the part of a plant that cannot be digested. Thus, it adds virtually no calories to the diet. However, there are many important roles that fiber may play in overall health. A high-fiber diet helps reduce the production of cholesterol, increases cholesterol excretion, and reduces blood pressure, all of which will, in turn, help to lower the risk of heart disease.

It is recommended that adults consume 35 g of fiber per day. In order to ensure adequate fiber intake, an individual should be certain to obtain 50% to 60% of the daily energy intake from complex carbohydrates. Any dietary changes that may result in a substantial increase in dietary fiber intake should be made gradually in order to provide the body with adequate opportunity to adjust.

There are two types of fiber—those that are water soluble and those that are insoluble in water. The two types have different sources and functions:

• **Water-soluble fiber.** Water-soluble fiber plays a very important role in lowering cholesterol levels. Products that contain oat fiber can be labeled heart healthy. Water-soluble fibers also slow the rate of glucose absorption, which is especially important for people with diabetes. Some sources of soluble fibers are fruits (apples, pears, citrus, strawberries), vegetables, dried beans and peas, nuts and seeds, brown rice, and barley, oat, and rice bran. Bulky, high-fiber foods may also help with weight control because fiber, when

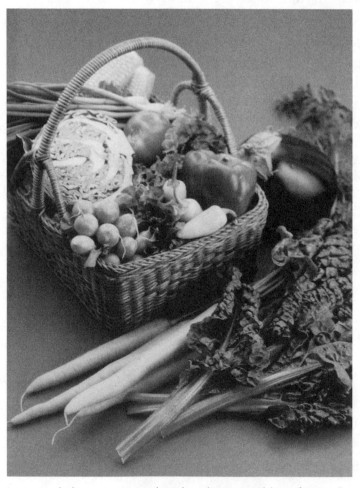

In general, the more intensely colored a vegetable or fruit is, the more nutrients it packs. Choose deeply colored foods such as the carrots, purple cabbage, green and yellow peppers, Swiss chard, and tomato pictured here.
© Photodisc

saturated with water, gives people the sense that they are full without adding calories. Foods with fiber also take longer to chew, which helps to slow the rate at which people eat.

- **Insoluble fiber.** Insoluble fiber promotes regularity because it keeps products moving through the digestive tract. It is thought to reduce the incidence of colon cancer. Insoluble fiber may also alleviate some digestive disorders. Some sources of insoluble fibers are wheat and corn bran, whole-grain breads and cereals, vegetables, fruit skins, and nuts.

Protein

Protein is essential at any age, but in the later years of life it plays an integral role in the maintenance of body tissue and is critical to the body's immune system.

Insufficient protein intake may result in an accelerated loss of muscle tissue, increased risk of infection, and a decreased ability to provide for support during periods of trauma and infection. The need for protein is likely similar for old and young adults. Thus, men and women over the age of 50 should consume 60 to 70 g of protein per day, or 0.8 to 1.0 g of protein per kilogram of body weight. In general, with age the energy demands of an individual decrease due to a lower level of activity and a decrease in lean tissue. Thus, the goal as one gets older is to pick foods that are higher in protein and nutrients and lower in fat and calories.

According to *Canada's Food Guide to Healthy Eating* (2007), adults should consume two to three servings of meat and alternatives, along with two to four servings of milk and milk products per day. This should supply adequate protein when combined with a proper diet of grains, which also supply small amounts of protein. Top protein sources include meat, poultry, fish, eggs, milk, cheese, yogurt, ice cream, peanuts, peanut butter, nuts, and seeds.

Minerals

- **Calcium** is an essential mineral used for building and maintaining strong bones, and it also plays a role in helping the muscles to contract and the heart to beat. In addition, calcium regulates processes such as blood clotting, cell division, and nerve impulses. Current statistics show that three of every four adult women in North America do not meet the recommended intake of 1,200 mg of calcium per day. This also may affect other vital nutrients, as diets low in calcium are often low in vitamins A, D, B_6, and B_{12}, as well as riboflavin, magnesium, potassium, and folate. Other facts to keep in mind about calcium are the following:
  - Calcium plays a role in the prevention and treatment of a number of diseases or conditions commonly associated with aging, including osteoporosis, hypertension, colon cancer, and kidney stones.

– The disease most commonly associated with insufficient calcium intake is osteoporosis (see chapter 6). Following menopause, the estrogen levels in women fall, which causes a decline in bone strength. Adequate calcium intake may prevent additional bone loss and help build new bone when combined with weight-bearing activities such as walking, dancing, tennis, and golf (without the golf cart) and also strength training.

– For lactose-intolerant individuals, lactose-free milk products, as well as calcium-fortified foods such as breakfast cereals and nutrition bars, are good replacements.

• **Zinc** deficiency is very common. More than 90% of elderly individuals suffer from this malady, due to reductions in absorption (often due to medications). This deficiency further complicates nutritional concerns because zinc deficiency depresses appetite and blunts sense of taste, which often leads to very low energy intakes. Most of the zinc in the typical diet comes from animal products, such as meat, liver, eggs, and seafood, especially oysters. Zinc is also available from other food sources such as legumes, whole-grain cereals, wheat germ, and nuts. However, zinc from these sources may not be absorbed as well as zinc from animal products.

• **Iron** deficiency can usually be avoided if one eats the major source of this nutrient, which is animal organs. If this is not possible (e.g., because of distaste for this source), the active older person should concentrate on iron-fortified foods. Iron deficiency is frequently less common in elderly women because iron losses due to menstruation cease. However, iron losses can occur in elderly men and some women due to

– low-energy diets,

– chronic blood loss from ulcers or hemorrhoids,

– poorer absorption due to reduced stomach acid secretion,

– excessive antacid use (interferes with iron absorption), and

– use of medicines that increase blood loss (anticoagulants, arthritis drugs).

The major source of iron is animal organs, although many foods are now fortified with iron.

Antioxidants

Antioxidants are vitamins, minerals, and other compounds found in foods or taken as pills that can help slow down or prevent the oxidation process, and thus help prevent or repair damage done to the cells of the body by free radicals. Antioxidants have also been shown to increase immune function and possibly decrease risk of infection and cancer. Both macular degeneration and cataracts have been associated with diets that are low in fruits and vegetables. Some examples of vitamin and mineral antioxidants are carotenoids (beta-carotene), copper, magnesium, selenium, vitamin C, vitamin E, and zinc.

Water

Dehydration is one of the most frequent causes of hospitalization among people over the age of 65. Dehydration is a common concern in elderly people because with age, the thirst mechanism becomes imprecise, the ability of kidneys to retain fluid decreases, and there are lower amounts of total-body water. These physiological changes may result in a variety of problems such as muscle weakness, mental confusion, inability to tolerate high environmental temperatures, and intestinal distress. Some of the early signs of dehydration are dry mouth, flushed skin, fatigue, headache, increased breathing and pulse rate, and dizziness.

Benefits of Exercise and Healthy Eating

While the importance of healthy eating combined with regular physical activity is well recognized by both the lay public and the health care system, only 24% of older adults are active enough to gain the desired health benefits. And only one in eight seniors over the age of 65 consumes the recommended five servings of fruit and vegetables per day. The implications of poor dietary habits are equally well known, yet a significant portion of the elderly community obtains less than optimal nutrition. Healthy eating is the consumption of a variety of foods in adequate amounts (both quantity and quality are important) to result in good nutritional health.

Canada's Food Guide to Healthy Eating is recognized worldwide as a gold standard for guidance to healthy nutrition. Figure 5.1 shows a personalized program that a 60-year-old woman created for herself using the version of the guide found on the Health Canada Web site. The four food groups (grain products, fruits and vegetables, milk products, and meats and alternatives) are pictured along with sample foods chosen by the woman in question. Each food group provides a set of key nutrients. The "other foods" category, which includes those high in sugar, fat, salt, and beverages, offers fewer nutrients than the main four food groups and is therefore not included. What is important for the aging population is that as the total energy requirements decrease, the total nutrient requirements be maintained.

The guide can be ordered in hard copy as well. It is user friendly, printed in bold colors on matte paper, and features large fonts, making it easy for seniors to use. The URL for this guide is www.healthcanada. gc.ca/foodguide.

At the same time *Canada's Physical Activity Guide to Healthy Active Living for Older Adults* (the style is similar to that of the food guide) explains the need for regular physical activity for seniors. Activities are broken down from simple to more complex, and the material is easy to read and understand. The guide recommends levels of activity that will help reduce the risk of developing some of the diseases mentioned in previous chapters. As well, the guide

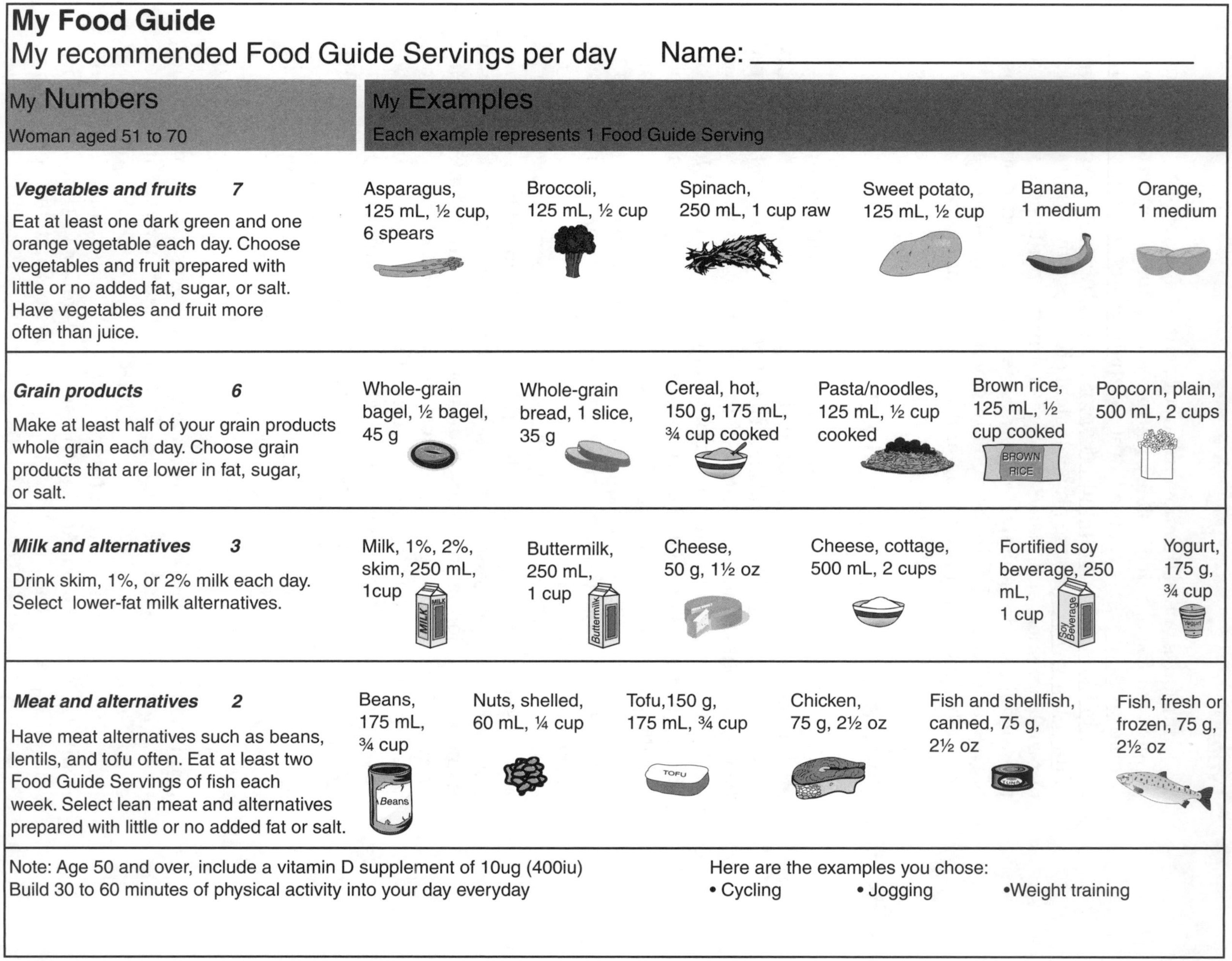

My Food Guide
My recommended Food Guide Servings per day   Name: _____

My Numbers	My Examples
Woman aged 51 to 70	Each example represents 1 Food Guide Serving

Vegetables and fruits   7

Eat at least one dark green and one orange vegetable each day. Choose vegetables and fruit prepared with little or no added fat, sugar, or salt. Have vegetables and fruit more often than juice.

Asparagus, 125 mL, ½ cup, 6 spears

Broccoli, 125 mL, ½ cup

Spinach, 250 mL, 1 cup raw

Sweet potato, 125 mL, ½ cup

Banana, 1 medium

Orange, 1 medium

Grain products   6

Make at least half of your grain products whole grain each day. Choose grain products that are lower in fat, sugar, or salt.

Whole-grain bagel, ½ bagel, 45 g

Whole-grain bread, 1 slice, 35 g

Cereal, hot, 150 g, 175 mL, ¾ cup cooked

Pasta/noodles, 125 mL, ½ cup cooked

Brown rice, 125 mL, ½ cup cooked

Popcorn, plain, 500 mL, 2 cups

Milk and alternatives   3

Drink skim, 1%, or 2% milk each day. Select lower-fat milk alternatives.

Milk, 1%, 2%, skim, 250 mL, 1cup

Buttermilk, 250 mL, 1 cup

Cheese, 50 g, 1½ oz

Cheese, cottage, 500 mL, 2 cups

Fortified soy beverage, 250 mL, 1 cup

Yogurt, 175 g, ¾ cup

Meat and alternatives   2

Have meat alternatives such as beans, lentils, and tofu often. Eat at least two Food Guide Servings of fish each week. Select lean meat and alternatives prepared with little or no added fat or salt.

Beans, 175 mL, ¾ cup

Nuts, shelled, 60 mL, ¼ cup

Tofu,150 g, 175 mL, ¾ cup

Chicken, 75 g, 2½ oz

Fish and shellfish, canned, 75 g, 2½ oz

Fish, fresh or frozen, 75 g, 2½ oz

Note: Age 50 and over, include a vitamin D supplement of 10ug (400iu) into your day everyday

Build 30 to 60 minutes of physical activity into your day everyday

Here are the examples you chose:
- Cycling
- Jogging
- Weight training

Figure 5.1   An example of Canada's Food Guide for Healthy Living completed for a 60-year-old active woman.

Source: Canada's Food Guide, Health Canada, 2006. Adapted with the permission of the Minister of Public Works and Government Services, Canada, 2007.

covers the components of exercise, including strength, endurance, balance, and flexibility.

In the United States, a leadership role concerning the effects of good nutrition on healthy aging has been taken by the American Academy of Family Physicians. Reference to the work of this organization can be found in chapter 11 and appendix B. With respect to the effects of exercise and aging, the American College of Sports Medicine (ACSM) is the unequivocal leader. The college took a position stand in 1998 on the effects of physical activity on older adults. The ACSM is internationally recognized and considered the final voice on this matter. The college followed up, in 2000, with guidelines for exercise testing and prescription. In the following year, ACSM published these guidelines in a text that is now used worldwide. Unquestionably, ACSM has become the world leader as a resource in exercise testing, prescription, and risk factors for all age groups. References for these resources are cited in chapters 7 and 8.

Regular physical activity and healthy eating are an inseparable team if one wishes to maintain a healthy quality of life as aging progresses. Unfortunately these domains are seldom explored together. The positive effects of healthy eating and regular physical activity are obvious and include positive effects on several chronic diseases and the maladies of aging. An excellent test of nutritional status from the Nutritional Screening Initiative is found in appendix B. It can be used easily by laypeople to assess the nutritional status of any older individual.

Diabetes

Diabetes is an international health problem. Nearly 25 million North Americans suffer from diabetes, and approximately one-third of these cases are not diagnosed. Diabetes is a serious disease with life-threatening complications. Most people with diabetes, especially those with the disease going undiagnosed for a long period of time, will develop long-term complications. A lack of physical activity and poor dietary habits lead to the early onset of type 2 diabetes. And because the process is sometimes lengthy, type 2 becomes prevalent in the senior population. The human toll is reflected in reduced life expectancy, increased stress on individuals and families, increased school and work absences, career disruption, and personal hardship. In fact, health care costs for diabetes and its complications are estimated to approach $100 billion annually in North America alone.

Diabetes is characterized as a metabolic disease in which the body is unable to properly store and use glucose for energy expenditure. Under normal circumstances, in order to use glucose appropriately,

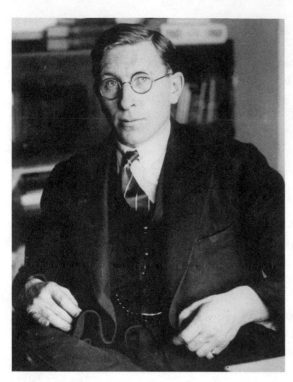

Sir Frederick Banting, the discoverer of insulin (circa 1930).

© Getty Images

the body requires insulin. With the onset of diabetes, the body either is unable to produce insulin (type 1) or is unable to use the insulin it produces (generally type 2). The unused glucose then resides in the bloodstream or is passed in the urine. The symptoms of glucose retention are then presented in direct proportion to the blood concentration. Thereafter, initial direct medical intervention is necessary; and if the diabetes is permitted to progress unabated, chronic and finally acute results will occur.

The discovery of insulin by Sir Frederick Banting is one of the most important medical discoveries to date. Banting began his work in 1920 at the University of Western Ontario in London, Canada, and completed the first successful use of endocrine on a human subject in 1922 at the University of Toronto with the able assistance of coworkers Best, Collip, and McLeod.

Today, it is well known that there are three types of diabetes; their symptoms are rather similar, but the etiology of each is distinctly different. These types of diabetes are known as type 1, type 2, and gestational. Because gestational diabetes occurs only in pregnancy, it will not be discussed here.

- **Type 1** diabetes is also known as juvenile-onset diabetes or insulin-dependent diabetes mellitus (IDDM). The individual's own immune system attacks the beta cells of the pancreas that are responsible for the production of insulin, and as a result the pancreas is no longer able to produce insulin. This results in elevated blood glucose levels, as insulin is the hormone responsible for transporting the glucose in the blood to the body tissues. Thus, the individual must administer regular insulin injections in order to manage blood sugar levels effectively. Approximately 10% of people with diabetes have type 1.

- **Type 2** diabetes is also known as adult-onset diabetes or non-insulin-dependent diabetes mellitus (NIDDM). This disease usually affects people over the age of 30. Either the pancreas is unable to produce enough insulin or the body does not use the insulin that is produced effectively, often as a result of reduction of receptor and cell sensitivities to insulin. Consequently, blood glucose levels become elevated. In many cases, proper diabetic diet, weight management, and regular exercise can control type 2 diabetes. However, medication and insulin are often required after the disease has been present for an extended period of time, or as a result of poor management of the disease. See table 5.1 for a summary of common medications for type 2 diabetes.

Only type 2 diabetes is pertinent to the topic of this book, as type 1 and gestational diabetes cannot be controlled by diet and exercise. We do refer to type 1 in this chapter to clarify how it differs from type 2.

TABLE 5.1 **Action of Common Medications for Type 2 Diabetes**

Class of medication	Brand names	Action
Sulfonylureas	Diabeta, Diabinese, Diamicron	These stimulate the pancreas to produce more insulin. When one is taking these pills, it is very important to eat three regular meals a day.
Biguanides	Glucophage	These help the body to use sugar more efficiently.
Acarbose	Prandase	This type of medication prolongs the absorption of carbohydrate after a meal. One must consume food in order for these pills to work.
Thiazolidinediones	Actos, Avandia	These medications control blood glucose by making the muscle cells more sensitive to insulin.

Reprinted, by permission, from P. Tiidus, 2008, *Skeletal muscle damage and repair: Mechanisms and interventions* (Champaign, IL: Human Kinetics).

Glucose Transport

Glucose is taken into the muscle by means of a transport system. This transport system is triggered when the muscles are exposed to insulin or if the muscles contract. When glucose is in the bloodstream, insulin and a transporter are required to help it move into the cell where it is to be utilized. This transporter is called GLUT-4. Once the insulin and insulin receptor complex is formed, the glucose transporter proteins (GLUT-4) carry the glucose into the muscle cell (see figure 5.2).

When a muscle contracts, more of the GLUT-4 transporters are brought to the surface of the cell and the transporters also work more efficiently; thus more glucose can be brought into the cell at this time.

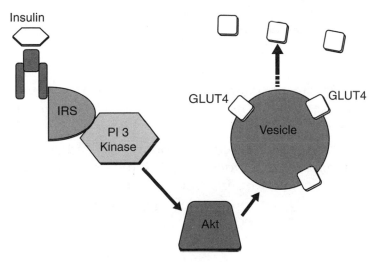

Figure 5.2 The transport of glucose into the muscle cell.
Data from AAFP.

Risk Factors, Symptoms, and Diagnosis of Diabetes

Type 1 and Type 2 diabetes have several common risk factors and symptoms, but they are distinct from one another. The next sections describe these in detail. If these risk factors and symptoms are present in an individual, three blood tests can diagnosis diabetes.

Risk Factors

The risk factors for types 1 and 2 diabetes are distinctive:

• **Type 1 diabetes** has a definite relationship to race or ethnicity (diabetes is more prevalent in people of Aboriginal, African, and Latin

American descent). Those with a family history of diabetes have been shown to be particularly susceptible to the disease.

• Age is a primary factor for the incidence of **type 2 diabetes.** All individuals over 45 should have annual checkups for this disease. A second primary risk factor is obesity. The number of people with this type of diabetes who are in an unhealthy weight range is double that in the population without diabetes. Other factors, which are perhaps less apparent, include

- high cholesterol;
- a sedentary lifestyle;
- family history;
- high blood pressure;
- Aboriginal, African, Latin American, or Asian ethnic ancestry;
- having given birth to a large baby (over 4.0 kg, or 9 lb); and
- previous diagnosis of impaired glucose tolerance.

Symptoms

Though types 1 and 2 diabetes have many symptoms in common, the constellations of symptoms are quite distinct:

• **Type 1.** Type 1 diabetes presents with frequent high-volume urination, unusual thirst, extreme hunger, unusual weight loss, extreme fatigue, irritability, nausea, vomiting, and sweet-smelling breath (acetone).

• **Type 2.** Type 2 presents with frequent infections; cuts and bruises that are slow to heal; tingling or numbness in the hands or feet; itchy skin; recurring skin, gum, or bladder infections; frequent urination; unusual thirst; extreme hunger; unusual weight loss; extreme fatigue; irritability; nausea; vomiting; and sweet-smelling breath; and additionally, in women, frequent vaginal yeast infections.

Diagnosis

Diabetes is diagnosed by means of a blood test measuring blood sugar. Blood glucose levels are affected rapidly by food intake, so the timing of the test is critical.

A simple test for diabetes is to assess the casual plasma glucose. This test is taken without regard to the time of the last meal. A second test is the fasting plasma blood glucose (FPG), administered when the individual has not eaten in at least 8 hr. Impaired fasting glucose shows values of 6.1 to 6.9 mmol/L, whereas the diabetic condition would present as 7+ mmol/L.

A third test is the oral glucose tolerance test (OGTT). This measure, taken after an 8 hr fast, is often used for postpartum testing and research. It is a measure of the body's ability to metabolize carbohydrate.

Subjects are given a standard dose of glucose, and blood and urine glucose concentrations are measured at regular intervals. Subjects with diabetes will have plasma blood glucose levels of >11.1 mmol/L 2 hr after receiving a 75 g glucose load.

Treatment of Type 2 Diabetes

Type 2 diabetes can generally be controlled with a combination of exercise and diet. Individuals with Type 2 diabetes must be vigilant about nutrition and exercise because the dangers are great if this control isn't maintained. However, if type 2 diabetes is controlled, people with diabetes can lead healthy lives, enjoying many of their favorite foods and exercise.

Type 2 Diabetes and Nutrition

One of the most important tools in the treatment of type 2 diabetes is nutrition. The primary goals for diabetics are to monitor their energy intake, maintain a healthy weight (often there is a great need for weight loss), and control blood glucose levels. Decreasing the body weight to an acceptable level improves insulin sensitivity. With careful planning, one can still enjoy a wide variety of one's favorite foods. The matter is primarily one of how much and how often to eat. The Canadian Diabetes Association (CDA, 2000) recommends that people adhere to the following easy steps (and often with the assistance of a registered dietician):

- Eat three meals per day and allow 4 to 6 hr between meals.
- If you do have snacks between meals, keep them small.
- Have some starchy food at each meal (bread, pasta, or potato or rice).
- Include a food from each of the food groups at each meal.
- If you are overweight, eat smaller portions.
- If you are thirsty, drink water (avoid too many fruit juices).
- Avoid an overabundance of pop, candy, chocolate, and other sweets.
- Avoid fatty foods such as French fries, ice cream, deep-fried foods, processed meats, and high-fat dairy products.

It is important for people with diabetes to closely monitor the intake of carbohydrate, as this is the macronutrient that has the greatest effect on blood glucose levels (complex carbohydrates break down into simple sugars). One can do this very simply by using the *carbohydrate exchange system*. The exchange system is a plan that allows for a specific amount of carbohydrates, in measured serving sizes, throughout the day in order to ensure stable blood sugar levels. There are two types of carbohydrates: starches (complex) and sugars (simple). Starches include cereals, bread, pasta, and many vegetables. Sugars include candy, fruits, most juices, pastries, cakes, and cookies.

Type 2 Diabetes and Exercise

Aging is associated with the development of impaired glucose tolerance. Type 2 diabetes is very common in adults over the age of 65. It is unknown whether impaired glucose tolerance is a primary effect of aging or of other age-related changes such as increased body fat, decreased muscle mass, and decreased physical activity. It is known that regular exercise can help reverse the usual decrease in insulin sensitivity normally associated with aging. The person with diabetes is susceptible to atherosclerosis, blood vessel and nerve damage, and infection.

The role of exercise is often not emphasized enough in the treatment of diabetes. Regular activity can significantly lower the likelihood of obesity, along with improving body composition (decreasing body fat). Regular exercise has many additional physical benefits including cardiovascular conditioning, decreased blood pressure, improved lipid profile (more high-density lipoprotein, less low-density lipoprotein, lower total cholesterol levels), and an increased effect of insulin. The beneficial effects of insulin include increased insulin sensitivity, increased insulin action, and increased insulin binding. These effects are due to a combination of the acute effects of exercise and of short-lived adaptations. Therefore, diabetic patients must maintain a physically active lifestyle in order to preserve the acquired benefits.

According to the CDA (2000), being active is one of the most positive influences on diabetic health, as physical activity

- lowers blood pressure,
- lowers blood glucose levels,
- helps one to lose weight,
- improves heart and lung health,
- improves general well-being, and
- improves muscle tone and strength.

It is most important to remember that exercise helps glucose transport and the regulation of blood glucose concentrations. Regular monitoring of these levels is valuable especially if one is involved in any high-intensity physical activity.

Glucose Control

A major focus in any diabetes management plan is to ensure that the blood glucose levels are under control. Exercise that is regular and of sufficient duration and intensity can positively affect glucose levels. It is important to ensure that the levels are monitored regularly to protect against a drop in blood glucose, known as hypoglycemia, as well as to indicate the unhealthy rise in blood sugar known as hyperglycemia. Here are the basics one should understand about each of these conditions:

- **Hypoglycemia.** Hypoglycemia can occur when the glucose levels in the blood fall below the accepted normal range due to the increased energy demand that is placed on the body during exercise.
  - Blood glucose testing and sufficient carbohydrate intake, prior to activity, can aid in the prevention of hypoglycemia.
  - The warning signs of hypoglycemia include shakiness, dizziness, light-headedness, sweating, uncontrollable hunger, blurred vision, mood change, irritability, fatigue, irrational and unclear thinking, pounding heart, headache, nervousness, and anxiousness.
  - The causes of hypoglycemia include late or missed meals; exercising without monitoring blood glucose and controlling glucose levels with food; too much medication or insulin; illness; or stress.
  - The best treatment for hypoglycemia is to administer fast-acting carbohydrates (sugar). Orange juice, candy, sugared soda, raisins, and fruit punches are some good examples.
- **Hyperglycemia.** The majority of complications that are associated with diabetes occur as a result of high blood glucose levels and their impact on the body.
  - Some of the signs that a person with diabetes may be in a hyperglycemic state include frequent urination, extreme thirst, fatigue, irritability, blurred vision, and sweet-smelling breath.
  - The causes of hyperglycemia include excess food (especially carbohydrates), too little exercise, forgetting medication, illness, and unusual stress.
  - As treatment, the blood glucose levels should be tested to give an accurate reading, and insulin or medication should be administered when required.

Complications of Diabetes

Diabetes is one of the most insidious diseases known. Complications can lead to the onset of other severe diseases, which are described next. These vary in intensity from mild hypoglycemia to cardiovascular distress and can lead to amputation of limbs and eventually death if the person is not monitored daily and treated properly. Selected complications are listed here also.

- **Microvascular (small blood vessel) damage.** Three major areas of microvascular disease are associated with diabetes:

– **Retinopathy** is the impairment or loss of vision due to blood vessel damage in the eyes. Retinopathy is the sole cause of blindness in 86% of type 1 diabetics and 33% of type 2 diabetics. Of all new cases of adult blindness, 12% are caused by diabetes.

– **Neuropathy** is primarily demonstrated by nerve damage and foot problems due to blood vessel damage to the nervous system. Among people with diabetes, 40% to 50% are affected by neuropathy. Lower extremity amputation is 11 times more frequent for people with diabetes than for people without diabetes, due to poor lower limb circulation resulting from the neuropathy.

– **Nephropathy** is a kidney disease, the etiology of which is blood vessel damage in the kidneys. Twelve percent of seniors with diabetes suffer from kidney disease. Nephropathy is a major cause of illness and early death for people with diabetes and is the number-one cause of end-stage renal failure in North America.

• **Macrovascular (large blood vessel) damage.** Two major problems related to diabetes result in macrovascular distress:

– **Cardiac problems.** The risks of heart disease, high blood pressure, and stroke are increased twofold in men and three- to fourfold in women

– **Hypertension** (high blood pressure). Seniors with diabetes are more likely to develop hypertension than those without diabetes.

• **Other complications.** The diabetic state leads to many other physiologic complications in humans, including the following:

– **Infection.** People who have diabetes are more susceptible to infections (mouth, gums, urinary tract, lower extremities, incisions after surgery) if blood sugar levels are not monitored and controlled. Even with proper treatment, prolonged diabetes can result in lower limb amputation.

– **Impotence.** Among men with diabetes, 50% to 60% experience impotence.

– **Increased risk of developing type 2 diabetes later in life, for both mother and child.** This occurs in women who have experienced gestational diabetes.

Programming Recommendations

It is most important to inform people with diabetes who wish to begin an exercise regimen that the first step is always to consult a physician who specializes in diabetes, if possible. With the possibilities of serious complications because of the disease, people with diabetes should seek exercise partners just to be safe. The regularity of the devised exercise program need not differ from that of a program engaged in by others. Exercise has so many positive benefits that the types of exercise, the frequency, and the duration should be modestly adjusted to take diabetes into account.

Check the principles of exercise for older subjects outlined in chapter 7, and adapt them to meet the needs of persons with diabetes. Remember, start slowly, monitor blood glucose before and after exercise, and use the principles of warm-up and cool-down, as these are important for people with diabetes. Keep the glucose concentrations as constant as possible. Contraindications for exercise include the following:

- On one's doctor's advice
- If one is in pain or feeling ill
- If one's blood sugar is too low
- If control is poor and the blood sugar level is above 16 mmol/L
- If there are ketones in the urine
- If temperature extremes are severe (i.e., heat or cold, excessive humidity, or pollution alerts)

Summary

In this chapter we have reviewed the three types of diabetes and discussed type 2 diabetes in detail. The causes of diabetes, the risk factors, and the effects on diabetes of aging, nutrition, and exercise were discussed. As well, the physiological mechanism behind the transport of glucose from the blood to the muscle cell was briefly explained.

We have emphasized the need for healthy eating, combined with regular physical activity, to assist with the quality of life to be enjoyed as one ages. Specific nutrients pertinent for the senior population were explained. As well, the positive effects of regular physical activity on amelioration of several maladies and diseases were touched upon. The take-home message is that healthy eating and regular exercise in tandem will enhance the quality of life for the senior population. The chapter included the symptomology of diabetes and the beneficial effects of regular exercise when combined with dietary regulation.

Questions to Consider

1. Why are certain nutrients more important for the aging population than for younger people?

2. Are vitamin supplements necessary in the majority of older citizens? If so or not, explain why.

3. Why is regular physical activity important for the aging population?

4. Do the dietary requirements of older women differ from those of older men?

5. Describe a healthy three-day diet for an elderly couple.

6. Which is more important for the elderly population—a healthy diet or regular exercise?

7. Describe the causes of the three types of diabetes found in humans.

8. What are the symptoms and risk factors associated with diabetes?

9. What are the benefits of regular exercise for those who have type 2 diabetes?

10. What are the rules for eating and nutrition for diabetics?

11. Is glucose transport different in people who have diabetes than in others?

12. How does glucose transport differ in type 1 and type 2 diabetes?

13. What are the major problems related to microvascular disease? To macrovascular disease?

14. What is the incidence of diabetes in North America?

15. Outline an exercise program for a 65-year-old adult who has type 2 diabetes and who has never been involved in a regular regime of exercise.

16. What nutritional advice would you give the person described in question 15? Any other advice?

chapter 6

Bone Health and Osteoporosis

Dr. Darien Lazowski-Fraher, BSc, MSc, PhD, BScPT

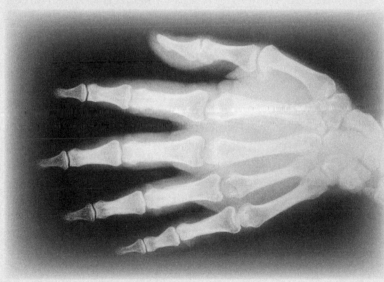

© Photodisc

This chapter primarily deals with bone and osteoporosis, a disorder of bone metabolism resulting in weak, porous bone that can fracture with minimal trauma. Factors that affect bone and osteoporosis such as nutrition, activity, and menopause are discussed. Several beneficial exercise routines are identified, including walking, running, swimming, weight training, sports, and dance. Ways and means for exercise to assist with reducing fracture risk are highlighted, as well as specific exercises that are safe and those that are contraindicated.

Bone Function and Structure

Bone is one of the most important, complex, and fascinating organs in the human body. Bones have been used throughout time for myriad functions as tools, vessels, weapons, decorations, and jewelry, and bone is often cited in poetry and literature as a result. The skeleton is an image recognized by even the youngest children and conveys many different meanings in various cultures all over the world.

Function

The most well-known function of the bones is to form the skeleton—to provide structure, stature, movement, and protection. The rigidity of the skeleton allows for movement; its flexibility allows for breathing; and its structure preserves the integrity of the organs. The skeleton provides a support structure for the muscles to attach to; provides protection for vital organs such as the heart, lungs, brain, and spinal cord; and is the largest reservoir for calcium in the body, making it vital to calcium homeostasis. On the inside, bones provide a safe, protected, rich environment for the bone marrow containing the valuable stem cells and immune cells.

Bones are often taken for granted, until one breaks. It is then that their importance is recognized. Maintaining healthy bones is a lifelong endeavor that begins at conception. It can be hard work to build a healthy skeleton and even harder to maintain it throughout life; but the rewards, especially in the later years, far outweigh the effort.

Structure

Bone is a dynamic, living, growing tissue that is made up mostly of collagen, a protein that provides a soft framework, and calcium phosphate, a mineral composite that adds strength and hardens the framework. This combination of collagen and calcium makes bone strong yet flexible (Davison et al., 2006). More than 99% of the body's calcium is contained in the bones and teeth. The remaining 1% is found in the blood and interstitial fluids (Rosen et al., 1999).

Two types of bone are found in the body: cortical and trabecular. Cortical bone is dense, compact, and organized into concentric layers surrounding blood vessels. It forms the outer layer of the bones. Trabecular bone makes up the interior of bone and has a spongy, honeycomb-like structure. It is the trabecular structure and integrity that give bones most of their strength. Different bones have varying proportions of cortical and trabecular bone. The long bones in the body have more cortical bone, and the spinal bones consist mainly of trabecular bone (Rosen et al., 1999).

Bone Remodeling

Bone is continually being renewed through a process known as bone remodeling (Parfitt, 1996). This process consists of two stages, resorption and formation, and is orchestrated by the cells in the basic multicellular unit (BMU) of bone, the osteoclasts and osteoblasts. During resorption, the large multinucleated osteoclasts break down and remove the old or damaged bone tissue from the system. Growth factors released during resorption and produced by osteoblast progenitor cells stimulate the production of mature osteoblasts, which initiate new bone formation (Jilka, 2003). The functions of osteoclasts and osteoblasts are closely linked and under endocrine regulation by several hormones including calcitonin, parathyroid hormone, vitamin D, estrogen (in women), and testosterone (in men), among others.

The staff at the Mayo Clinic suggest that one might "think of bone as a bank account, where you 'deposit' (formation) and 'withdraw' (resorption) bone tissue. During childhood and the teenage years, new bone is added to the skeleton faster than old bone is removed. As a result, bones become larger, heavier and denser. Bone formation continues at a faster pace than removal until peak bone mass (maximum bone density and strength) is reached around age 30. Remember, in order to be able to make 'deposits' of bone tissue and reach your maximum peak bone mass (PBM), you need to get enough calcium, vitamin D and exercise—important factors in building bone" (Bailey et al., 1996; Bass et al., 1998; Welten et al., 1994). (Refer to www.osteoporosis. mayoclinic.com.)

After peak bone mass is attained, bone "withdrawals" can begin to exceed "deposits." Generally speaking, bone loss can be minimized if people practice good bone health—continuing to get enough calcium, vitamin D, and weight-bearing exercise. Tobacco and excessive caffeine or alcohol use must be avoided (Hernandez-Avila et al., 1991). One is more likely to develop osteoporosis if the peak bone mass achieved during the bone-building years was lower than it needed to be (Brown and Josse, 2002).

Osteoporosis

Osteoporosis is a disease of the bones whereby they weaken and are prone to fracture (figure 6.1). The affected bones become thinner and structurally weaker and more susceptible to breakage. It is important to note that any bone can be affected, but the bones most at risk for fracture are those in the wrist, hip, and spine (Kanis et al., 1994).

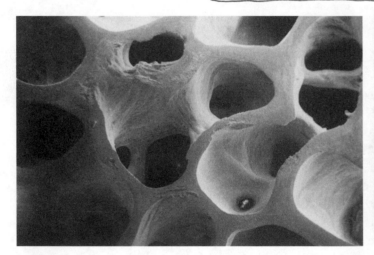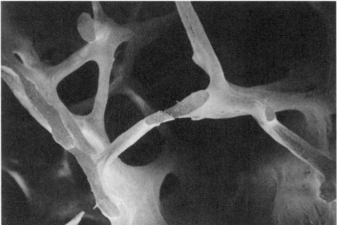

Figure 6.1 Osteoporosis is a condition of weak bone caused by a loss of bone mass as well as a change in bone quality.

Reproduce from Dempster, D.W. et al., 1986 A simple method for correlative light and scanning electron microscopy of human iliac crest bone biopsies: Qualitative observations in normal and osteoporotic subjects, Journal of Bone and Mineral Research 1: 15-21. American Society for Bone and Mineral Research, Washington DC, USA, pp. 129-137 with permission of the American Society for Bone and Mineral Research.

Definition and Causes

Osteoporosis is often called the "silent thief" because there are no symptoms with bone loss, and the condition may come to one's attention only after a fracture. Osteoporotic fractures can occur even after a minor injury, such as a fall from standing height or lower, or after no apparent trauma. Many spinal fractures occur without pain. In some instances back pain may be interpreted as a muscle strain or spinal disc problem. In these cases a spinal fracture is neither suspected nor investigated, and osteoporosis is diagnosed as an incidental finding on X-ray (Ismail et al., 1999; Jackson et al., 2000; Giangregorio et al., 2006; Lentle et al., 2007).

Risk Factors

Many factors will increase one's risk of developing osteoporosis and suffering a fracture. Some of these risk factors can be changed, while others cannot. Recognizing one's personal risk factors is important in order to prevent the continued development of osteoporosis or to take steps to minimize bone loss and fracture risk.

Osteoporosis Canada published the world's first evidence-based guidelines for osteoporosis in the 2002 "Clinical Practice Guidelines for the Diagnosis and Management of Osteoporosis in Canada" (Brown and Josse, 2002). This document specifies major and minor risk factors that identify people who should be assessed for osteoporosis. A bone mineral density measurement is recommended for people who have at least one major or two minor risk factors (table 6.1).

TABLE 6.1 **Risk Factors for Osteoporosis**

Major risk factors	Minor risk factors
Age >65	Rheumatoid arthritis
Vertebral compression fracture	Past history of clinical hyperthyroidism
Fragility fracture after age 40	Chronic anticonvulsant therapy
Family history of osteoporotic fracture (especially maternal hip fracture)	Low dietary calcium Intake
Systemic glucocorticoid therapy of >3 months duration	Smoking
Malabsorption syndrome	Excessive alcohol intake
Primary hyperparathyroidism	Excessive caffeine intake (>4 cups coffee per day)
Propensity to fall	Weight <57 kg
Osteopenia apparent on X-ray film	Weight loss >10% of weight at age 25
Hypogonadism (reduced estrogen in women or testosterone in men)	Chronic heparin therapy
Early menopause (before age 45), either natural or surgical	

Causes of Bone Loss

Bone loss is multifactorial in nature. Age-related bone loss occurs in both men and women after peak bone mass has been achieved (usually between the ages of 20 and 30) and continues throughout life (Rosen et al., 1999).

In women, the rate of bone loss increases for 5 to 15 years at menopause due to the loss of ovarian hormones that have a bone-preserving effect. It is this accelerated phase of bone loss, combined with a lower average peak bone mass, that puts women at higher risk of osteoporosis and fracture than men (Seeman, 2002).

Nutritional factors can have deleterious effects on bone mass and bone strength. Some of these are insufficient dietary calcium and vitamin D; inability to absorb calcium from the diet (as in Crohn's disease or ulcerative colitis); excessive caffeine, alcohol, or salt intake; eating disorders; weight loss diets; and gastrectomy or gastric stapling (Rosen et al., 1999).

Bone loss also occurs with lack of weight-bearing physical activity (Jonsson et al., 1992). Weight-bearing activities produce biomechanical stresses on the bones, initiating a cascade of events to cause bone remodeling (i.e., to make the bone strong in the direction of the stresses imposed upon it) (Kannus et al., 1995). To maintain strength, bone needs continual stimulation, of sufficient magnitude to enable it to withstand the stress of physical activities in a gravity-dependent atmosphere. A sedentary lifestyle, or exercise deficiency, causes bone loss because the skeleton is no longer stimulated to remodel bone to keep it strong (Henderson et al., 1998).

A combination of low peak bone mass, hormone deficiency, calcium or vitamin D deficiency, a sedentary lifestyle, and advancing age leads to the rapid onset and progress of osteoporosis (Brown and Josse, 2002).

Demographics and Cost

Osteoporosis is more common in older individuals and non-Hispanic white women than in other groups, but can occur at any age, in men as well as in women and in all ethnic groups (Brown and Josse, 2002).

In the United States, total acute care costs of osteoporosis are $15 to $20 billion a year. One in three women over 50 will experience osteoporotic fractures in her lifetime, as will one in five men. Mortality is significant and largely unrecognized. Most women fear developing breast cancer far more than they do osteoporosis. Research shows, however, that the lifetime risk of hip fracture (1 in 6) is much greater than the lifetime risk of breast cancer (1 in 9), and the death rate associated with hip fracture is higher. In addition, about 50% of women who have had a hip fracture are unable to return to their former functional level in daily activities, and 20% require long-term care (Brown and Josse, 2002; Lofman et al., 2002).

Around the world, the incidence of osteoporosis varies across racial groups. Caucasian and Asian people are most likely to experience osteoporosis and osteoporosis-related fractures (Johnell et al., 2001). Hispanic and non-Hispanic black people can also develop osteoporosis and related fractures, but have a lower risk when compared to Caucasians and Asians. The reasons for the varying susceptibility to osteoporosis and fractures among different racial groups are complex. Genetics are certainly a factor; but lifestyle, cultural habits, diet, and

Osteoporosis and Spinal Fractures

Spinal fractures are often silent. At least 60% of spinal fractures are painless and are discovered only as an incidental finding on an X-ray that was taken for another reason. For example, a chest X-ray for suspected pneumonia may reveal a spinal or rib fracture. Spinal fractures can also be misinterpreted as a pulled muscle or herniated disc. A spinal fracture, often referred to as a compression fracture, is defined as a reduction in the height of the vertebra by 20%. Consequently, there can be more than one fracture in each spinal bone. The fracture can occur in the front (anterior) of the bone, causing a wedge-shaped compression. Fractures can also present as a collapsing of the middle of the bone (vertebral end plates) or as a complete crush such that the height of the entire vertebra is severely reduced. Because of the shape of the spine and the fractures, the spine curves forward, resulting in a spinal deformity called a thoracic kyphosis or a "dowager's hump" (figure 6.2). The good news is that osteoporotic fractures are largely preventable.

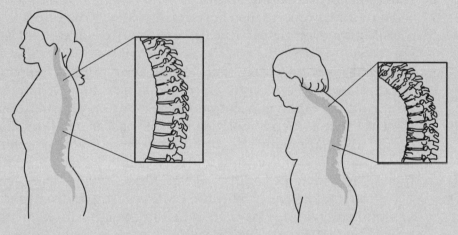

Figure 6.2 As the bone of the spine thins, fractures can occur that cause a loss of height and a forward curvature of the spine.

habitual work and physical activity patterns also play a role (Brown and Josse, 2002).

Women have a higher incidence of osteoporosis and fractures compared with men because, on average, they have smaller, thinner bones and lower peak bone mass and because they can lose bone tissue rapidly in the first 5 to 15 years of menopause due to the sharp decline in estrogen, a hormone produced by the ovaries that has a protective effect on bone. Menopause usually occurs between ages 45 and 55. By age 60 to 65, the rate of bone loss declines and approaches that in men. While men do not undergo the equivalent of menopause, a decrease in the production of the male hormone testosterone may occur and can lead to increased bone loss and a greater risk of developing osteoporosis eventually (Khan et al., 2007).

Diagnosis

Bone mineral density (BMD) can be readily measured and can help determine the incidence of osteoporosis. Presently, dual-energy X-ray absorptiometry (DEXA or DXA) appears to be the best measure of BMD. The test is quick and painless; it is similar to having an X-ray taken, but uses much less radiation. Even so, to avoid any risk of damaging the developing fetus, pregnant women should not have this test done.

The World Health Organization (WHO) definition of osteoporosis is widely used around the world and is based on comparing an individual's BMD with the mean for a normal young adult population of the same sex and race (WHO, 1994, 1998) (table 6.2). The "T-score" is the number of standard deviations (SD) above (+) or below (–) the mean BMD for normal young adults.

Many BMD reports also specify a Z-score. This refers to the number of SD above or below the mean BMD for age- and sex-matched controls.

As originally proposed, this classification applies to postmenopausal white women. There is still no consensus on how to define normal and abnormal in other populations. The relationship between BMD and fracture risk in men is not well understood due to limited clinical trial data. This relationship may be different from that in women due to bone size, peak bone mass, differences in bone remodeling, and habitual type of activities (Lohman et al., 1995).

Certain factors can modify the BMD reading. Extremes of body weight or significant change (over 10%) in body weight can have unpredictable effects on BMD and affect serial measurements.

Factors that result in *apparent increased BMD* include the following:

- **Hip:** excessive or inadequate internal hip rotation, osteoarthritis, metal artifact, focal skeletal sclerosis
- **Spine:** osteophytes, focal skeletal pathology (i.e., sclerosis, metastasis, Paget's disease), vertebral compression fractures, vascular

TABLE 6.2 **The World Health Organization (WHO) Classification of Bone Mass and Osteoporosis**

Classification	T-score
Normal bone mineral density (BMD)	Between +2.5 and −1.0 (the BMD is between 2.5 SD above and 1 SD below the young adult mean)
Osteopenia	Between −1.0 and −2.5, inclusive
Osteoporosis	Below −2.5
Severe osteoporosis	Below −2.5 and associated with a fragility fracture*

*A fragility fracture is defined as a fracture that occurs from a force equivalent to a fall from a standing height or less.

calcifications, metal, radiology contrast, stones, calcium tablets, or other artifact overlying spine

Factors other than osteoporosis resulting in *apparent decreased BMD* include these:

- **Hip:** artifact overlying soft tissue, lytic lesions
- **Spine:** artifact overlying soft tissues, rotoscoliosis, laminectomy, lytic lesions

Treatment

Since osteoporosis is multifactorial, the best means of treating it is to identify individual risk factors and target the therapy appropriately. For example, treatments will be very different for a 30-year-old woman with anorexia nervosa, irregular menses, and low estrogen; a 60-year-old woman with rheumatoid arthritis (Adachi et al., 2000); and a 75-year-old man with a hip fracture (Rosen et al., 1999). It is important that treatment begin as early as possible and be designed to ensure retention or enhancement of bone mass and preservation of the structural integrity of the skeleton to prevent fragility fractures.

Pharmacologic interventions have been aimed at reducing resorption and are largely effective in reducing fractures. Newer therapies aimed at increasing formation are currently under development and study.

- **Bisphosphonates:** Etidronate (Didrocal), alendronate (Fosamax), and risedronate (Actonel) are antiresorptive agents that exert their effects on osteoclasts by interfering with osteoclast recruitment, differentiation, and action as well as enhancing osteoclast apoptosis. These medications help slow down bone loss and have been shown to decrease the incidence of vertebral and nonvertebral (hip, wrist, rib, humerus) fractures.

- **Calcitonin (Calcimar, Miacalcin):** This medication is a naturally occurring peptide. As a peptide, it cannot be given orally since it would not survive digestion. It is usually administered in a nasal spray or, less commonly, by injection. Because calcitonin from fish is more potent in humans than the human form, recombinant salmon calcitonin is usually used. Calcitonin is an antiresorptive agent that interferes with osteoclast activity. Calcitonin has been shown to be effective in reducing vertebral, but not nonvertebral, fractures and to reduce pain associated with acute vertebral fractures.

- **Ovarian hormone therapy (OHT) or hormone replacement therapy (HRT):** Estrogen in combination with another hormone, progestin/progesterone, has been shown to decrease the risk of vertebral and nonvertebral fractures and decreases the risk of colorectal cancer. On the downside, OHT/HRT taken for more than five years has been associated with a small but significant increase in the relative risk for coronary artery disease (heart attacks), breast cancer, stroke, and venous thromboembolism (blood clots). Given the complexity of this issue, it is important for women to consult with their doctors about whether hormone replacement therapy is appropriate, as the risks may outweigh the benefits.

- **Selective estrogen receptor modulators (SERMs):** These medications, such as Raloxifene (Evista), mimic estrogens by binding to estrogen receptors. In some tissues they have agonist effects and in others antagonist effects. In bone this type of medication results in reducing spinal fractures. It lowers low-density lipoproteins (LDL, the "bad" cholesterol) in the blood, reduces the risk of heart attacks and stroke in women with cardiovascular disease, and significantly reduces the incidence of breast cancer. On the downside, it has not been shown to reduce nonvertebral fractures, can result in increased hot flashes and leg cramps, and can increase risk of venous thromboembolus (blood clots). Currently, raloxifene can be used only for prevention or treatment in postmenopausal women.

- **Iproflavone:** Iproflavone is a synthetic phytoestrogen, a weak estrogen-like compound produced by plants (soybeans, flax seed, fruits, and vegetables). It has been shown to help maintain BMD in the spine in postmenopausal women but not to prevent fractures in women with osteoporosis. Because of the lack of evidence for effectiveness or safety in long-term use, it is not recommended as a treatment for osteoporosis.

- **Teriparatide (Forteo):** Teriparatide is a recombinant form of parathyroid hormone (hPTH 1-34) that helps increase BMD in the hip and spine (Cranney et al., 2006) and reduces vertebral and nonvertebral fractures in postmenopausal women, in men, and in people with glucocorticoid-induced osteoporosis. It is given as a daily injection under the skin and is approved for use in postmenopausal women and in men at high risk for osteoporotic fracture.

Nutrition for Bone Health

Good nutrition plays an important role in maintaining good bone health over the life span. A well-balanced diet is just as important to bone health as it is to cardiovascular fitness, weight control, glucose regulation, and general health. The following sections address specific nutrients important for good bone health.

Calcium

To maintain good bone health it is important to ensure sufficient dietary calcium intake (Specker, 1996): 1,000 mg per day of calcium for women and men before the age of 50 and 1,500 mg per day for women and men over the age of 50 (Brown and Josse, 2002).

The most calcium-rich foods available are dairy products. In addition to calcium they contain many essential nutrients, are a good source of protein, and are low in fat—even full-fat milk contains only 3.25% milk fat. There are many good nondairy sources of calcium, such as tofu chelated with calcium, almonds, and beans. Calcium-fortified soy milk is also a good alternative. Many different brands and flavors of soy milk are now available, and the quality and flavor have improved greatly over the past few years due to the increase in popularity of soy products.

Plant foods are a less concentrated source of calcium than dairy products, and it is difficult to ingest sufficient calcium through plant sources alone. Consider the following food selections containing roughly the same amount of calcium: 1 cup of milk (including chocolate milk), 1.5 oz of cheddar cheese, 1.5 cups of milk-based soup, 2 cups of baked beans, 1/3 cup of tofu chelated with calcium, six sardines, 12 figs, or 18 spears of broccoli. Three servings of any of these is equivalent to about 1,000 mg of calcium (Webb and Lazowski, 2006). Osteoporosis Canada has a section on its Web site that helps individuals calculate calcium intake from the diet. Visit www.osteoporosis.ca.

If adequate calcium cannot be obtained through the diet, calcium supplements are a good alternative. Many types of calcium can be useful. The two most common supplements are calcium carbonate and calcium citrate. Calcium carbonate is inexpensive; it needs to be taken with food; the total dose should be divided up throughout the day; and it can be associated with gastrointestinal side effects such as constipation, bloating, and gas. Calcium citrate is more expensive but does not need to be taken with food and produces fewer side effects. Natural-source calcium made from oyster shells or ground bone should be avoided because of the risk of lead poisoning.

Vitamin D

Vitamin D is essential for calcium regulation and bone health. Vitamin D stimulates the production of calcium-binding protein (CBP) in the intestine to facilitate absorption of calcium from the diet. It also binds to osteoblasts to mobilize calcium stores from the skeleton. Apart from intestine and bone cells, there are vitamin D receptors (VDR) in cells of the immune system, brain, heart, skin, pancreas, breast, and colon. Vitamin D is a regulator of cell growth and maturation and modulates the function of macrophages and activated T- and B-lymphocytes (Holick, 2005).

In the United States the recommendations for daily vitamin D intake are 200 IU up to age 50, 400 IU for age 51 to 70, and 600 IU for those over 70. In Canada the recommendations have recently been updated as indicated by evidence-based research to 400 IU per day until age 50, and then 800 to 1,000 IU per day after age 50 (Brown and Josse, 2002). Natural dietary sources of vitamin D include fatty fishes such as salmon and mackerel, cod liver oil, and sun-dried mushrooms. Milk is supplemented with vitamin D in Canada and the United States. Some yogurts, margarines, orange juice, cereals, and breads are also fortified with vitamin D (Holick, 2005).

The most potent natural source of vitamin D is exposure of the skin to sunshine. Tanning beds that emit ultraviolet type B (UVB) radiation are also very effective in producing vitamin D in the skin. Melanin reduces vitamin D production, and therefore dark-skinned individuals require more sun exposure than fair-skinned people to produce the same amount of vitamin D. Ensuring adequate daily sun exposure (at least 15 min per day on unprotected skin—face, hands, and arms) maximizes the body's own production of vitamin D. People who live north of the 37th parallel do not get adequate exposure in the fall and winter because of the oblique angle of the sun and decreased UVB photons; hence they are unable to produce sufficient vitamin D in the skin during these months. Many older adults living in institutions are vitamin D deficient partially due to lack of exposure to sunshine. Supplementation is necessary when sun exposure is limited (Holick, 2005).

Factors associated with vitamin D deficiency are aging, obesity, sunscreen use, and increased skin pigmentation. The result of vitamin D deficiency in bone is rickets in children and osteomalacia in adults. Both conditions are unfortunately on the rise in Canada and the United States because of inadequate sun exposure, excessive sunscreen use, and inadequate intake in the diet (Holick, 2005). Vitamin D deficiency has also been linked to colon, prostate, breast, ovarian, and other cancers (Grant, 2002). Supplementation of the diet with vitamin D has been shown to improve muscle strength (Bischoff-Ferrari et al., 2003, 2004a) and bone density (Bischoff-Ferrari et al., 2004b; Tangpricha et al., 2004), as well as to decrease the risk of developing multiple sclerosis (Embry et al., 2000), rheumatoid arthritis (Merlino et al., 2004), hypertension (Kohrt et al., 1995; Rostand, 1979), heart disease (Zitterman et al., 2003), and diabetes (Hypponen et al., 2001).

Protein, Caffeine, and Sodium

Maintaining adequate protein intake is important to bone health and may become a problem for older adults who find it difficult to eat enough. On the other hand, excessive protein intake when calcium intake is low can interfere with calcium absorption and metabolism. Excess caffeine and sodium are also associated with bone loss (Hernandez-Avila et al., 1991). Caffeine is contained in significant amounts in coffee, tea, and cola beverages. Most of the sodium in the North American diet is hidden in food additives and preservatives. It is advisable to avoid excess caffeine (more than four cups of coffee per day) and sodium (>2,400 mg/day: equivalent to 1 teaspoon). More than four cups of coffee per day or equivalent is associated with increased risk of hip fracture in both men and women.

Micronutrients

A healthy and nutritious diet is an important part of a healthy lifestyle. There is limited existing evidence that supplementing the diet with essential fatty acids, fiber, magnesium, copper, zinc, iron, phosphorus, or manganese will have any beneficial effect on bone health or osteoporosis (Brown and Josse, 2002).

Physical Activity for Bone Health

Physical activity, especially weight-bearing exercise, is associated with a stronger skeleton and reduced risk of hip fractures in later life (Coupland et al., 1988). Osteoporosis Canada recommends that children, especially those entering and passing through puberty, be encouraged to participate in impact exercises or sports (mainly field and court sports) (Brown and Josse, 2002). Throughout life, both men and women should be encouraged to participate in physical activity, particularly in weight-bearing exercises that include impact as a component. For older men and women at risk of falling, or who have fallen, tailored programs that are based on individual assessment, that include exercises to improve strength and balance, and (where necessary) that are multidisciplinary, should be made available (Ecclestone et al., 1995; Nelson et al., 1994).

Osteoporosis Prevention

Osteoporosis is avoidable for most people. Prevention of this disease is very important because, while there are treatments for osteoporosis, there currently is no cure. Table 6.3 outlines strategies that can help prevent osteoporosis (Brown and Josse, 2002).

True prevention of this disease requires a societal awareness and practice of good bone health that must be maintained throughout life. Unfortunately, because osteoporosis is multifactorial and has a genetic component, it is not always possible to avoid bone loss with diet, exercise, and good bone health. Many people who present with osteoporosis have tried to prevent it by exercising well and maintaining a good body weight and a nutritious diet. The diagnosis of osteoporosis can be especially discouraging in these cases. However, the bone loss and morbidity resulting from the disease would likely be much greater if a healthy lifestyle had not been followed. Observing good bone health throughout life will maximize bone health, minimize bone loss, and reduce the morbidity and mortality of osteoporosis if it does occur.

TABLE 6.3 **Strategies to Reduce the Risk of Osteoporosis**

Strategy	Guidelines and recommendations	Benefits
A well-balanced diet rich in calcium and vitamin D is important throughout life. Ensure adequate calcium (1,000-1,500 mg/day) and vitamin D (400 IU daily for people under 50; 800-1000 IU for those over 50).	• The best source of calcium is food. Vitamin D comes from food and exposure to sunshine. • *Calcium supplements* can help if the recommended intake cannot be met with diet. • *Vitamin D supplements* are necessary for those who live north of the 37th parallel, those who do not go outside, or those who always wear sunscreen.	• A diet rich in calcium gives the body the material it needs to build strong bones and ensures that when the body needs calcium for metabolic processes it does not take it from the skeleton. • Vitamin D helps the body absorb calcium from the diet.
Weight-bearing exercise	• >30-60 min per day, at least 3 days per week. • High-impact exercise is more effective than low impact. • Incorporating more weight-bearing activity into daily activity (10,000 steps/day) is a successful strategy and will be effective throughout life.	• Improves bone mass. • Signals the body to produce more bone where it experiences more stress.
Balance exercise	Exercises need to be weight bearing and challenge existing level of balance. Both static and dynamic exercises should be included.	Reduces the risk of falling and fractures.
Healthy lifestyle	Avoid: • Smoking • Excessive alcohol intake (>2 drinks/day) • Heavy caffeine ingestion (>4 cups of coffee/day) • High salt intake (<2,400 mg of sodium/day) • High protein intake with low calcium • Sedentary lifestyles	• Smoking affects collagen synthesis and results in wrinkled skin and weaker bones. • Alcohol increases fall risk. • High caffeine, salt, protein, and carbonated beverages result in removal of calcium from the skeleton.
Bone mineral density testing	People who should be tested: • Men and women over 50 with one major or two minor risk factors • Younger people who experience a fragility fracture (fracture resulting from a force equivalent to a fall from a standing height) • Long-distance runners (>20 miles/week) • Young female athletes who stop menstruating due to heavy physical activity	Identifies people at risk for fracture or in need of medicines to strengthen bones (or both).

General Bone Health

Physical activity is "vital at every age for healthy bones and is an important part of an osteoporosis prevention and treatment program. Not only will exercise improve bone health, but it also increases muscle strength, coordination, balance and leads to better overall health." (See www.nlm.nih.gov/medlineplus/osteoporosis.html.)

Exercise has many roles in the prevention and management of osteoporosis (Dilsen et al., 1989). Table 6.4 outlines the key benefits of exercise.

Many modes of exercise are beneficial in combating the insidious effects of osteoporosis (Forwood and Burr, 1993; Nelson et al., 1994). The best exercise for bones is weight bearing (Kerr et al., 1996; Kohrt et al., 1995). This type of exercise involves supporting the body weight against gravity. Examples include walking, hiking, jogging, running, stair climbing, tennis, bowling, badminton, basketball, soccer, and dancing. The types of activities and exercises that are best are based on the individual's goals, overall health status, degree of bone loss, and enjoyment.

The following are the most appropriate types of exercise for those attempting to postpone the onset or to delay the progress of osteoporosis. People with osteoporosis and fractures have special needs due to the fragility of their bones and risk of fracture.

- **Walking.** Walking, when done properly, is an excellent form of exercise that is feasible for most people to incorporate into their daily lifestyles (Nelson et al., 1991). Walking also has a positive impact on fitness, strength, functional independence, cardiac health, lipid profile, glucose regulation, and weight. To be effective, a walking program must

TABLE 6.4 **The Role of Exercise in the Prevention and Management of Osteoporosis**

Benefits of exercise for bone health	References
Maximizing bone mass	Dalsky et al., 1988
Preventing bone loss associated with inactivity	Rikli and McManus, 1990; Smith et al., 1989; Snow-Harter et al., 1992
Maintaining strength, balance, endurance, coordination, flexibility, aerobic fitness, and functional independence	Chow et al., 1987, 1989; Helmes et al., 1995; Lazowski et al., 1999; Nelson et al., 1994; Rikli and Busch, 1986
Strengthening postural muscles and reducing fracture risk	Lazowski et al., 1994, 1995; Sinaki et al., 1989
Correcting muscle imbalances, reducing pain, and improving mobility	Webb and Lazowski, 2001, 2006
Reducing risk of falling, diabetes, and heart disease	Campbell et al., 1997; Gillespie et al., 2003

be based on the overload principle, as with any exercise. Walking with a toddler, shopping, and pushing a stroller are not effective (unless the stroller is an exercise stroller that will allow the pusher to walk briskly or run). Walking a dog can be an excellent motivator but is beneficial only if the dog allows one to walk at a good pace for at least 30 min without stopping. Walking has to be brisk and done regularly (three to four times per week) for 30 to 60 min (Brooke-Wavell et al., 1997; Ebrahim et al., 1997). Carrying handheld, wrist, or ankle weights should be discouraged because of the risk of joint damage or injury. The pace should be set so that the person is able to talk but not carry on a conversation while walking. As this varies greatly between individuals, it is important for people to walk with others who match their pace. Many shopping malls have walking programs in the mornings before the stores open. These programs provide a safe and supportive environment for people to exercise year-round.

• **Running.** Running or jogging is becoming more and more popular. Many people start running in their 40s, even those who did not run when they were younger. Running can be safe for people with osteoporosis as long as it is done under the supervision of a physiotherapist or appropriately trained kinesiologist, who can address muscle imbalance and pain problems immediately as they arise and who will educate the client on posture and safety. People can start with 10 s intervals of running separated by 2 to 3 min walks, working up through very gradual progression over five or six months to running four or more 5 min intervals separated by 1 min walks. Eventually they can work up to 20 to 30 min runs. Posture, good footwear, supervised training, immediate physiotherapy for any problems that develop or require modification of the program and correction of muscle imbalances, gradual progression, and maintaining run-walk intervals and a slow, gentle pace are the keys to success.

• **Swimming.** Swimming and resistance training in the water are not bone-building exercises but will strengthen muscles, reduce pain, and improve mobility and flexibility and may have an indirect effect on bone. The bones may become stronger because of the increased forces placed upon them in the reduced-gravity environment provided by the water. However, functionally the bones will not necessarily be stronger in a gravity-dependent weight-bearing position. Swimming does have many other benefits and provides an excellent mode of exercise for those who cannot exercise on land due to arthritis or other concomitant conditions (Simmons and Hansen, 1996). Swimming should not be discouraged; however, it should not be advocated as a bone-building exercise, and clients should understand its benefits and limitations.

• **Weight training.** Weight training may or may not be effective in improving bone mass (Snow-Harter et al., 1992) and could be dangerous if not done correctly. If a person has osteoporosis or low bone mass, all flexion moments with weights should be strictly avoided, as this increases compression forces on the spine and fracture risk.

- **Sports.** Some sports are not recommended for people with osteoporosis. This is especially true for sports that entail a risk of falling (e.g., skiing, skydiving, skating, in-line skating) or trauma (e.g., hockey and other contact sports) or those that impart a large flexion moment to the spine (e.g., rowing, curling, bowling, golfing). If people have been inactive and want to start exercising or competing in a sport they used to do when they were younger, caution is warranted in recommending an appropriate activity. It is important for people to avoid flexion forces and risks of falling.

- **Dance.** Dance is a good exercise activity. It has the benefits of being weight bearing and is easy on joints, as well as being good for balance and aerobic fitness (Heinonen et al., 1998). Any kind of dance can be recommended—for example, line, square, round, ballroom, and tap dancing, Irish dancing, Scottish country dancing, or clogging. The participants should be warned to include no flexion moments, to maintain good posture, and to be aware of the probable risks of falling.

Programming Recommendations

People with osteoporosis and fractures have common problems, including these:

- Bone fragility, risk of fracture
- Postural abnormalities (thoracic kyphosis)
- Back or hip pain (or both)
- Reduced strength and endurance
- Impaired balance, increased risk of falling
- Decreased functional independence
- Decreased mobility

Appropriate, individualized programs of physical activity are a vital part of helping individuals with osteoporosis to minimize and deal with these difficulties.

General Recommendations

People with osteoporosis have special exercise requirements because of the fragility of their bones. There are general principles and precautions, but the individual's specific problems must be assessed and their exercise program targeted to address their issues. Just as cardiovascular exercise is recommended for people following a heart attack, weight-bearing, strengthening, and balance exercises are crucial to the rehabilitation of people with osteoporosis and fractures.

Exercise programs need to be tailored to the individual, but in general the strategies listed in table 6.5 are useful.

TABLE 6.5 **Benefits of Different Types of Exercise to Bone Health and Osteoporosis**

Type of exercise	Benefits
Weight-bearing aerobic exercise	Builds/maintains bone mass; improves physical fitness, dynamic balance, core strength, endurance, and functional capacity (Helmes et al., 1995; Kerr et al., 1996; Kohrt et al., 1995; Lazowski et al., 1995; Nelson et al., 1994; Prince et al., 1991).
Balance exercises, tai chi	Improves balance, reduces fall incidence (Campbell et al., 1997; Gillespie et al., 1998).
Muscle strengthening	Improves function, may strengthen bones, reduces falls and fracture risk. Strengthens lower extremity muscles in a weight-bearing position. Resistance can be provided by elastic resistance, free weights, weight machines, or water (Hartard et al., 1996; Helmes et al., 1995; Nelson et al., 1994).
Stretching	Improves flexibility and posture, reduces pain (Webb and Lazowski, 2001, 2006).
Deep breathing	Expands the rib cage, facilitates spinal extension and improved posture (Webb and Lazowski, 2001, 2006).
Back strengthening	Improves posture and endurance in activities of daily living and reduces fracture risk by reducing spinal compression forces (Nguyen et al., 1993; Webb and Lazowski, 2001, 2006; Francis et al., 2004).
Abdominal strengthening (without spinal flexion)	Improves core stability, reduces spinal compression, and stabilizes the spine and pelvis (Nguyen et al., 1993; Webb and Lazowski, 2001, 2006; Francis et al., 2004).

*Contraindications: Loading the spine in a flexed or twisted position and loading the hip in torsion (Francis et al., 2004).

Good Posture

Forward bending increases the compression forces in the spine (Adams et al., 2006; Bouxsein et al., 2006). When the bones are weak as in osteoporosis, this can be enough to result in a fracture (Francis et al., 2004). Good posture reduces the compression of the spine and therefore the risk of fracture (Nguyen et al., 1993). Good posture is most important during normal daily activities that place stress on the spine. Spinal extensor muscles need to be strong and need to have the endurance to maintain good posture throughout the day. Abdominal muscles need to be strong to support the spine and stabilize the pelvis during movement (Webb and Lazowski, 2006). Postural correction exercises should progress as follows:

- Ability to attain erect or more erect posture
- Ability to maintain the corrected posture for a functionally useful period of time
- Ability to coordinate breathing with corrected posture

- Ability to maintain the corrected posture with breathing during movement
- Ability to maintain the corrected posture with breathing during functional activities

An essential component of fracture prevention is training in safe movements during dangerous activities such as lifting grocery bags, opening windows, cleaning the bathtub, moving objects in and out of cupboards, making or changing the bed, backing up the car, taking items out of the trunk of the car, doing laundry, and carrying things up and down stairs (Webb and Lazowski, 2001).

A consultation with a physiotherapist or occupational therapist in the client's home environment can be beneficial for reducing fracture risk.

Specific Activities

The following are instructions to keep in mind when patients or clients are engaged in selected activities:

- **Long-distance running.** Running distances has the most benefit for those who run up to 15 to 20 miles per week (MacDougall et al., 1992). Running more than 20 miles per week results in little further benefit and can actually result in bone loss (Hetland et al., 1993). This effect is likely due to nutritional factors and low body weight or low BMI (body mass index) (Bilanin et al., 1989).

- **Weight training.** People should weight train with specificity of function in mind. Functional exercises are better than isolated movements. Stabilizing muscles should be worked isometrically in a functional position, whereas muscles that provide movement should be worked isotonically (Webb and Lazowski, 2001). Weight training should be done in a weight-bearing position. Good posture must be maintained, and the weights should not surpass 30° anterior to the frontal plane. Moment arms must be kept short, abdominal muscles contracted, back straight, and knees unlocked. It is especially important that hip strengthening be carried out in a standing position because the hips need to be strong enough to support weight during activities against gravity. Closed kinetic chain exercises are functionally superior to seated or lying open kinetic chain exercises both for muscle strength and to provide the desired effect on bone (Webb and Lazowski, 2001).

- **Sports.** An older adult who has been or is a runner or skier, or performs any other sport or activity that would not be recommended for people with osteoporosis, should not immediately be told to give up the activity. Individuals who have been performing a sport on a regular basis for a long period of time have developed a certain level of skill and the muscle strength to safely perform that activity. Over the years, through progressive adaptive bone remodeling, their bones have developed the strength needed to resist forces placed upon them during the activity. They will be less likely to fracture than a person with the same bone density who has not previously performed the given activity. They must, however, be counseled regarding the risk of high-impact movements, the importance of maintaining good posture during the activity, movements that put them at risk of fracture, and their higher risk of fracture if they fall. For older adults, the benefits of performing a sport that they enjoy regularly far outweigh the risks of falling and fracture. And if they do fracture, they will recover much more quickly than a sedentary deconditioned person (Webb and Lazowski, 2001).

Summary of Precautions for People With Osteoporosis

Sometimes your client or patient can't avoid certain movements, such as bending forward or reaching overhead. Instruct such clients to use caution and practice good posture and body mechanics to decrease the risk of injury. Here are some specifics:

- **Forward bending.** Avoid activities and exercises that involve bending forward excessively at the waist because they increase the risk of vertebral compression fracture.
- **Heavy lifting.** Avoid heavy lifting, especially when bending forward at the waist. This may include lifting loads of laundry, bags of groceries, or exercise weights.
- **Twisting.** Twisting movements can place unusual force on the spine. Golfing and bowling are two common sports that involve twisting and may be harmful.
- **High-impact activities.** Activities that involve higher-impact movements, sudden stops and starts, and abrupt weight shifts may put too much stress on the spine and can lead to falls and injuries.

Summary

Bone is a live, dynamic tissue that provides the body with protection, support, strength, and an intrinsic source of calcium. Maintenance of good bone health is multifactorial. Some factors are fixed and not under our control; however, many are modifiable. Physical activity, nutrition, hormonal status, and lifestyle all affect the maintenance of good bone health. Health habits that help build and maintain strong bones should start in childhood and continue throughout life. Physical activity and adequate calcium and vitamin D are important components in this process. Other lifestyle factors such as smoking, alcohol, and caffeine intake also have an impact on bone health.

It is important to recognize that exercise, diet, and lifestyle, although important to bone health, are not the only determinants of bone strength and the likelihood of developing osteoporosis and fractures. Both women and men need to be aware of the other risk factors that can lead to bone loss such as genetics, hormone status, other medical conditions, and medications. There are many medical treatments that can help increase bone mass and reduce the risk of fracturing when bone loss becomes a problem.

It is never too late to make healthy changes to improve your bones. For older people, exercise not only helps to maintain bone strength, but also improves balance and coordination, which reduces the risk of falling. Other benefits of exercise are improvements in strength, flexibility, posture, weight control, and general fitness. These factors are important to help older adults reduce pain, improve functional capacity, and maintain independence over their lifespan.

Questions to Consider

1. How early in life does a person need to think about building strong bones?

2. What is the difference between normal and osteoporotic bone?

3. Why are osteoporotic bones more prone to fracture?

4. What is the best exercise for building bone?

5. How much exercise is needed to maintain strong bones?

6. Does a recreational runner have to give up running after being diagnosed with osteoporosis?

7. How can long-distance running actually result in bone loss?

8. What are the benefits of being physically active throughout life?

9. John has had a physically demanding job all his life. He has just retired at the age of 60 and wants to relax and take it easy from now on. How would you counsel him? What are the risks for his bones and general health? How could you help John incorporate physical activity into retired life?

part III

Physiologic Adaptability to Training and Physical Activity

Part III includes chapters 7 through 11. This section of the text adds another unique dimension to the study of exercise physiology that is not generally found in standard texts, which seldom address aging. Exercise results in adaptive responses by the various physiologic systems of the body. In people who are elderly, however, these adaptations are confounded by the process of aging, and this calls for additional adaptive responses in older adults.

In chapter 7 we look at the principles of exercise for older adults. Although the basic principles do not differ from those applied by younger individuals, they must be adjusted or adapted for older subjects; additionally, other guidelines such as more stringent safety measures must be followed. In chapter 7 we take a functional approach, which is most important for older people involved in formal exercise classes and programs in particular. The FITT program is outlined and described in some detail. The chapter refers readers to the important programs initiated and supported by the American College of Sports Medicine.

Chapter 8 explores exercise for elderly people from a more specific perspective: training for aerobic and anaerobic fitness. We look at the physiological and functional benefits but stress the health benefits, which are even more important to consider for the older population because of the combined deleterious effects of the aging process. Although many of the effects of exercise for young and older subjects are similar in direction, they are definitely different in magnitude. Therefore, we emphasize the ways and means to safely maintain appropriate levels of fitness in our aging population.

Over the past two decades, considerable research has shown that older individuals can benefit from resistance training to produce superior levels of muscular fitness. In chapter 9 we set guidelines for older adults who are "pushing lead." Programs delineating specificity, frequency, the number of "reps," concurrent training, and safety are outlined. Resistance training is a "new" need that leads to a healthier lifestyle for many seniors.

Chapter 10 contains information seldom included in exercise physiology texts. One must remember that older adults are all suffering from the aging process. They have certain diseases of aging, along with debilitating side effects, that gradually lead to a low quality of life and eventually death. It is of the utmost importance that we realize the reasons for attrition from exercise programs. In this chapter we emphasize the need and reasons for exercise adherence on the part of older subjects, and at the same time we stress the need for particular safety measures when one is dealing with this population.

Chapter 11 is a most important and interesting chapter of this book. In this chapter we consider elite athletes from the older population, the masters athletes. The chapter raises some physiological questions but as well brings to the forefront some philosophical issues. The present international stand against the use of drugs by athletes is well known, especially in view of the recent banning of several Canadian and American world champions and world-record holders and their coaches. Nevertheless, the issue of how to deal with masters athletes who use drugs is a very recent phenomenon. Older athletes in many cases rely upon certain banned drugs to maintain life. This presents a most interesting dilemma for readers of the book to consider.

In chapter 11 we describe, define, and explain many drugs and drug families currently in use throughout the world by older adults (as well as by younger athletes). Numerous examples of abuse are also identified. In each case we note the problems associated with abuse or potential abuse of these drugs. Each section also covers problems related to abuse of prescription drugs. The final section of the chapter deals with the use of supplements, the necessity for using them, and potential abuse problems for older athletes.

chapter 7

A Functional Approach to Exercise

Denise M. Connelly, BSc(PT), MSc(PT), PhD

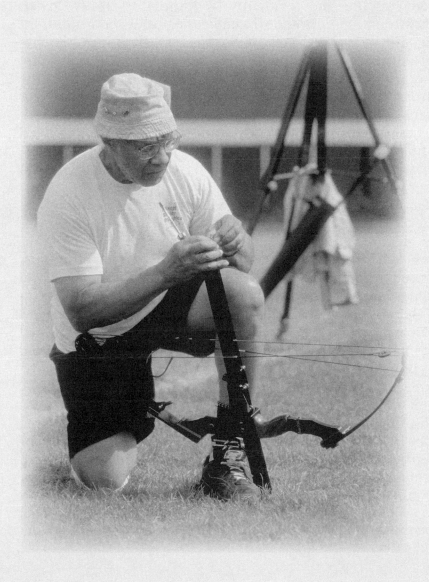

An older adult participating in an exercise program desires to maintain or improve his or her ability to be independent. What it means to be independent is different for each person. To maintain independence in their daily lives, many older adults are challenged to choose among the activities of daily living on which they will spend their energy. Exercise can increase their energy resources and help them function independently by improving upper, lower, and core body strength; endurance; balance; flexibility; coordination; pain control; and mood and self-confidence. These same benefits of exercise are available to young adults; however, for older adults, these improvements can make the difference between living at home or not, requiring assistance with basic activities of daily living, or walking independently. The range of movement, intensity, duration, progression, timing, equipment, and type of exercise can be modified on an individual basis to enable participation. With knowledge, care, and planning, almost all older adults can participate in some form of exercise.

Other issues that need to be considered for an older adult participating in an exercise program—issues that are often not barriers for young adults—include transportation, psychosocial factors, community resources, scheduling of exercise programs, costs of programs, risks of exercise participation, safety precautions for various medical conditions, types of exercise, and knowledge and experience of exercise leaders. Older adults are resilient. That's how they became older adults, but their proximity to the various physiologic and functional thresholds for independent living leaves less room for recovery from injury or inappropriate or ineffective exercise. Maximal return for the exercise completed is a priority.

This chapter provides guidelines for application of the principles of exercise to promote independence at whatever level of function is available to an older individual. In discussing exercise programs for older adults, the chapter describes a functional, applied approach that incorporates these principles. The framework that is outlined for developing exercise programs and promoting increased daily activity for older people includes five components: client-centered exercise; goal-driven exercise; measurable outcomes; functional activities; and screening and safety.

Principles of Exercise

Older adults often manifest physical changes that require specific knowledge and understanding on the part of the exercise leader. Many resources are available that provide this type of information. The next section provides information on selected resources that readers can consult to supplement the material presented in this chapter. These address specific health conditions, suggest exercise modifications, and discuss topics on exercise implementation that are not covered here. The subsequent section presents seven principles of exercise in order to provide a framework for the application of an exercise intervention. Using these principles and this framework for the prescription of exercise, an exercise leader can systematically reflect on the exercise goal or the intention of the exercise (anticipated outcome) and adjust the type, volume, and pace of exercise.

The *FITT* approach (frequency, intensity, time, and type of exercise) is a recipe-like method for ensuring that one includes all the necessary ingredients when designing and implementing an exercise program. Additionally, FITT can function as a reminder for communicating the details of an exercise program to a client. Without knowledge of the details of FITT, an individual would be unable to independently complete prescribed exercise. The basics of exercise-related knowledge are outlined here, but readers should note that whole textbooks, in some cases, are needed to provide the depth and breadth of knowledge required for supervising and prescribing exercise for older adults with chronic health conditions, or for modifying exercise position or type, for example, to enable exercise participation by older adults with a range of abilities.

Resources

Every textbook on the topic of exercise includes a chapter on the principles of exercise. Entire textbooks have been written to address the principles of exercise testing and prescription. The American College of Sports Medicine (ACSM) published a seventh edition of *ACSM's Guidelines for Exercise Testing and Prescription* (2005) and a fifth edition of *ACSM's Resource Manual for Guidelines for Exercise Testing and Prescription* (2006). These texts present a comprehensive approach to exercise involvement including screening, testing, and prescription; they also provide information on the application of exercise for chronic health conditions, on health behavior modification, and on program management. In addition, some resources focus entirely on the application of exercise for people with chronic conditions, for example, *ACSM's Exercise Management for Persons with Chronic Diseases and Disabilities* (2003); *ACSM's Resources for Clinical Exercise Physiology: Musculoskeletal, Neuromuscular, Neoplastic, Immunologic,* and *Hematologic Conditions* (2002); and *Exercise Testing and Exercise Prescription for Special Cases: Theoretical Basis and Clinical Application* (1993). These texts address many age-related chronic conditions as well as other health conditions across the life span.

One of the first comprehensive resources to present guidelines for exercise by older adults was "American College of Sports Medicine Position Stand: Exercise and Physical Activity for Older Adults" (Mazzeo et al., 1998). This publication summarizes the physiological responses to exercise in older adults and recommendations for exercise programs in this population. Jones and Rose recently published a textbook, *Physical Activity Instruction of Older Adults* (2005), that promotes the application of exercise across the spectrum of older adults—those who are the "healthy" older and those who have medical conditions that require additional knowledge on issues of safety and modification of exercise. Morris and Schoo, in *Optimizing Exercise and Physical Activity in Older People* (2004), describe the benefits of physical activity for older adults and discuss health promotion and the management of chronic health conditions with physical activity.

Other textbooks, such as *Therapeutic Exercise: Techniques for Intervention* (2001) by Bandy and Sanders and *Therapeutic Exercise: Moving Toward Function* (1999) by Hall and Brody, address the application of exercise for the rehabilitation of injuries, surgery-related conditions, and functional decline as well as health issues related to older adults. Brill, in *Functional Fitness for Older Adults* (2004), describes a functional approach to activity for healthy older adults and for older adults with chronic health conditions. Brill's book presents detailed program guides according to specific impairments relevant to older adults. Frail older adults and those with special needs are the focus of Best-Martini and Botenhagen-DiGenova's *Exercise for Frail Elders* (2003). These last two textbooks provide detailed information on exercise instruction of older adults, specific guidelines for a number of chronic health conditions and functional impairments, and modifications of exercise movements for seated exercise.

These textbooks illustrate the spectrum of available resources on the principles of exercise and their application—from those that focus on the physiology of exercise testing and prescription to those that describe a functional approach. An understanding of the physiology of exercise is critical when one is leading or supervising older adults during exercise, and the resources listed in this chapter are excellent.

Foundational Principles of Exercise and Prescription

Exercise training for improved ability is based on several principles or firmly held beliefs. Central to beliefs about exercise training is the idea that adaptation will occur in a physiological system when it is exposed to a training stimulus; this is *the principle of adaptation* (ACSM, 2001). To promote an adaptation in a system, one must routinely impose a training stimulus on the system above that to which it is accustomed—*the principles of threshold* and *overload.* Threshold is the level of performance capacity beyond which one does not normally work. Loading or pushing the body to complete an activity at an intensity above what it is accustomed to is overload. Through a methodical approach over time, the body will respond to the stimulation and perform at a higher level; this is adaptation. Continual increases in the level of work required of the system must occur in order for the system to undergo further adaptations—*the principle of progression.* Gradually, through multiple progressive levels of stimulation, the desired performance can be achieved.

Improvements from training within a physiological system can be maintained if an adequate stimulus is sustained *(the principle of maintenance).* However, gains will be lost if the training stimulus is below the level of work to which the system has grown accustomed, and the rate of loss will correlate with the reduction in the training stimulus *(the principle of regression).* Generally, improvements can be made or lost at any level of physical fitness. Finally, the stimulus applied to the physiological system must be specific in order to effect the desired change in the system—*the principle of specificity.* According to this principle, exercise should relate as closely as possible to the activities the older adult wants to participate in (ACSM, 2001). These seven principles are the fundamental components of prescribed exercise to specifically address the participant's goals and activities, regardless of the participant's age or ability.

Combinations of changes in the components of exercise will promote an increase in fitness and improved physiologic responses to an exercise stimulus. One must guard against prescribing an exercise program for an older adult that includes too large a stimulus, which may result in injury, overtraining, or refusal by the client to continue. Too small a stimulus may fail to produce any training effect (Thomas, 1995) and promote withdrawal from the program because the participant is not seeing any results. The client's current physical capacity and goals will guide the choices for exercise specificity, frequency, intensity, and duration. Generally, previously sedentary older adults should start with an aerobic, strength, or flexibility exercise similar to a movement required to complete a daily task, at a low intensity (50% of $\dot{V}O_2$max) and moderate frequency (three to four sessions per week) and for a short duration (10-15 min) (Thomas, 1995). Duration should be increased before intensity (i.e., working for a longer time, increasing the number of repetitions, or prolonging a static stretch); once an adequate exercise duration is attained, then intensity can be increased (i.e., working at a higher metabolic equivalent [MET] value (Ainsworth et al., 1993), increasing the load, working through a greater range of movement, graduating from an isometric to an isotonic contraction, progressing from a concentric to an eccentric contraction, or altering body position to increase the difficulty of a stretch). Changes in intensity or duration should not increase the total volume of exercise by more than 10% every week (Thomas, 2005). A guideline for increasing duration is 5-10 min per session once a week, and intensity should be gradually progressed from 50% to 85% of age-predicted maximal heart rate (ACSM, 2001).

The FITT Approach

A complete prescription for an exercise program requires guidelines for exercise intensity, frequency, duration, type, and progression. All of these components are neatly packaged in the well-known FITT approach to creating an exercise program. The acronym FITT represents

- F, frequency of exercise sessions per week;
- I, intensity of the exercise;
- T, time or duration of the exercise session; and
- T, type of exercise.

A suggested range for each of these components of an exercise program is necessary to guide adults of any age. Progression of exercise is inherent in the framework and requires adjustment of the FITT components. The FITT structure provides a great amount of freedom in the design of programs to provide a training stimulus. Altering any one of the four components—frequency, intensity, type, and time—will provide variations in the program and introduce a new stimulus to the exercising individual. The FITT approach is flexible and can be applied to aerobic, strength, balance, and flexibility types of exercise.

The basic types of exercise are common to both young and older adults—aerobic exercise to tax the cardiorespiratory system, resisted exercise to overload the musculoskeletal system, balance exercises to stress the neuromuscular system, and agility and flexibility activities to challenge joint range of motion and coordination. The differences between exercise programs for young and older adults may be in the activities of interest, motivation for exercise involvement, adaptations of exercise positioning, equipment choices, rate of progression, or range of exercise intensity. The abilities of individuals, their personal goals, and their interests will guide the form of an exercise program. Chronological age is not as relevant as physiological age to participation in exercise; assumptions about the format and style of a program should not be based on age. Rather, the individual and what makes that person unique will guide the development of his or her exercise program and participation in exercise activities.

Implementing FITT

The exercise literature suggests a range of values for exercise of any type—aerobic, resisted, balance, or flexibility. This often leaves one confused and unsure when prescribing exercise, especially for older adults. Suggested guidelines are provided in order to allow one to "start somewhere" when faced with clients who are just beginning, returning to, or continuing with an exercise program. Time and experience working with older adults in multiple settings will provide the confidence and knowledge for prescribing exercise. Generally, it is better to begin with caution when formulating exercise volume (that is, the sum total of exercise frequency, intensity, time, and type) because of age-related health conditions that increase susceptibility to muscle or joint pain, fatigue, and perhaps reduced self-efficacy. Exercise volume can readily be increased; but it is almost impossible to take away the pain, stiffness, or sense of defeat following exercise completed at a level that is too high for the individual.

Training Zones for Endurance Exercise

Providing an exercise program for a client without explaining how to implement the program or how to monitor the effects is rather like giving someone a car without teaching them the rules of driving. Once the program has been designed according to the basic principles of exercise and the FITT approach, the exercise leader must give clients the knowledge and tools to exercise within a target range of intensity appropriate to their fitness level. For endurance exercise, this target range is defined by a percentage of age-predicted maximal heart rate. Training zones have been described in a couple of different ways. One method characterizes training zones according to the target heart rate range of the participant, and another categorizes training zones by the health benefits that can be achieved in the given range of training intensities. Categorization by target heart rate range would be suitable for older adults. A beginner or low fitness level suggests an exercise intensity of 50% to 60% of age-predicted maximal heart rate; average fitness level corresponds to about 60% to 70% of age-predicted maximal heart rate; and a high fitness level corresponds to 75% to 85% of age-predicted maximal heart rate. These percentages should be converted to a target heart rate range specific to the exerciser using the equation by Tanaka (2001), $208 - (0.7 \times age)$.

The second method provides target training zones based on the person's goals or motivation, or the anticipated outcomes from participating in an exercise program (http://walking.about.com/cs/fitness walking/a/hearttraining_2.htm). The terms for these target training zones may differ from one source to another, but the training outcomes are similar. The "healthy heart zone" is at 50% to 60% of age-predicted maximal heart rate. This is the easiest zone and probably the best zone for people just starting a fitness program. Exercise in this zone can be used as a warm-up for those who are already consistently exercising. Exercise at this intensity has been shown to promote the loss of body fat and to maintain or improve healthy blood pressure and cholesterol levels. Such exercise carries a low risk of causing degenerative joint diseases and a low risk of injury. The body burns 85% of calories from fat, 10% from carbohydrates, and 5% from protein when in this zone. The "fitness zone," at 60% to 70% of age-predicted maximal heart rate, provides the same benefits as exercise in the healthy heart zone and uses fat (85%), carbohydrates (10%), and protein (5%) as fuel. However, at this higher intensity, an exerciser can burn more total calories in the same amount of time. This zone has been described as "fat burning." The "aerobic zone" is at 70% to 80% of age-predicted maximal heart rate. Exercise in the aerobic zone improves cardiovascular and respiratory system function and increases heart muscle strength. This is the preferred zone for people who are training for an endurance event. At this exercise intensity, 50% of calories burned are from fat, 50% are from carbohydrates, and less than 1% are from protein. There are two more zones, anaerobic (80-90%) and red-line (90-100%), but neither are suitable for the general population of older adults. These zones are unsuitable because of the increased risk of adverse events at these exercise intensities. The client's goals, choice of exercise interests, and fitness level will direct the selection of the applicable training zone. Issues of safety as they apply to each of the FITT components will be discussed later. The skills to monitor training intensity are also described later in this chapter.

Sets and Reps for Resisted Exercise

Specific guidelines for muscular fitness are not as well defined and accepted as those for aerobic fitness (Bryant et al., 2001). One can determine the amount of weight an individual should lift during a resisted exercise program by using either a 1-repetition maximum (1-RM), a 6-repetition maximum (6-RM), or a 10-repetition maximum (10-RM). A 1-RM is defined as the amount of weight an individual can lift only once using good form (ACSM, 2000). Given that this load may cause injury in an older adult who has not been lifting weights regularly, a 6-RM or 10-RM, or the amount of weight that can be lifted either six or 10 times using good form, respectively, may be a better option. The difficulty with using a 10-RM load is that manipulating the weights to determine the 10-RM value takes time and may cause fatigue and injury. Three or four attempts to determine either a 1-RM or a 10-RM value would be the maximum to avoid excessive fatigue and increased risk for injury. A description of the technique for 1-RM testing is provided in *ACSM's Guidelines for Exercise Testing and Prescription* (2000). Once the maximal weight is ascertained, the intensity of the resisted exercise can be determined based on the individual's health status, physical fitness level, goals, and limitations. A moderate intensity of resisted exercise (~50-60% 1-RM) has been shown in the literature to be effective in improving muscle strength and endurance in community-dwelling older adults (Brandon et al., 2004), and residents of long-term care centers (Connelly, 2000).

Appropriate resisted exercise for older adults should be based on a number of guidelines and principles, including a warm-up prior to exercise, correct form during lifting and lowering weights, and a focus on multijoint work to promote functional muscle fitness (Bryant et al.,

2001). At least one set of 8 to 12 repetitions of each exercise should be completed just until fatigue. The exercises should address the major muscle groups of the body, preferably during multijoint movements. Lifting and lowering the weights should be done in a slow, controlled manner to avoid any ballistic movements. To avoid a Valsalva maneuver, people should be instructed to breathe out during the lift portion while keeping a normal breathing pattern and rhythm. Exercise should be performed within a pain-free range of motion. Exercisers should progress by increasing the number of repetitions to 15 or 20 per set before increasing the amount of weight. The amount of weight should be increased slowly at approximately 5% increments (Bryant et al., 2001).

Stretch and Hold for Flexibility Exercise

Stretching should be incorporated into the warm-up prior to and cool-down following physical activity. Opinions differ about how long a stretch should be sustained; the ACSM (2000) suggests a 10 to 30 s hold per stretch. People can accomplish a static stretch independently with minimal, if any, equipment. The static stretch is a slow, smooth, sustained movement that never involves bouncing, and focuses on one major joint at a time. Stretches should be prescribed for every major joint in the body, including the knee, hip, upper and lower back, neck, shoulder, and elbow (ACSM, 2000). A stretch (e.g., sit-and-reach or shoulder flexion) should not be painful, should not push beyond the normal range of the joint, should not result in soreness lasting >24 hr, should not be done in a fractured limb until 8 to 12 weeks after the injury, and should be done, if at all, very cautiously by individuals who have a known or suspected diagnosis of osteoporosis (ACSM, 2002). As a starting point, all of the major muscle groups should be stretched a minimum of four times during a session, starting with a 10 s hold and progressing to four repeats of the stretch and holding each for 30 s, two to three days per week (ACSM, 2000).

Static and Dynamic Techniques for Balance Exercise

Balance, or control of our center of gravity, requires training when any of the somatosensory, visual, or vestibular systems, or self-confidence are impaired. A key reference for balance training exercises is the text by Rose (2003), *Fall Proof! A Comprehensive Balance and Mobility Training Program.* In this text, chapters are dedicated to each of the following types of exercise: 1) center of gravity (COG) control training; 2) multisensory training, outlining specific exercises to isolate each of the somatosensory, visual, and vestibular systems, and including exercises to address balance and eye-head coordination; 3) postural strategy training, isolating the hip, ankle, and step strategies to adjust for perturbation through specific exercises; and 4) gait pattern enhancement and variation training, with exercises requiring altered base of support, directional challenges, and environmental and task demands. Other types of effective balance training exercises that fit within a functional approach to exercise for older adults include Tai Chi (Li et al., 2004), square-stepping exercise (Shigematsu and Okura, 2006), and dance (Federici et al., 2005).

The belief or self-confidence that older adults have in their capacity of balance—or their fear of falling—is just as important as their actual ability to move around safely. Li et al. (2003) found that the relationship ($r = -0.20$, $p < 0.001$) between activity restriction and fear of falling, using the Survey of Activities and Fear of Falling in the Elderly (SAFFE), indicated that those older adults with higher fear scores participated in fewer activities. As well, the group of older adults categorized as the high fear group had significantly poorer SF-12 mental and physical health scores compared to the low fear group. Bruce et al. (2002) found that fear of falling was common (33.9%) in their sample of healthy, high-functioning older women (n = 1,500, aged 70-85 years) and was independently associated ($p = 0.003$) with self-imposed reduced levels of particpation in recreational physical activity. Baker et al. (2007) found that reduced depressive symptoms were significantly related to compliance (attendance rate $r = -0.57$, $p = 0.009$; 1RM workload $r = -0.59$, $p = 0.02$; total volume of aerobic training $r = -0.54$, $p = 0.01$), and improved hip muscle strength ($r = -0.50$, $p = 0.002$). Exercise may have an important role in promoting balance confidence and quality of life for an older adult.

Exercise Prescription

A functional approach to exercise for older adults is practical, incorporates the specificity principle of exercise, and attaches meaning to the exercise. Exercise that promotes the repetition of movements required to complete daily activities is functional, practical, and time efficient. A high priority for many older adults is to remain as independent as possible in their daily activities for as long as possible. Exercise that mimics some or all of the components of daily activities, including whole-body endurance, speed, or power, is a priority. A program in which one practices the specific sequences of individual or combined movements for a daily activity will optimize one's success in completing the targeted daily activity and promote independence. Because this approach to exercise addresses the specificity principle, it maximizes the gains from training.

Exercise for older adults should be designed within the "bigger picture" of a person's life. The bigger picture comprises the daily activities people need to complete, their interests or hobbies, their support system, their living situation, and the demands they must fulfill each day. Providing a context for the exercise gives the activity meaning and reinforces the relevance and importance of the exercise, thereby improving compliance and adherence. Exercise that involves functional activities can be incorporated more easily than other forms of exercise into a person's daily life.

Defining the Functional Approach

What exactly does it mean to say that the focus of exercise for older adults should be functional? The term *functional* refers to those basic and instrumental activities of daily living that are required to care for ourselves and others; engage in meaningful activities, whether they involve work or leisure; and move around in our environment. A list of basic activities of daily living can be found in the Barthel Index (Mahoney and Barthel, 1965). Daily living activities include personal hygiene, bathing self, feeding, dressing, toileting, bowel and bladder function, chair–bed transfers, ambulation, and stair climbing. Seven categories of instrumental activities of daily living, as originally formulated by Lawton and Brody (1969), have been reframed within the context of home care needs of community-dwelling older adults (Carriere et al., 1996); these include meal preparation, general housekeeping, ability to handle finances, grocery shopping, heavy domestic work, mobility outside the home, and social life.

Functional exercise often engages the whole body. Use of the whole body incorporates the three primary systems of the body, the musculoskeletal, the cardiorespiratory, and the neurological. These three primary systems cannot work independently from each other, and a decline in one of the systems has an impact on the capacity of the others. For example, an older adult who has sustained a hip fracture, an injury to the musculoskeletal system, will limit the amount and distance of ambulation; this limitation in turn causes a decrease in cardiorespiratory function and may affect balance, a function of the neurological system. The focus on functional activity for exercise with older adults requires the combined use of two or three of the primary body systems. The use of multiple body systems is an effective approach for recruiting strength, endurance, or balance as often as possible. Repetitive use of the systems and their components produces a training effect if the demand exceeds what the system or component is accustomed to. Specific exercise does have a place in rehabilitation of an injury or in recovery from surgery, for example. Specific exercise, though, would be used in these situations in addition to functional exercise that incorporates the basic and instrumental activities of daily living.

Active Living

Fundamental to promoting a functional approach to fitness was the idea that completing daily activities—choosing stairs instead of the elevator, or parking farther away from the movie theater and walking more, for example—could be considered exercise. Completing daily activities for exercise has been described as *active living*. One of the first mentions of the term "active living" in the literature was in a study on the intention of people to incorporate physical activity into their everyday activities (Collette et al., 1994). The results suggested that a social marketing campaign should promote walking every day for 15 min and educate people about the health benefits they would derive from such a program.

Active living, a functional approach to fitness, has been advocated for the general population and older adults. A debate about the effects of active living versus exercise is ongoing in the literature. A review by Shephard (1997) showed that active daily living was largely effective in providing cardiovascular and health rewards previously sought through vigorous aerobic fitness programs. In a review, Hardman (2001) stated that improvements in the cardiorespiratory fitness of middle-aged sedentary women, as measured by maximal oxygen uptake, were as effectively accomplished by exercise in short sessions as by longer continuous sessions. Pescatello and colleagues (2000) reported that habitual physical activity was a stimulus sufficient to lower blood lipid or lipoprotein levels and enhance blood glucose level control in older adults (74.2 ± 0.5 years) living at home, independent of abdominal and overall adiposity. Other results, however, indicated that 2.5 hr per week of heavy housework was not associated with reduced odds of being overweight in a group of women age 60 to 79 years (Lawlor et al., 2002). Further research is required to delineate the effects of active living on health outcomes.

Active living has been promoted through the media. Advertisements on Canadian television for *ParticipACTION* have been replaced with *BodyBreak,* in which middle-aged adults demonstrate an exercise or are shown participating in a daily activity while discussing the benefits of good eating habits and of doing some exercise on a daily basis.

In a recent announcement, the Canadian government has decided to renew *ParticipACTION* to motive people of all ages and abilities to be active in sport and physical activity (www.hc-sc.gc.ca/hc cs/media/nr-cp_e.html). In addition, a new Web site has been launched (www.HealthyCanadians.ca) to help Canadians develop healthier lifestyles.

Canada's *Physical Activity Guide to Healthy Active Living for Older Adults* (www.phac-aspc.gc.ca/pau-uap/paguide/) advocates incorporating physical activity into the daily routine. Suggested activities include vacuuming, gardening, walking, washing the floors, or climbing stairs in the house or apartment building. The guide advocates a goal of 30 to 60 min a day, which one can accomplish by adding up the time for all of the individual activities completed throughout the day. This active living approach is attractive in that all of the activity does not need to be done in one big chunk of time; several blocks of at least 10 min of activity are recommended. A mix of endurance (four to seven days a week), flexibility (daily), and strength and balance (two to four days a week) activities is provided as a guideline for the frequency of exercise. A handy checklist in the guide enables people to record and tabulate activities done during the day. Additionally, a personal goals page and space for writing down the next steps for further action are provided in the guide book to motivate and guide the uptake of more daily physical activity and to promote the new habit of daily participation in physical activity.

Similar recommendations are made in the National Institute on Aging (NIA) AgePage publication, "Exercise: Getting Fit for Life" (www.niapublications.org/agepages/PDFs/Exercise_and_Physical_Activity_Getting_Fit_for_Life.pdf), and in a publication titled *Exercise for Older Adults* from the National Institutes of Health (NIH) (www.nihseniorhealth.gov/exercise/toc.html). The NIH Web site, which has been described as "senior friendly," gives the viewer options for large type and higher visual contrast, as well as a "speech" option that reads the text aloud for older adults with visual impairment. A thoughtful approach has been taken in the design of these tools to provide information about and encourage the adoption of physical activity among older adults. An exercise program must be designed so that people will experience success early on in the process. Continued success throughout the process is necessary to establish the habit of daily exercise and to promote maintenance of exercise participation.

Defining Exercise

Our idea of what constitutes exercise should not be limiting. The word "exercise" conjures up images of a weight room, a cardio or spinning class, or people using the treadmill or elliptical machines. Exercise should be thought of as physical activity, as daily activity, as active living. When exercise is approached in this broadest sense, a functional, person-oriented, goal-driven program can be conceptualized that meets the individual needs of the participant. In keeping with a functional approach to the principles of exercise, equipment should be chosen carefully. Modifying the environment or equipment to promote success will enhance the exercise experience for an older adult.

Activities that older adults engage in will depend on their interests, physical abilities, and living situations. For example, interacting with grandchildren can be an excellent form of exercise. Many "young-old" adults can sit on and get up from the ground, reach, carry, swim, and run with their grandchildren. Such activities promote and preserve good hip flexibility for sitting and reaching, the ability to get up from and down to the ground, and a level of lower extremity strength and aerobic fitness sufficient for running to keep up with the child. Seated activities such as rocking a great-grandchild and playing tickle and peek-a-boo—or even a short game of chase—may be embraced by older adults described as "old-old" (those in the "fourth age"). Such activities require balance, upper and lower body strength, and aerobic fitness above the threshold necessary for community living. Participating in these fun activities is not likely intentional "exercise" for these older adults, but does require energy expenditure above what they may normally do, as well as providing loving feedback through affectionate interaction and laughter.

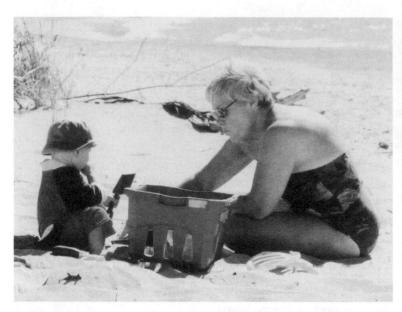 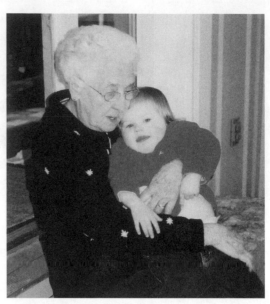

(left) Playing with one's grandchild at the beach is an active living type of exercise that may appeal to the healthy young-old. *(right)* The "old-old" will enjoy activities such as rocking a great-grandchild, engaging in sitting play, and walking (sometimes rather fast!) hand in hand.

Courtesy of Denise M. Connelly

The window of opportunity for exercise for an older adult may be limited by time, energy, finances, transportation, or capability. Efficient delivery of targeted exercise is important. With limited energy resources, older adults must engage in exercise that provides the largest return for the cost. From this perspective, whole-body exercise is required more often than simple single-joint exercise. Most daily activities that an older adult participates in require a combined effort of many body structures and functions. Walking, for example, requires strength, balance, and coordination. Getting up from a chair requires lower extremity power, flexibility in the ankle joint, and balance. Practice of an activity using multiple body systems simultaneously will be most beneficial to an older adult who wants to maintain independence. Performance is limited by the weakest system. All the systems of the body are linked and have an effect on each other. For example, for people who have a balance impairment, the problem within the neuromuscular system will have an effect on endurance and strength because they will limit their mobility, resulting in deconditioning of the other body systems. Improvement in any one of the three main body systems will have a positive impact on the others.

Exercise Programming

A functional approach to the principles of exercise requires the transfer of knowledge and skills for exercise programming and motivation for participation onto the individual participant. With this approach, the participant is educated using lay language to apply the principles of exercise. Canada's *Physical Activity Guide to Healthy Active Living for Older Adults* is a prime example of how to achieve this transfer of knowledge. The *Physical Activity Guide* presents scientific evidence written in lay language, with visually appealing figures, defined categories of exercise, and examples of the different types of exercise, as well as providing clear and concise instructions on the ranges of adequate frequency and duration.

However, the *Physical Activity Guide* does not address practical methods—methods that can be used by individuals themselves—to select the appropriate level of exercise intensity, determine progression, or write measurable functional outcomes. This chapter outlines practical methods of monitoring exercise intensity, guidelines for progressing an exercise program, and ways to develop measurable goal-driven outcomes. These methods are suitable for older adults to implement within their daily activities. Also suggested are selected practical outcome measures that an exercise leader or an older adult can use to track changes in physical function over time. A paradigm of empowering individuals

- shifts the power onto individuals so that they are responsible for their participation and the outcomes of an exercise program and have a source of knowledge they can draw on;
- creates a locus of control;
- promotes involvement in the process;
- develops a sense of commitment;
- provides the tools people will need;
- orients the process toward the individual;
- structures the activity according to the person's interests;
- achieves "buy-in" from participants;
- tracks their progress over time; and
- defines what they have done to achieve the original goal.

Building on the *Physical Activity Guide,* five suggested areas of focus will guide exercise participation, screening, prescription, and testing. The five components guiding a functional approach to exercise are client-centered exercise, goal-driven exercise, measurable outcomes, functional activities, and screening and safety. The foundation for an exercise program comprises the fundamental principles of exercise: adaptation, threshold, overload, progression, specificity, maintenance, and regression. These principles are inherent to any program designed to improve the performance of body systems and function, including the summation of chunks of daily activity to achieve an exercise effect. The proposed components for a functional approach to the principles of exercise provide an opportunity to involve the individual in the design and implementation of an exercise program.

Success is a powerful motivator. People naturally gravitate toward activities that they are good at. Taking a client-centered approach to the application of the principles of exercise enhances participation because it gives older adults the opportunity to choose the activities they want to participate in, for how long, and at what time of day. For many older adults, exercise composed of lifting weights, riding a stationary bicycle, or jogging on a treadmill was not part of their experience growing up. This is why promoting daily, functional activities at an appropriate dose–response level seems like a good approach. Additionally, the idea of active living may be less intimidating to this segment of the population than the idea of "exercise." Fear of injury from exercise is common among older adults and acts as a barrier to participation (Lees et al., 2005). Providing simple measures of safety that do not require equipment and can be incorporated into any activity will support older adults as they participate in exercise activities. As in the *Physical Activity Guide,* specific goals focus individuals on their target and provide them with the motivation to continue. Goals should be very specific, should be suggested by the older adult, and should be measurable. For example, an older adult with knee osteoarthritis may have as his or her goal to independently climb the six steps up to the front door of the home using the railing. Another older adult with chronic obstructive pulmonary disease may cite that his or her goal is to walk 100 m in 5 min with only some shortness of breath.

These goal examples incorporate what is important to the individual *(client centered),* relate to daily activities *(functional activity),* minimize fear of injury or of exacerbating an existing health condition *(safety),* include specific targets for completion *(goal driven),* and can be objectively measured *(measurable outcomes).*

Client-Centered Exercise

A client-centered approach includes the client's goals, expectations, needs, and abilities as the focus of all interventions. To achieve this focus requires open communication between the health care provider and the older adult client. In conversing with older adults, one can identify their interests, preferred activities, daily activities engaged in to take care of themselves or others, individual challenges to exercise participation, and long- and short-term goals. Table 7.1 lists typical adherence-related problems uncovered by such discussions, along with effective strategies for addressing them.

Another issue that the exercise professional should consider is the client's mental preparedness to commit to exercise. Table 7.2 provides a summary of six stages that often describe a client's state. It is useful to know what the client's attitude and stage of commitment are, because these will affect the choice of approaches that will be most effective in overcoming emotional and mental obstacles to regular exercise. The table provides brief statements of strategies one can use with clients depending on what their current attitudes toward consistent, ongoing exercise may be.

TABLE 7.1 Effective Problem Solving to Improve Adherence

Client information	Problem-solving strategies
Overweight clients may have to struggle more and may have unrealistic expectations about what can be accomplished.	• Be honest and help client form realistic goals. • Provide monitoring techniques that clearly show their progress. • Avoid positive feedback that is undeserved, but look for opportunities for recognition of progress. • Use social support systems such as "buddies" or a personal trainer if good rapport is present.
Clients need to be aware of the benefits and costs of their fitness program.	• Help your clients list the benefits they hope to experience and also the inconveniences and difficulties they may encounter. • Discuss how they will deal with these.
Smokers have difficulty sticking with exercise.	• Give permission to feel winded and less energized after exercise. • Avoid making smoking a big issue, but have literature available.
A client's personality problems or mood may affect attendance.	• Don't assume that you are responsible for how your clients feel or for the fact that they often miss sessions because of mood disturbances.
Improvement of health is often given as a reason for initiating exercise.	• Point out the specific health benefits that may be expected from their type of prescription. • Use screening tools (e.g., *Par-Q* or *FANTASTIC Lifestyle Checklist*) to assure clients that they are ready for exercise and increase their health-related awareness.
There are large differences in goals and activity for specific ages and sexes. In one study, competition was seen as a benefit for young men and health for young women, whereas health was seen as a barrier for older men and women (De Bourdeauhuij and Sallis, 2002).	• Emphasize to seniors that improved health should reduce that barrier. • Use careful monitoring and appropriate prescription to keep activities manageable and safe.
Satisfaction with you as an exercise specialist is an important issue for many clients.	• Seek your clients' input on many aspects of goal setting, techniques of training, variations in routines, and satisfaction. • Give your clients feedback about their progress and solicit their feedback about your abilities as a trainer. • Provide support and be available.

Clients often have trouble getting past common road blocks.	• Consider the following responses, as suggested by Patrick and colleagues (1994):
	  (a) If time is the barrier: "We're aiming for three 30-min sessions each week. Do you watch a lot of TV? If so, maybe cut out three TV shows a week."
	  (b) If enjoyment is a problem: "Don't exercise. Start a hobby or an enjoyable activity that gets you moving."
	  (c) If exercise is boring: "Listening to music during your activity keeps your mind occupied. Walking, biking, or running can take you past lots of interesting scenery."

Adapted, by permission, from J.C. Griffin, 2006, *Client-centered exercise prescription*, 2nd ed, (Champaign, IL: Human Kinetics), 51.

TABLE 7.2 **Strategies for Change Process**

Stage	Client behavior	Change process strategy	Counseling strategies
Precontemplative	Is somewhat aware of the message	Consciousness raising	• Increase awareness of imporatance. • Start a dialogue. • Increase "pros" for activity.
Contemplative	• Is aware and interested in the message • Recognizes the problem	• Consciousness raising • Contingency management	• Increase intention to action by addressing ambivalence, highlighting personal benefits, and building self-confidence. • Create a relationship of understanding and acceptance.
Preparation	• Identifies a course of action • Is ready to take action	• Consciousness raising • Contingency management • Self-liberation	• Help the client plan (e.g., set date, location). • Focus on the "pros." • Strengthen self-confidence. • Provide helpful resources (e.g., knowledge and skills).
Action	• Makes a decision to implement a course of action • Tries the activity • Makes short-term adoption	• Contingency management • Self-liberation • Helping relationships	• Teach client how to deal with lapses. • Promote social support. • Deal with lapses; reevaluate next action step. • Provide encouragement.
Maintenance	• Makes long-term commitment • Achieves permanent lifestyle change	• Helping relationships • Counterconditioning • Stimulus control	• Refine and add variety to program. • Prepare in case of relapse. • Provide support in maintaining behavior to prevent relapse.

Adapted, by permission, from J.C. Griffin, 2006, *Client-centered exercise prescription*, 2nd ed, (Champaign, IL: Human Kinetics), 43.

Goal-Driven Exercise

The identification of specific goals by the participant, with the assistance and guidance of the exercise leader, will provide a structure for the development of an exercise program. The broad goals of physical activity participation, including improved physical, psychological, and social functioning, may not be meaningful to an older adult (Thomas, 1995). Specific, more tangible goals relevant to the person's current living situation, interests, or hobbies will be more meaningful and provide motivation, direction, and purpose. Seeking specific information in order to set goals will help ensure that the goals are realistic and relevant (Thomas, 1995). These specific goals will identify any particular deficits that the participant would like to decrease or overcome; provide a context for the participant's specific impairments and the impact they have on daily living; determine the appropriate mode, intensity, and frequency of exercise; provide meaning for the specific exercise activities; and encourage ownership on the part of the client for his or her goals and responsibility for completing the exercise program.

The SMART goal approach has been frequently used to assist in the goal-setting process (Gowland and Gambarotto, 1994). SMART is an acronym for the components that must be included in developing and writing a goal that will be useful within an exercise program; SMART stands for *specific, measurable, action oriented, realistic,* and *time.* Additionally, any specific resources or requirements to accomplish the goal (e.g., a person, piece of equipment, specific set-up, location, or program) could be added to the SMART goal as "R." The acronym would then be a SMARTR goal to improve function and independence of an older adult.

Having a specific goal means that participants know exactly what they are striving for in enough detail to clearly define what they want to achieve from the exercise program. A measurable goal includes concrete criteria for measuring progress. By measuring progress participants can stay on track, reach their target dates, and experience the gratification of achievement. Asking the participant "How will you know when you have reached your goal?" will provide the words needed to write a measurable goal. An action-oriented goal produces results because the steps needed to reach the goal are included in the written goal. A realistic goal is one that is practical and can be achieved. The exercise leader coaches clients toward a goal that is within their range of abilities in order to set them up for success. However, the client's ambition should not be squashed in this process. Guiding the client to seek completion of smaller chunks of the original goal may be an appropriate strategy if the goal is beyond the person's current abilities. The goal should represent an objective that both the exercise leader and the participant are willing and able to work toward (see "Six Steps for Designing and Achieving Exercise Goals," p. 134). Finally, the goal should have a definite deadline and be based on the limits of available resources.

Measurable Outcomes

To provide a measure of baseline function prior to the start of an exercise intervention, one should use a reliable and valid outcome measure to quantify the functional tasks relevant to the participant's exercise goals. This same measure can then be used to assess for changes in the activity following an exercise intervention. The focus here is on field-based tests of functional activities for use with older and frail adults.

Six Steps for Designing and Achieving Exercise Goals

The process for designing and achieving exercise goals can be summarized as follows:

- Begin with the end in mind.
- Write down the SMARTR goal as a statement that includes all of the components.
- Break down larger or more difficult goals into manageable steps.
- Maintain the motivation and commitment of the client to his or her goals.
- Remind clients of their goals to keep them on track.
- Review the goal statements periodically with clients and reassess their progress.

College of Physiotherapists of Ontario. *Professional Portfolio Guide*, 2004, p.14.

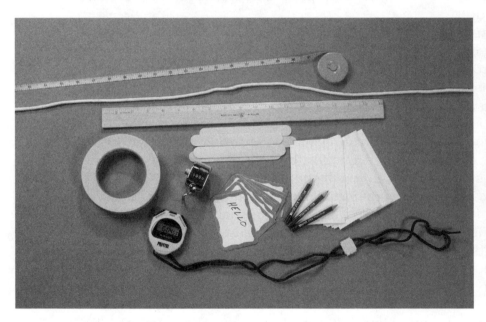

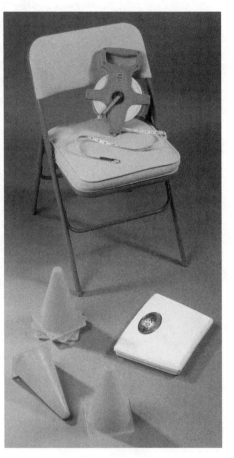

The required equipment for assessing seniors' fitness across the range of exercise experience and performance can be minimal, simple, and inexpensive.

Outcome Measures

Several outcome measures have been developed to assess specific physical activities and have been used for testing with older adults, for example walking speed in a 10 m walk test (Connelly et al., 1996), a 400 m walk test (Chang et al., 2004), a 2 min walk test (Connelly et al.,

1996), or a 6 min walk test (American Thoracic Society, 2002; Butland et al., 1982; Steffen et al., 2002), depending upon the participant's level of function. Questionnaires addressing activities of daily living relevant to older adults provide an opportunity to capture a broad assessment of an older participant's current physical activity habits (see Thomas, 1995), including, for example, the Yale Physical Activity Survey (DiPietro et al., 1993), Physical Activity Scale for the Elderly (PASE) (Washburn et al., 1993), and Late-Life Function and Disability Instrument (Sayers et al., 2004). Several measures of balance performance have been developed for older adults, including the Timed Up & Go test (Podsiadlo and Richardson, 1991), the 14-item Berg Balance Scale (Berg et al., 1989, 1992), and the 10-item Fullerton Advanced Balance Scale (Rose, 2003).

The outcome measure should be carefully chosen in order to allow room for the participant to demonstrate improvement and see success. The "floor" and "ceiling" characteristics of an outcome measure, the appropriateness of the tool for the participant, and the anticipated use of the data from the outcome measure should all be considered. Tests that relate as closely as possible to the activities the older adult wants to perform should be selected. For example, a walking test is most appropriate for those who plan on a walking program, and an upper extremity muscular endurance test would be the most representative measure for those who propel their own wheelchair.

Senior Fitness Test

The Senior Fitness Test was developed to measure the basic physical abilities required to perform functional activities of daily living, as well as functional mobility (Rikli and Jones, 1999). The Senior Fitness Test is currently the only functional fitness test battery that has national norms and has established reliability and validity for adults aged 60 to 94 years. Each of the six test items is a functional measure of a combination of physical parameters, including muscle strength/endurance, aerobic fitness, flexibility, balance, coordination, speed/agility, and power (Rikli and Jones, 1997). The Senior Fitness Test Kit is a comprehensive package including a manual, instructional videotape, and computer software for recording and analyzing the test results (Rikli and Jones, 2001). The scores of a client on the Senior Fitness Test can be compared to those of others of the same sex and age using the provided norm-referenced standards for American older adults. Evaluation of the client's performance as it relates to his or her peer group provides additional information that is useful for interpretation of the client's scores. The *Senior Fitness Test Manual* describes the performance, measurement, and scoring of each test item in detail. In the appendixes of the *Senior Fitness Test Manual*, several sample forms are available for the exercise leader to copy and use as part of exercise programs for older adults. These include informed consent, accident report, scorecard to summarize test results, station signs for group testing in a circuit format, and age-group percentile norms and performance charts for each of the six test items.

Functional Exercise Activities

In response to the question "What are you having difficulty with?" most often older adults respond by describing a functional activity, for example climbing stairs, getting into and out of the bathtub, or picking an item up from the floor. Sometimes they respond with a complaint about a physical parameter. They may say, for example, that they feel their legs are weak or tired; or that they are experiencing joint, muscle, or regional pain; or that they feel stiff. Most likely with further questioning older adults can link their physical discomfort with a functional activity. For example, they experience back pain when they walk, or they feel so stiff that they cannot put their socks on. The functional activity of interest and the physical parameters required to complete that activity can then be used to guide and direct the development of an individualized, client-centered exercise program.

The trend toward including and practicing functional activities in an exercise program for older adults is evident from the information in Canada's *Physical Activity Guide to Healthy Active Living for Older Adults*, the NIH *Exercise for Older Adults*, and the Senior Fitness Test. From a client-centered and goal-driven approach to exercise prescription for older adults, inclusion of functional activities in an exercise program seems appropriate. Further, the inclusion of functional activities in an exercise program addresses the principle of specificity, according to which exercise targeting a specific activity promotes improvement in the performance of that activity. Measurement of performance of the specific functional activity or a highly related activity will inform the exercise leader and the participant of the gains that have been made with the exercise program to reach the target goal.

Screening and Safety Measures

Providing information about how to know when it is safe to begin or return to exercise further empowers individuals to be responsible for their health and to become active participants in the exercise program. Not knowing if it is okay to exercise would stop someone at the contemplation stage, the second of six stages in the Transtheoretical Model/Stages of Change developed by Prochaska and DiClemente (1982). The Transtheoretical Model can be very helpful in "labeling" people's "stage" of behavior and thereby promote an understanding of what they may be going through as they begin, continue, or stop exercising, as well as what type of support they may need at each particular stage of behavior and thinking. Further, exercise leaders must have appropriate training to ensure that, first and foremost, older adults can safely participate in exercise and that the exercises are safe for older adults. As Hippocrates wrote, "As to diseases, make a habit of two things—to help, or at least to do no harm" (*Of the Epidemics*, Bk. I, Sect. XI, 400 BCE).

Exercise Readiness and Health History

A well-known measure to assess whether an individual is ready for an exercise program is the Physical Activities Readiness Questionnaire, or PAR-Q (www.csep.ca/forms.asp). This form can be used by individuals themselves, exercise leaders, or health care providers to determine if there are any indications that the family physician should be consulted before exercise is begun for the first time (see appendix B). The guidelines for use of this form indicate that the PAR-Q is applicable to people aged 15 to 69 years of age (www.csep.ca/forms.asp). The instructions suggest that individuals over the age of 69 years who are not used to being very active should make an appointment with their physician to review whether they are okay to begin an exercise program. Older adults who respond with a yes answer to any of the questions on the PAR-Q should be advised to see their family physician. Applying the Physical Activity Readiness Medical Examination (PARmed-X) (see appendix B) can help the physician determine the patient's readiness to exercise safely (www.csep.ca/forms.asp). In addition to the PARmed-X results, older adults should ask their physician to describe any risks or precautions relevant to their participation in an exercise program. Knowledge of risks for exercise and suggested modifications to an exercise program would be valuable for the exercise leader in designing the individualized exercise program.

Chronic disease becomes more prevalent with age, and the safety of older adults in exercise programs becomes an increasing concern. A systematic approach in completing a medical history for an exercise participant—addressing the cardiorespiratory, neurologic, metabolic, and musculoskeletal systems as well as overall function—should be taken prior to any exercise involvement. A comprehensive assessment of health and activity developed by the Canadian Center for Activity and Aging (www.uwo.ca/actage/), the Health History and Activity Questionnaire (see appendix B), is available in the text by Jones and Rose (2005). Examples of assessment tools for some common age-related impairments and health conditions are provided in table 7.3. This list of examples of potential impairments or health conditions in an older adult population is not comprehensive. In general, screening is done to determine what type of exercise is appropriate and if any modifications are required to ensure an individual's full participation. Medical conditions should not preclude participation in exercise but rather guide the application of exercise to provide full benefit to the participant. For a comprehensive list of precautions and

TABLE 7.3 **Suggested Screening Tools to Be Used Prior to Exercise Participation, Organized According to Impairments Within Body Systems**

System	Example of impairment or health condition	Example of outcome measure*
Cardiorespiratory	Heart condition	PAR-Q[a]
	Dizziness	PAR-Q
	High blood pressure	PAR-Q
Neurologic	Balance	Berg Balance Scale[b]
	Memory	FAB Scale[c]
	Loss of sensation, tingling	Mini-Mental State Exam[d]
		Health History and Activity Questionnaire[e]
Metabolic	Diabetes	BMI[f]
		Blood glucose level[g]
Musculoskeletal	Osteoporosis	Bone density[h]
	Arthritis	WOMAC[i]
Overall function	Mobility	TUG[j]
	Fear of falling	Senior Fitness Test[k]
		PPT[l]
		ABC scale[m]

*These outcome measures can also be used to chart the progress of the participant during the exercise program.
[a]Physical Activity Readiness Questionnaire (PAR-Q). www.csep.ca/forms.asp.
[b]Berg Balance Scale.
[c]Fullerton Advanced Balance (FAB) Scale. D.J. Rose, 2003, *FallProof: A Comprehensive Balance and Mobility Program* (Champaign, IL: Human Kinetics).
[d]Mini-Mental State Exam (MMSE). www.alzheimers.org/caregiving/challengepdfs/mmse.pdf.
[e]Health History and Activity Questionnaire. G.J. Jones and D.J. Rose (Eds.), 2005, *Physical Activity Instruction of Older Adults* (Champaign, IL: Human Kinetics), pp. 69-73.
[f]Body mass index (BMI). www.consumer.gov/weightloss/bmi.htm.
[g]Blood glucose level. G.J. Jones and D.J. Rose (Eds.), 2005, *Physical Activity Instruction of Older Adults* (Champaign, IL: Human Kinetics), pp. 342-344.
[h]Bone mineral density. G.J. Jones and D.J. Rose (Eds.), 2005, *Physical Activity Instruction of Older Adults* (Champaign, IL: Human Kinetics), pp. 46-47.
[i]Western Ontario McMaster Arthritis.
[j]Timed Up & Go (TUG) test.
[k]Senior Fitness Test. R.E. Rikli and C.J. Jones, 2001, *Senior Fitness Test Manual* (Champaign, IL: Human Kinetics).
[l]Physical Performance Test (PPT). www.umshp.org/pt/geritool/Physical-Performance-Test-original.rtf.
[m]Activities Balance Confidence Scale (ABC scale).

contraindications to exercise participation, the reader is referred to a publication by the ACSM (2000). For specific considerations in special cases, such as osteoporosis, rheumatoid arthritis, hypertension, chronic obstructive respiratory disorders, or low functional capacity, the reader is referred to Skinner (1993). Further, specific effects of exercise on several chronic conditions and suggestions for exercise programming for these chronic conditions can be found in a text by Durstine and Moore (2003).

Exercise Instructor Education and Training

Exercise leaders must be aware of safety and knowledgeable about the promotion and implementation of safety guidelines for older adults participating in exercise programs. Older community-living adults have a desire to participate in exercise programs; however, often not enough qualified exercise instructors are available (Lachenmayr and Mackenzie, 2004). The Canadian Centre for Activity and Aging (CCAA) has implemented the Senior Fitness Instructor Course (SFIC). The SFIC was developed to address a need for training leaders and disseminating information about appropriate physical activity programs for older adults. It is a certification program for anyone (older and young adult volunteers) who wants to learn how to design and lead effective fitness classes for seniors (www.ccaa-outreach.com/show_course.php?coursetypeid=1).

In 2004, international guidelines, titled *International Curriculum Guidelines for Preparing Physical Activity Instructors of Older Adults*, were presented at the 6th World Congress on Aging and Physical Activity (www.seniorfitness.net/international_curriculum_guidelines_for_preparing_physical_activity_instructors_of_older_adults.htm). *International Curriculum Guidelines for Preparing Physical Activity Instructors of Older Adults* represents consensus of many experts in the field of physical activity for older adults and the World Health Organization (WHO) Active Ageing Policy Framework. The document describes the major content areas that should be included in an entry-level training program for physical activity instructors who will work with older adults. The suggested topics for each of the nine training modules can be found in appendix A of the text by Jones and Rose (2005). The importance of knowledge, experience, and skill in the application of physical activity programming for older adults is evident from the number and stature of the contributors to this initiative in developing *International Curriculum Guidelines for Preparing Physical Activity Instructors of Older Adults*.

Programming Recommendations

This section describes measures to ensure the safety of an older adult as they pertain to the FITT approach to exercise participation. Injury can result from participation in aerobic, strength, flexibility, or balance exercise too frequently, at too high an intensity, or for too long; from using improper form during exercise; or from progressing the parameters for exercise too quickly. Delayed-onset muscle soreness from exercise activity should last no longer than 48 hr and should not limit joint function or range, the ability to complete activities of daily living, or restrict mobility. Soreness from exercise beyond this time frame indicates that the volume of exercise was too great for the individual. The following sections outline safety guidelines for each component of the FITT approach.

Frequency

The end goal is for an exercise participant to engage in a particular volume of exercise activity. To achieve the prescribed volume of exercise, any one or all of the FITT components can be altered to provide a sum of exercise activity equal to a targeted volume. For example, a similar volume of exercise can be attained with 1) a low exercise intensity paired with a higher frequency for a longer duration, or 2) exercise at a high intensity, short duration, and lower frequency. Canada's *Physical Activity Guide to Healthy Active Living for Older Adults* provides distinct guidelines for exercise frequency by category of exercise type, that is, endurance, flexibility, and strength and balance (www.paguide.com). The range in number of exercise sessions on a weekly basis represents the targeted total. For older adults who are beginning an exercise program, the number of exercise sessions in each of the four categories of exercise should be progressed from a low number to the target range over a period of time, that is, four to seven days a week (endurance), daily (flexibility), and two to four days a week (strength and balance). A method of monitoring the effects of exercise to guide the frequency of sessions is to attend to the body's symptoms. The symptoms that will reflect whether the body is tolerating the exercise program include muscle pain, joint pain, muscle or joint stiffness or both, fatigue, exacerbation of an existing health condition, decreased range of motion, and a prolonged (>24 hr) return to pain-free function.

Intensity

Several methods can be used by exercise participants to monitor their exercise response to the intensity of exercise. A target heart rate range to be reached and maintained during aerobic exercise can be calculated to monitor exercise heart rate response. The Karvonen formula is one example of how to calculate an age-specific target heart rate zone (Karvonen and Vuorimaa, 1988). This method of calculating the target heart rate training zone is based on an age-related maximal heart rate and the individual's resting heart rate. To determine the resting heart rate, people should be instructed to take their resting pulse three mornings in a row, just after waking up and before getting out of bed. The pulse can be felt on the wrist (radial pulse) or on the side of the neck (carotid pulse). People should be instructed to use the site at which they can feel the pulse most easily and to count the number of beats, starting with zero for the first beat, for 1 min. People who do not have a stopwatch or a clock with a second hand can measure their pulse in the time it takes for the minute number to change on a digital clock—that is, find the pulse and start counting when the minute number changes the first time and stop counting when it changes again. Clients should be reminded to use the pads of their first or middle fingers and not their thumb. As well, they should rest the pads of the fingers on the carotid or radial site and not apply too much pressure. Using the thumb or pressing too hard on the artery can inhibit obtaining an accurate pulse count. Once three measures of the morning resting pulse are obtained, the client should add the three numbers and then divide by three to calculate the average pulse. Then, with use of the Karvonen formula, the target training zone can be calculated.

For example, we will calculate the target training zone for an older adult who has a resting pulse of 60 beats per minute, is 70 years of age, and wishes to exercise at a moderate to high intensity (60-70%). The first step is to calculate the age-related maximal heart rate (maxHR) using the formula 220 – age for men and 226 – age for women. Then to calculate heart rate reserve (HRR), use the formula maxHR – resting heart rate. In this example, the training range heart rate (training range %) is calculated using HRR × 60% for the lower range and HRR × 70% for the higher range. The target heart rate for training is (training range % + resting heart rate) at 60% and is calculated again at 70%. The range in target heart rates is the suggested heart rate training zone for the individual. For example, a man who is 70 years old with a resting heart rate of 60 beats per minute when exercising at 60% to 70% intensity should maintain his exercise heart rate between 114 and 123 beats per minute. To monitor the exercise intensity, the client should be instructed to take his pulse during exercise starting with the first beat as zero (i.e., 0-1-2-3-4 . . . 12, for 10 or 15 s) and then multiply by 6 or 4, respectively, to obtain pulse in beats per minute. The exercise heart rate should fall within the target training zone. If the heart rate is lower than the range, the exercise intensity can be increased; exercise intensity should be lowered if the heart rate is above the target zone. Alternatively, Polar heart rate monitors (www.polarca. com/), for example, worn against the skin around the chest during exercise calculate heart rate instantaneously and relay the values to a special wristwatch so that wearers can easily see their target heart rate without having to calculate it themselves.

The Borg Rating of Perceived Exertion Scale (Borg RPE scale), a 10-point category-ratio scale, is another method of monitoring intensity of exercise (Borg, 1998; Shigematsu et al., 2004). This is a subjective method that allows exercise participants to rate how hard they feel they are working during the exercise. Rating of perceived exertion can be the primary means of measuring exercise intensity if a client does not have typical heart rate responses to exercise. These people include those on beta-blocking medications, some cardiac and diabetic patients, pregnant women, and others who may have an altered heart rate response. On a scale of 0 to 10, clients rate how they are feeling during the exercise in terms of body fatigue and how they feel both physically and mentally. This scale has been validated in older adults (75.5 ± 3.8 years) as a means to safely monitor exercise intensity (Shigematsu et al., 2004). The target range for maintaining submaximal exercise intensity on the 10-point Borg scale is between an RPE of 4 (somewhat strong) and 5 or 6 (strong) (figure 7.1).

0	Nothing at all	"No P"
0.3		
0.5	Extremely weak	Just noticeable
1	Very weak	
1.5		
2	Weak	Light
2.5		
3	Moderate	
4		
5	Strong	Heavy
6		
7	Very strong	
8		
9		
10	Extremely strong	"Max P"
11		
⌇		
●	Absolute maximum	Highest possible

Borg CR10 scale
© Gunnar Borg, 1981, 1982, 1998

Borg RPE scale

Figure 7.1 This continuum of numbers and related words is the category-ratio 10-point scale for ratings of perceived exertion (RPE) developed by Borg. The category-ratio scale was devised so that the terminology would be more easily understood by exercise participants; this provides the tester with a better assessment of the exercise intensity in order to conduct the exercise session.

Reprinted, by permission, Borg G. *Borg's Rating of Perceived Exertion and Pain Scales.* Champaign, IL: Human Kinetics, 1998.

The Talk-Test Method (Persinger et al., 2004), like the RPE, is subjective and can be used in conjunction with taking a pulse. The talk test is quite useful in determining a comfort zone of aerobic intensity, especially if the client is just beginning an exercise program. Older adults who are able to talk during their workout without a great deal of strain are most likely in their comfort zone, or working at a submaximal level. As another way to describe this, people should increase the speed or resistance of their activity to the point at which they first hear themselves breathing and conversation is still possible. They should work at an intensity that allows them to breathe comfortably and rhythmically throughout all phases of the workout. This will ensure a safe and comfortable level of exercise.

Time

Canada's *Physical Activity Guide to Healthy Active Living for Older Adults* (www.paguide. com) advocates starting slowly on a new exercise program and building up gradually. An accumulation of 30 to 60 min of moderate physical activity on most days is recommended. The *Physical Activity Guide* suggests participating in 10 min blocks of functional activity throughout the day and adding the minutes up to reach the 30 to 60 min target duration of completed activity. A gentle progression in the block of time spent engaging in functional activity will promote longer segments of exercise. The duration of exercise should be increased until the target duration is reached. After a sufficient duration is attained, the exercise intensity can be increased. Attention should be paid to symptoms indicating that the body is not tolerating the exercise. Muscle pain, joint pain, muscle or joint stiffness or both, fatigue, breathlessness, and exacerbation of an existing health condition can occur during an exercise session if it is too long or at an intensity that is too high.

A warm-up period of approximately 5 to 10 min is often used to prepare the body for exercise. This is a strategy to promote safety in an exercise program and can be achieved in various ways. During a warm-up an older adult is advised to stretch the arms, legs, and back and to limber up the major joints of the body by walking slowly, swinging the arms, and reaching to touch the alternate toes, for example. Another safety suggestion is to incorporate a cool-down of about 5 min, or the duration of time required for the heart rate to return to its resting level. During the cool-down an older adult would be advised to replicate the activities of the warm-up period. During the cool-down the exercise leader can monitor participants' physiological responses to the exercise program; allow participants some time to interact with others within a group exercise situation; or provide participants with the opportunity to assess their pulse and reflect on how they feel, what went well during the exercise, or what they might change in the exercise next time, for example.

Type

All three modes of exercise are advocated, including endurance (aerobic), flexibility, and strength and balance. Safety during endurance exercise is determined by heart rate and guided by the same methods to measure heart rate as listed in the section on intensity. Exercise participants should be instructed in how to monitor their heart rate response to exercise and remain within the target heart rate zone during exercise participation. If a client's heart rate response to exercise is an inappropriate measure, secondary to heart rate–controlling medication, for example, clients should be taught how to monitor their exercise response with the Borg RPE scale. Finally, the talk test may be a useful and fun way to monitor exercise intensity if the older adult has a friend to exercise with.

For strength and flexibility, older adults can protect themselves from injury by paying close attention to the position of their limbs and the timing of movements. Whether resistance to a movement is provided by the client's body weight (for example, in repeated rising from a low chair without using the arms, to increase leg strength) or comes from an external source (as in completing arm curls with a large soup can), the movements should be performed slowly without jerking. A guideline for resisted movement is that one should perform the movement during a count of 3 s while breathing out during the effort, or "lift," and return to the start position during a 3 s count while breathing in. Emphasizing breathing during resisted movements helps to prevent a Valsalva maneuver, or breath holding. Breath holding during resisted movement elevates blood pressure and can lead to serious injury. Stretching movements should be performed slowly and smoothly, within a pain-free range, and should be held for 10 to 30 s at a time. This length of hold will allow time for the connective tissue and other inert tissues to benefit from being stretched. It is suggested that stretches then be repeated four times for both sides of the body.

The effects of weather should be considered depending on the type of exercise. Walking is a favorite activity among older adults, and cold and hot weather effects need to be considered. In hot, humid weather, an older adult needs to be educated about the benefits of being well hydrated and the importance of maintaining fluid level. Dehydration can be very dangerous for an older adult with a heart condition, for example.

The techniques for appropriate dressing, largely the importance of layering clothes, to keep the body warm in winter or allow the body to cool in summer should be described to an older adult. In extremes of weather, the options for indoor activity should be investigated. Mall walking is a popular alternative for older adults when the weather is not optimal. This alternative supports participation in exercise whatever the outdoor temperature. Another aspect of the environment for exercise is the water temperature of the pool used for aquatic exercise programs. Pool temperatures tend to hover around the high 80s or low 90s when older adults are participating in aquarobics or swimming. Older adults with joint arthritis find that the buoyancy and temperature of the water provide pain relief and enable them to participate in exercise at an intensity that is not often possible on land.

Summary

A functional approach in designing exercise programs for older adults is important. Equally paramount is practicing a client-oriented approach in choosing the activities of an exercise program and in guiding the exercise intervention. The use of a broad-minded definition of exercise is suggested to encourage an inclusive approach to structuring activity programs for older adults across the spectrum of ability for participation. Any stimulus for movement greater than what the body is accustomed to should be considered exercise. Using the FITT approach will ensure a complete prescription to increase the activity level of an older adult. Prescribing exercise or activity that is functional, in relation to the client's needs, and is client centered, to address the individual's goals, will promote clients' participation in and adherence to increased physical activity in their daily life.

Questions to Consider

1. List the principles to guide exercise prescription for older adults.

2. Provide a rationale for why each principle is important.

3. Describe how each principle may affect exercise participation by an older adult.

4. Propose what you think would be one meaningful outcome (i.e., client centered) for each of the following scenarios: (a) an older client who is recovering from a stroke and wishes to propel his own wheelchair; (b) an older client who is recovering from a hip fracture and wishes to bring the groceries in from her car by herself; (c) an older client who wishes to walk to the retirement home dining room by herself in less than 15 min; and (d) an older client who is planning to complete the Father's Day 5K with his son but can walk only 4 km (2.5 miles) on the treadmill.

5. Apply the FITT approach to each of the previous scenarios and design a client-centered, individualized exercise program for these older adults.

chapter 8

Training for Aerobic and Anaerobic Fitness

Tom Overend, BPE, MA, PhD, BSc (PT)

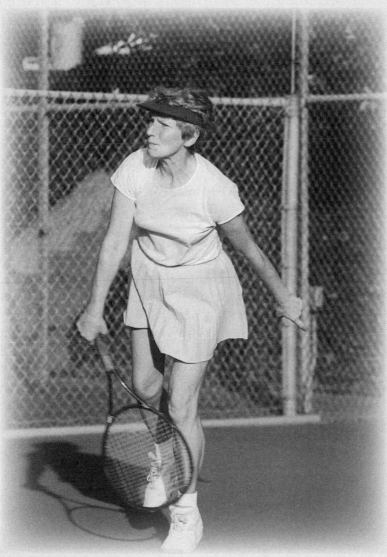

© Photodisc

The purpose of this chapter is to describe the rationale and methods for training to improve aerobic and anaerobic fitness in older adults. Previous chapters in this book have outlined the effects of aging and the benefits of exercise training for older adults, and subsequent chapters address the specific training challenges related to masters athletes and the frail elderly. The target population for this chapter is thus the "average" older adult who has started to exercise and now wishes to do some specific training to build aerobic or anaerobic fitness, or both.

The chapter starts with a brief review of exercise physiology as it relates to aerobic and anaerobic metabolism and fitness. It then moves on to answer the question "Why train to improve aerobic and anaerobic fitness?" before discussing how older adults should train to develop both types of fitness. The benefits of improved aerobic and anaerobic fitness are listed, and the chapter concludes with a short discussion regarding maintenance of fitness.

Review of Exercise Physiology

What is aerobic fitness? The word "aerobic" means "in the presence of oxygen." Aerobic fitness is best described as the ability to carry out endurance-type exercise, such as walking, jogging, running, swimming, cycling, rowing, and cross-country skiing. In endurance activities, exercise intensity is submaximal, and energy to carry out the work is supplied primarily through the aerobic breakdown of fuels in the body. "Aerobic breakdown" means that oxygen is used to metabolize the fats and carbohydrates stored in the liver and skeletal muscle, thus producing energy for exercise. This oxygen is provided through the joint efforts of two physiological systems in the body: the respiratory and the cardiovascular system. The respiratory system brings oxygen into the body and transfers it into the blood. The cardiovascular system is composed of the heart, which pumps this *oxygenated* blood to the working muscles, and the blood vessels: arteries (which bring blood to the muscles), capillaries (which take blood inside the muscles to the muscle fibers), and veins (which return blood to the heart). Aerobic breakdown of fuels is quite complete—producing only energy, water, and carbon dioxide.

Aerobic energy can be produced for long durations (i.e., the system *capacity* is large), but the *rate* of energy supply is limited. Exercise can continue only as long as the demand of the working muscles for oxygen does not exceed the capacity of the cardiovascular system to provide oxygen. When exercise intensity rises and the oxygen demand of the working muscles is greater than the supply, energy to continue exercise cannot be fully provided through the aerobic breakdown of fuels in the body. In these situations, the body turns to *anaerobic* metabolism to supply the additional energy required for exercise.

The word "anaerobic" means "in the absence of oxygen." Stored carbohydrates in the body can be broken down to produce energy without the use of oxygen, but the body pays a price for this. The *rate* of energy supply via anaerobic breakdown is very high, but the *capacity* of this energy supply system is quite limited. Thus anaerobic exercise can be continued only for minutes, rather than the hours of exercise enabled by aerobic breakdown of fuels. And the consequence of anaerobic breakdown of fuels is that by-products are produced that will inhibit muscle contraction as they accumulate.

It must be realized that aerobic and anaerobic metabolism do not operate like light switches. Both energy production systems are always working to some degree to supply energy for the body. Thus, there is never a situation in which one system is on and the other is off. What is important to understand is that the *proportion of energy* provided by each system changes as exercise intensity increases. For lower- and moderate-intensity exercise, most of the energy required comes from the aerobic breakdown of fuel; thus ability to supply oxygen is the limiting factor. As the intensity of exercise increases, the contribution of anaerobic energy gradually increases; and at the highest exercise intensities, where exercise duration is quite short, nearly all of the energy is supplied by this system.

What, then, is anaerobic fitness? Anaerobic fitness is the ability of the body to carry out high-intensity, short-duration exercise, in which the energy is provided by anaerobic breakdown of fuels. Key determinants of anaerobic fitness are not related to the respiratory or cardiovascular system, but instead to the ability to generate and maintain high levels of energy production and to withstand the inhibiting influence of the anaerobic metabolism by-products.

Aerobic and anaerobic fitness are specific types of fitness; hence training methods to improve aerobic and anaerobic fitness are quite different. The goal of methods to improve aerobic fitness is to increase the ability of the respiratory and cardiovascular systems to provide oxygen to the working muscles. The more oxygen that is provided, the more energy can be produced via aerobic breakdown of fuel. This leads to an enhanced ability to perform endurance-type exercise (i.e., aerobic fitness).

On the other hand, the goal of methods to improve anaerobic fitness is to increase both the rate and capacity of anaerobic energy supply as well as to enhance the ability to neutralize or "buffer" the anaerobic metabolism by-products. The faster the rate, and the larger the capacity, the greater the ability to perform high-intensity exercise; that is, anaerobic fitness.

Benefits of Aerobic and Anaerobic Fitness

Both aerobic and anaerobic fitness decline as people age. Reasons for this decline are linked to the interactions between (1) biological aging, (2) lifestyle habits, (3) development of subclinical and clinically apparent disease, and (4) sex and genetic composition. Examples of these factors include (1) reduced maximal heart rate and reduced maximal cardiac output, loss of muscle mass and motor units, changes in key anaerobic and aerobic enzymes, and increased body fat, all leading to decreased maximal oxygen consumption ($\dot{V}O_2$max); (2) decreased intensity, duration, and frequency of daily physical activity; (3) increased prevalence of cardiovascular risk factors that reduce the functional capacity of the cardiovascular system; and 4) sex differences, with females typically having smaller hearts and less muscle mass and lower oxygen-carrying capacity (hemoglobin concentration) than males.

Aerobic fitness is lost at the rate of about 10% per decade in both men and women regardless of activity levels (Hawkins and Wiswell, 2003). While there is some evidence to suggest that the rate of loss may be less in extremely active older adults compared to sedentary older adults (Katzel et al., 2001; Pollock et al., 1997), both cross-sectional and longitudinal studies have supported the concept that aerobic fitness declines in a rather consistent manner with aging, between sexes, and across activity levels (Hawkins and Wiswell, 2003).

Anaerobic activities include those in which the energy demands are too great to be met by energy produced via the oxidative breakdown of fuels. Thus lifting weights, climbing stairs or hills, hurrying to catch a bus, "overhead" activities, and vigorous yard work or housework, as well as most intermittent and team sports (e.g., soccer, hockey, softball), can be considered anaerobic activities. Anaerobic fitness declines at a faster rate than aerobic fitness, likely due to a greater reduction in frequency of anaerobic activities compared to aerobic activities as people age (Charmari et al., 1995) and also to the significant losses of muscle mass (sarcopenia) associated with aging (Doherty, 2003). While there is a scarcity of literature in the area of anaerobic fitness in older adults, it has been suggested that women lose anaerobic fitness at a slower rate than men (Kostka et al., 1997; Bonnefoy et al., 1998).

Regardless of any differences between sexes or activity levels, losses of either aerobic or anaerobic fitness have been linked to losses of mobility (Lauretani et al., 2003) and independence (Paterson et al., 2004) in older adults as well as to increases in health care utilization (Mitchell et al., 2004; Weiss et al., 2004). Thus training to improve aerobic and anaerobic fitness is important for older adults. Training the aerobic system may enhance the ability to perform personal activities of daily living (dressing, grooming, self-care, etc.) as well as instrumental activities such as shopping, walking, cleaning, and socializing (Binder et al., 1999; Posner et al., 1995). Training the anaerobic system can

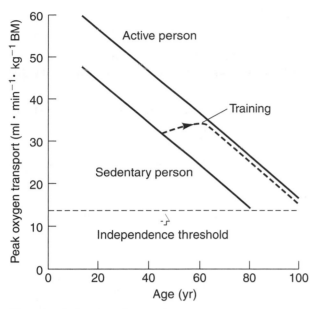

Figure 8.1 Regular endurance training increases the peak oxygen transport by 5 to 10 ml × min × kg⁻¹ body mass at any given age, thus taking the active individual 10 to 20 years longer for oxygen transport values to drop to the threshold where independence can no longer be sustained.

Reprinted from R.J. Shephard, 1993, "Exercise and aging: Extensive independence in older adults," *Geriatrics* 48(5): 61-64. By permission of R.J. Shephard.

reverse sarcopenia, which has been linked to an increased risk of falls (Moreland et al., 2004), as well as increased mobility (Ramsbottom et al., 2004). Together, training these two systems may extend the age at which people reach the "independence threshold," marked by a decline in exercise capacity to the point where assistance is needed with everyday activities (Shephard, 1993). Figure 8.1 shows the impact of aerobic training on extending the duration until the independence threshold is reached.

Improved Aerobic Fitness

Benefits of improved aerobic fitness result from the improved function of the cardiovascular and respiratory systems. From an overall perspective, these physiological systems are more efficient; the person has a higher functional level and is in better health.

- Physiological benefits
  - *Increased* stroke volume at rest and during exercise
  - *Increased* cardiac output during maximal exercise
  - *Decreased* heart rate at rest and during exercise
  - *Increased* blood volume
  - *Increased* blood flow to working muscles
  - *Increased* number of capillaries in working muscles
  - *Increased* extraction of oxygen by muscle tissue
  - *Increased* maximal oxygen consumption
- Functional benefits
  - *Increased* efficiency during physical activity
  - *Decreased* stress on the body for any given work rate
  - *Increased* maximal exercise capacity
  - *Increased* tolerance for submaximal activity at any given work rate
- Health benefits
  - *Decreased* risk of premature death
  - *Decreased* risk of coronary artery disease
  - *Decreased* risk of certain cancers (colon, breast)
  - *Decreased* risk of non-insulin-dependent diabetes mellitus
  - *Improved* body composition

Improved Anaerobic Fitness

Benefits of improved anaerobic fitness include increased resistance to fatigue during high-intensity exercise and increased capacity for and performance in high-intensity work. The most important benefit of anaerobic training is that it builds muscle mass, muscle strength, and muscle power to a greater extent than aerobic training. All three decline with age (Lexell et al., 1988; Frontera et al., 2000; Metter et al., 1997), and all three are linked to losses of function and mobility (Cahill et al., 1997; Doherty, 2003; Posner et al., 1995). Thus it is important for many older adults to include an anaerobic training component in their activity programs in order to maintain functional capacity and independent living capability.

Programming Recommendations

Up to now, this chapter has provided a brief review of exercise physiology and described why it is important for older adults to improve aerobic and anaerobic fitness, making reference to the benefits of improving each of these fitness components. Now it is time to describe *how* to train these energy systems, and how to train them effectively so that time spent training will yield measurable and lasting results.

Aerobic Fitness Training

There is a difference between exercise to improve general health status and exercise to improve aerobic fitness. Almost any physical activity practiced for a cumulative total of at least 30 min per day will improve health, but will do little to improve aerobic fitness if the exercise intensity is too low (ACSM, 1998a).

Effective training to improve aerobic fitness involves activities that primarily stress the respiratory and cardiovascular systems, since these two systems are the principal determinants of aerobic fitness. In general, then, aerobic fitness training for older adults involves low- to moderate-intensity exercise carried out for longer durations. The actual exercise can be performed continuously, as in a bike ride or long walk, or intermittently, following the principles of interval training whereby periods of exercise are interspersed with periods of rest (Billat, 2001a; Fox et al., 1980). Important characteristics of aerobic fitness training are frequency, intensity, duration, and mode of exercise. The American College of Sports Medicine (ACSM, 1998a) and the Centers for Disease Control and Prevention (CDC; Pate et al., 1995) have made the following recommendations regarding these parameters for aerobic training in healthy adults.

- **Frequency:** three to five days per week (for moderate- and higher-intensity aerobic exercise; low-intensity exercise can be carried out daily)

- **Intensity:** 55%-65% to 90% of maximal heart rate, or 40-50% to 85% of $\dot{V}O_2$ reserve or heart rate (HR) reserve (lower intensities are more appropriate for the least fit individuals and for those just starting to train)

- **Duration:** 20 to 60 min of continuous or intermittent aerobic activity (intensity is inversely related to duration; for interval-type aerobic training, work-to-rest ratios are typically 1:1 or 2:1, so that intensity is higher than for continuous exercise)

- **Mode:** any activity that uses large muscle groups, can be maintained continuously (or for numerous intervals), and is rhythmical and aerobic in nature (e.g., walking/hiking, jogging/running, cycling/bicycling, cross-country skiing, aerobic dance/exercise, rowing, stair climbing, swimming, skating)

Exercise intensity is a key factor in improving aerobic fitness. If intensity is too low, health benefits may be realized, but aerobic fitness will not improve (ACSM, 1998b). Table 8.1 shows how intensity can be classified using percentages of maximal heart rate, $\dot{V}O_2$max, HR reserve, and ratings of perceived exertion (RPE). How are these maximal values determined? Maximal heart rate can be determined during an exercise stress test or can be predicted using the equation HRmax $-$ 208 $-$ 0.7 $\times$ age (Tanaka et al., 2001). $\dot{V}O_2$max can be determined during a laboratory stress test or predicted from the results of different submaximal tests. Heart rate reserve is the difference between resting heart rate and maximal heart rate. Swain and Leutholtz (2002) have recommended using % HR reserve instead of % maximal heart rate because the range in actual maximal heart rate increases with age. Ratings of perceived exertion are made using a 15-point scale with anchors of 6 (no exertion at all) and 20 (maximal exertion) (Borg, 1998).

TABLE 8.1 Relationships Among Methods of Quantifying Exercise Intensity During Endurance Exercise

RELATIVE INTENSITY (%)				
HRmax	$\dot{V}O_2$max	HR reserve	Rating of perceived exertion	Classification of intensity
<35%	<30%	<30%	<10	Very light
35%-59%	30%-49%	30%-49%	10-11	Light
60%-79%	50%-74%	50%-74%	12-13	Somewhat hard
80%-89%	75%-84%	75%-84%	14-16	Hard
>89%	>84%	>84%	>16	Very hard

The ACSM and CDC guidelines do not include recommendations about the progression of intensity, frequency, and duration of aerobic exercise programs. The guidelines listed earlier set out the initial goals and ranges—older adults will start at different levels depending on their initial fitness level. For progression, Rogers and colleagues (2000) recommend keeping duration, intensity, and frequency at the low end of the range for the first four to six weeks (15-20 min per session, 60% of maximal heart rate, three sessions per week). This constrained introduction reduces the chance of injury and allows the body to accommodate gradually to the stresses of exercise. Over the next four to five months, intensity, duration, and frequency can all be slowly increased toward the higher end of each range.

The ACSM recommends progressing duration, intensity, and frequency for a six-month period and then establishing a maintenance program that can be followed on a continuing basis (ACSM, 2000). See table 8.2 for an example of a training progression for a healthy individual. As the medical and activity levels of older adults can vary considerably, progression must be prescribed individually. In general, the rate of progression is appropriate if older adults feel refreshed and not exhausted postexercise, if no undue fatigue is experienced the day after any given exercise session, and if there is no evidence of injury.

In any aerobic training program, most of the potential gains are realized in the first four to six months; and unless a person is interested in competing in aerobic events at a high level, there is little benefit to keep progressing the program. Doing so raises the risk of injury significantly, for very little increase in aerobic capacity.

TABLE 8.2 **Training Progression for the Apparently Healthy Participant**

Program stage	Week	Exercise frequency (sessions/week)	Exercise intensity (% HRR)	Exercise duration (min)
Initial stage	1	3	40-50	15-20
	2	3-4	40-50	20-25
	3	3-4	50-60	20-25
	4	3-4	50-60	25-30
Improvement stage	5-7	3-4	60-70	25-30
	8-10	3-4	60-70	30-35
	11-13	3-4	65-75	30-35
	14-16	3-5	65-75	30-35
	17-20	3-5	70-85	35-40
	21-24	3-5	70-85	35-40
Maintenance stage	24+	3-5	70-85	30-45

Adapted from ACSM's Guidelines for Exercise Testing and Prescription, 6th ed. Lippincott Williams & Wilkins: Baltimore, 2000, Table 7-4, p 154

Lemura and colleagues (2000) carried out a meta-analysis of the effects of such training programs on aerobic fitness in adults aged 46 to 90. Twenty-five of 27 studies in their analysis showed significant improvements in aerobic fitness ($\dot{V}O_2$max). Further, improvements were greater when the intensity was a minimum of 80% $\dot{V}O_2$max compared to intensities between 60% to 75% $\dot{V}O_2$max, and exercise durations of over 30 min produced greater improvements compared to durations less than 30 min. The authors concluded that despite the inevitable decline in $\dot{V}O_2$max with aging, aerobic exercise training imparted favorable adaptations in aerobic fitness in people well into their seventh and eighth decades of life. And in even older adults, Malbut and colleagues (2002) have shown that aerobic training of women with a mean age of 82 years produced a 15% increase in $\dot{V}O_2$max.

Since the recommendations for aerobic exercise parameters were established for healthy adults generally, some modifications are appropriate when one is applying them to those healthy adults who are older. Books written specifically on exercise in older adults consistently convey the same messages (Benyo, 1998; Friel, 1998; Goldstein and Tanner, 1999).

- Start at a lower intensity (30-40% of $\dot{V}O_2$max) and progress slowly.
- Increase intensity more slowly than frequency or duration.
- Get adequate rest between exercise sessions.
- Do a variety of aerobic fitness activities.
- Vary training duration, intensity, and volume from session to session.
- Do higher-intensity workouts infrequently.
- Pay attention to warm-up and cool-down.
- More is not always better.
- Train smart.

Anaerobic Fitness Training

As noted earlier, anaerobic activities include those in which the energy demands are too great to be met by energy produced via the oxidative breakdown of fuels. Thus, lifting weights, climbing stairs or hills, hurrying to catch a bus, "overhead" activities, and vigorous yard work or housework, as well as most intermittent and team games (e.g., soccer, hockey, softball, volleyball), can be considered anaerobic activities.

Training to improve anaerobic fitness involves higher-intensity exercise. This is more stressful than aerobic training, and thus is not recommended until the older adult has built a good base of aerobic fitness. Because of the higher intensity, an increased risk of injury is also associated with anaerobic training. Anaerobic fitness training should be considered more carefully than aerobic training by older adults who have preexisting musculoskeletal or cardiovascular disease. But it may be safely undertaken by most healthy older adults who follow recommended training practices. The decision to undertake anaerobic training should be based on need, such as a desire to improve sport performance, or a demonstrable decline in anaerobic capacity to the point where functional independence is at risk. There is a range of intensities in anaerobic training; programs for the average older adult should keep to the lower end of this range to minimize the physiological stress, muscular fatigue, and risk of injury associated with more intense anaerobic training.

Strength training represents one form of anaerobic training, but this topic is covered elsewhere in this book and will not be pursued here. Anaerobic training for running, swimming, cycling, and other such activities is most often accomplished by means of intermittent exercise, whereby periods of higher-intensity work are alternated with periods of rest. However, whereas interval exercise for *aerobic* training involves work:rest ratios of 1:1 or 2:1, *anaerobic* interval training work:rest ratios are typically much smaller, ranging between 1:3 and 1:6 (Fox et al., 1980). The longer the rest, the more intense the work period can be. Because of the high intensity level, prolonged fatigue, and need for recovery, it is recommended that anaerobic interval sessions be performed relatively infrequently—only once per week (Billat, 2001b) or once every two weeks (Goldstein and Tanner, 1999). And for the average older adult not interested in masters-level sport competition, the highest intensities of anaerobic training are not appropriate. Injury risk is increased while very few of our daily activities demand excessive anaerobic contribution.

Frequency, duration, and intensity of anaerobic training are much different than for aerobic training. General principles for anaerobic training include the following: (1) intensity must be above the upper limit of "steady state" exercise; (2) anaerobic exercise sets must be performed to near muscular exhaustion; and (3) recovery between bouts of anaerobic exercise must be incomplete. People achieve progression of anaerobic training by increasing the intensity of exercise, decreasing the rest periods between intervals, increasing the number of anaerobic repetitions, or some combination of these. Detailed guides for anaerobic interval training exist for various modes of activity as well as different sports (Billat, 2001b; Fox et al., 1980) and thus are not reviewed here.

For older adults not training for masters-level competition, not interested in formal interval programs, or just starting to get into anaerobic exercise, it is easy to add an anaerobic component to many activities simply by increasing the intensity for short periods. Activities such as climbing hills or stairs, exercising on an inclined treadmill, cycling on a stationary bike with increased resistance, pushing someone in a wheelchair, walking while wearing a backpack, or adding upper body exercise to lower body exercise each adds an anaerobic component to aerobic exercise without the formality of an interval training program. In fact, for most older adults, this may be the best way to improve anaerobic fitness.

Maintenance

Once aerobic and anaerobic fitness have been improved, the training goal changes to maintenance of these new levels. Both types of fitness will be lost if training stops or if it drops below the minimum needed for maintenance. This can be a challenge, as both aging and injury also have a negative influence on maintenance. However, any given level of fitness can be maintained with less training than was required to achieve it. One strategy for maintenance of any component of physical fitness is to maintain intensity while cutting back on duration and frequency. For example, someone riding an exercise bike five times per week for 40 min, at an intensity of 70% of HR reserve, could cut back to three sessions of 30 min at the same intensity. Another strategy is to cut back each component on some days and maintain the original prescription on others. Either way, the total training load is reduced, but the level of fitness is maintained.

Summary

The purpose of this chapter was to describe the rationale and methods for training to improve aerobic and anaerobic fitness in older adults. Aerobic and anaerobic fitness are important in maintaining function, mobility, and independence in older adults. However, older adults lose both aerobic and anaerobic fitness as they age; thus it is important to train to maintain and improve these fitness components. Aerobic fitness can be improved significantly in older adults provided that attention is paid to the important training parameters of frequency, duration, and intensity of exercise. Appropriate aerobic training will yield benefits including more efficient respiratory and cardiovascular systems and improved functional level and overall health status. Anaerobic training is more intense than aerobic training and carries a greater risk of fatigue and injury. Older adults thus need to be more careful with this type of training. Anaerobic exercise can be incorporated easily into aerobic exercise through the inclusion of brief bouts of higher-intensity exercise. Benefits of improved anaerobic fitness include increased capacity for high-intensity exercise as well as improved muscle mass, strength, and power. Maintenance of both aerobic and anaerobic fitness can be achieved with less training than was required to develop each type of fitness.

Questions to Consider

1. What are the two most important physiological systems for aerobic fitness?
2. Why is oxygen delivery important for aerobic activities?
3. What is the relationship between exercise duration and intensity?
4. How do the aerobic and anaerobic systems differ in the rate and capacity of energy production?
5. Explain the importance of maintaining a high level of aerobic and anaerobic fitness for older adults.
6. Describe the recommendations for frequency, duration, intensity, and mode of aerobic exercise.
7. Describe modifications of these recommendations for exercise in older adults.
8. What are the different measures for assessing exercise intensity?
9. Outline the physiological, functional, and health benefits from improved aerobic fitness.
10. What are the cautions associated with anaerobic exercise in older adults?
11. Compare the work:rest ratios for aerobic and anaerobic training.
12. How can older adults incorporate anaerobic exercise into aerobic exercise?
13. What is the main benefit of anaerobic training for older adults, and why is this important?
14. Describe two strategies for maintaining aerobic and anaerobic fitness.

chapter 9

Training for Muscular Fitness

Michel J. Johnson, PhD, Anthony A. Vandervoort, PhD

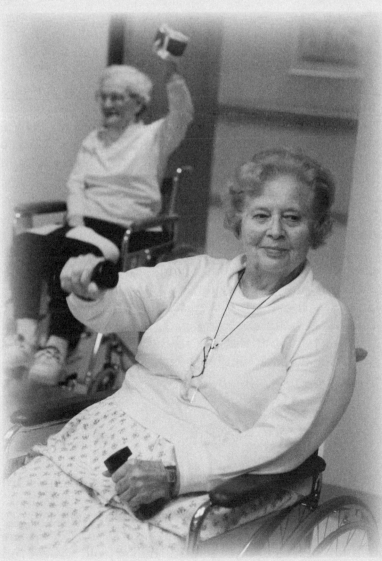

© Photodisc

Muscular fitness is made up of two components, strength and endurance. Muscular strength is the ability to lift a maximal weight, while muscular endurance refers to our ability to complete repeated muscular efforts. Both types of muscular fitness are important not only for recreational activities, but also for daily tasks at work or in the home. The terms *resistance, strength,* and *weight training* are all used to refer to conditioning modalities in which our muscles are asked to work against a resistive force, such as a dumbbell or barbell, body weight, elastic bands, or some other apparatus. We will use the term *resistance training* in this chapter when referring to training. Although commonly used in discussions of resistance training, the terms *weightlifting, powerlifting,* and *bodybuilding* in fact refer to specific sports.

Review of Exercise Physiology

Muscle strength seems to peak between 20 and 30 years of age and decreases with aging. Nonetheless, it is clear that elderly individuals can make substantial gains in strength in a short period of time, with two- to threefold gains observed in as little as three to four months (Mazzeo and Tanaka, 2001). Significant increases in strength have even been observed in individuals over 90 years of age (Fiatarone et al., 1990). The physiological impact of resistance training is a reflection of the individual (genetics, health status, goals, etc.) and the training program (frequency, intensity, type, time). Acute responses to resistance training typically include increased heart rate and blood pressure, slight or no changes in cardiac output and stroke volume, and no change in oxygen consumption. Chronic benefits attributed to regular resistance training include increased muscular strength, power, and endurance; increased muscle size (hypertrophy); reduced body fat; increased balance, coordination, and flexibility; increased bone mineral density; increased tendon and ligament strength; increased basal metabolic rate; greater insulin sensitivity and glucose tolerance; and enhanced well-being and self-esteem.

Neuromuscular Function

Although minor decreases in the strength of maximum voluntary contractions (MVC) of muscle begin to appear in middle age, important reductions do not become apparent until after the age of about 60 (figure 9.1). During isometric tests, healthy people in their seventh and eighth decades score on average about 20% to 40% less during maximal contractions than young adults, and the very old show even

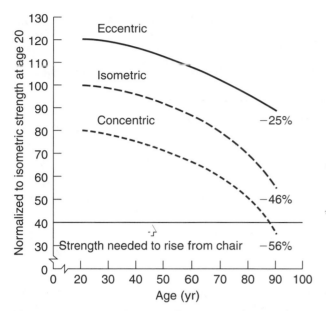

Figure 9.1 A schematic illustration of age-related loss of voluntary muscle strength that can contribute to frailty in old age. Note that the extent of these changes across the adult age range varies considerably for the three types of muscle activity, and in the case shown for knee extension strength can result in a lack of adequate concentric strength (muscle shortening) to perform an activity of daily living. The curves are based on the author's various studies during the past two decades on age-related changes in muscle force production.

greater (50% or more) reductions. Males and females appear to show similar patterns of age-related deterioration (Sale and Spriet, 1996; Doherty, 2003). Sedentary populations may also show greater loss in the lower limb musculature than the upper.

Results of strength testing of concentric muscle actions (in which the muscle is allowed to shorten) are also lower in older people than in young adults; at higher velocities of movement, the age-related deficit is quite marked. However, the amount of strength deficit with age is consistently less for the eccentric type of muscle action (lengthening) than during either isometric or concentric muscle activity; and in some situations there may be no difference at all (Porter et al., 1997). Although the explanation for this relative advantage in the muscles of older people during lengthening against resistance remains to be fully clarified, it is a phenomenon worth noting. Perhaps fatigue resistance for a given task would be improved if it could be performed during eccentric rather than concentric loading (i.e., the muscle would be able to work at a lower relative intensity of maximum capacity).

Age differences in MVC strength reflect either a reduced amount of muscle (atrophied muscle) or a reduction in muscle excitation via the descending motor pathways. The fullness of the motor drive was assessed by Vandervoort and McComas (1986) using a twitch interpolation technique: A brief percutaneous electrical shock was applied to the motor nerve during a well-practiced MVC of the ankle plantarflexors and dorsiflexors. Healthy elderly people, ranging in age from 60 to 100 years, were usually found to be able to activate their ankle muscles maximally in this simple isometric task, with the superimposed twitch stimulus adding little or nothing to their volitional force. Furthermore, older people have demonstrated quite reproducible isometric strength values in reliability studies, which provide additional evidence that they are highly motivated to achieve maximum strength scores. Thus, we concluded that the primary mechanism to explain the age-related declines in scores on simple strength tests must be a decreased excitable muscle mass. Indeed, there is good agreement between measures of strength loss and muscle atrophy in gerontology studies (Lexell and Vandervoort, 2002). However, as the interpolated twitch just described was applied only to a simple, isometric, single-joint task, it is still quite possible that a lack of central nervous system coordination is an important limiting factor during dynamic strength maneuvers involving many muscle groups.

Muscles of older people contract and relax more slowly than those of young adults. This slowing may stem from the reduced proportional contribution of type II fibers to the twitch contraction, together with an age-related change in the muscle's calcium regulatory mechanisms. Slowing of a muscle contractile response confers an adaptation of greater efficiency for the excitable membranes of the associated motoneurons and their muscle fibers; the more slowly a muscle contracts, the lower is the frequency of nerve impulses required to attain a given muscle tension or reach tetanic fusion. This benefit for the central nervous system, along with the fact that type I fibers take up more of the total muscle mass, may explain why even sedentary older people still demonstrate adequate fatigue resistance in their muscles. Indeed, healthy and fit older people could potentially experience less metabolic stress during a submaximal exercise bout than sedentary young adults because their muscles have undergone a natural adaptation toward tonic activity.

A key principle for exercise programming with frail older populations is that their tissues and organ systems retain a capacity to adapt to an appropriate therapeutic stimulus. The adaptive response will vary widely depending on factors such as the initial level of function present, plus the intensity and duration of the stimulus. Due to effects of aging, frail older people may not respond in the same manner as young adults to interventions, and care must be taken to tailor exercises to their present capacity and goals.

Resistance Training

Recently there has been a growing interest in the adaptive potential of the neuromuscular system in frail older populations, including those living in residential care facilities (Seynnes et al., 2004). Can muscle cells that have survived into old age still respond with hypertrophy to an "overload" stimulus? Can descending motor pathways adapt to increased demands and allow older adults to relearn the skill of coordinating a strong voluntary movement? Mounting evidence now supports the belief that cellular adaptation in both the muscular and nervous systems is possible at all ages. Until recently, for example, it was thought that strength increases in older people following a resistance training program resulted solely from increased neural drive, but significant hypertrophy of muscle cells has also now been demonstrated during such programs (Doherty, 2003). This finding, in turn, indicates that the cellular regulation of contractile proteins can still be stimulated to increase the production of myosin, actin, and other muscle constituents. At least some of the deleterious age-related change in body composition is reversible, given the appropriate biological stimulus. It is useful to remember, too, that seemingly small changes in activity can make an impact on strength and function, especially in very old people who start from quite low baseline levels (Connelly and Vandervoort, 1997; Seynnes et al., 2004).

Research on resistance training for seniors was given considerable impetus in the 1980s when Frontera and colleagues (1988) reported their findings involving both strength and muscle biopsy results from a heavy resistance training study in older men. The researchers observed striking improvements in leg muscle strength, as well as significant increases in muscle fiber sizes. Since then, an increasing number of studies have documented the benefits of resistance training for older men and women, including frail persons above the age of 90 years (see Latham et al., 2004, for a systematic review).

The typical duration of these resistance training programs has been 10 to 12 weeks, with a few studies going longer. Strength changes have been quite variable across studies; this is likely a reflection of key design factors influencing outcome, such as intensity of training, amount of direct supervision, baseline fitness level of the subjects, and age range of the sample. Muscle mass or muscle cross-sectional area (using various noninvasive techniques) has been measured before and after training, combined in some cases with morphometric analysis of the proportion and areas of different fiber types. Typical training-induced increases in muscle cross-sectional area have shown a relatively moderate effect of 5% to 10%. However, it should be remembered that above the age of 70 years, muscle mass is normally being lost each year, and simply maintaining the existing tissue at that age is considered a benefit. Tracy and colleagues (1999) used magnetic resonance imaging techniques to evaluate the effects of resistance training on quadriceps muscle volume in men and women ranging in age from 65 to 75 years. After nine weeks of resistance training, a 12% increase in quadriceps muscle volume was observed in both men and women. Notable, also, is the study of McCartney and coworkers (1996), who reported on an older group that continued to participate in a resistance exercise program for two years, showing progressive strength gains and also moderate muscle hypertrophy during the training. Benefits from strengthening programs need to be maintained with a continuing program, or rapid detraining will result. But these initial gains can be sustained with a reduced maintenance exercise frequency of even once per week.

Resistance Training Guidelines

Physical activity recommendations from the American College of Sports Medicine and the Canadian Society for Exercise Physiology include regular endurance, resistance, and flexibility activities (Adams et al., 1999; Mazzeo et al., 1998). Resistance training involves two types of muscular action: isometric and isotonic. Isometric (static) exercise involves muscular contraction without shortening of the muscle or movement of the limb. Isotonic (dynamic) exercise involves muscular contraction whereby the muscles shorten (concentric) and lengthen (eccentric). Current recommendations for resistance training suggest at least two sessions per week. However, data from the 2001 National

Health Interview Survey (NHIS) indicate that only about 12% of persons aged 65 to 74 years and 10% of persons aged >75 years participate in strength training activities two or more days per week (Centers for Disease Control and Prevention, 2004).

For specific suggestions on exercises to use with older adults, and for ways to progress their workouts, see "Programming Recommendations" (p. 165).

Training Principles

A number of basic training principles can assist in the design of an appropriate resistance training program for the older adult.

- **Individualization:** A successful program must take into account each individual's baseline abilities, resources, and goals. It is vitally important that preliminary information be gathered as part of the program design process.

- **Specificity:** Adaptations to resistance training reflect the muscle actions involved, speed of movement, range of motion, muscle groups trained, and energy systems solicited. Knowledge of the need to strengthen a muscle group for a particular activity or following an injury can assist in the selection and organization of exercises.

- **Progressive overload:** As we adapt to a given training routine, we require greater challenge for gains to continue. Too great an increase in intensity or volume can lead to serious injuries. A gradual increase is recommended for elderly individuals. Through monitoring of both the participant's physical activity and health status (injuries, disease, etc.), the overload can be adjusted accordingly.

- **Reversibility:** The benefits gained from a fitness program are reversible if activity is discontinued or substantially reduced.

Acute Program Variables

Adjusting acute program variables can customize the physiological impact of a resistance training program.

- **Choice of exercise.** The selection of the exercise as well as the equipment used is a reflection of the individual's goals, experience, and resources. In the earlier stages of training, the beginner might appreciate simpler exercises using weight machines, body weight, or elastic bands. With time, the participant will progress to more demanding multijoint exercises using free weights and greater resistance. Particularly for beginners, it is recommended that workouts consist of exercises that work the whole body. For specific suggestions, see "Programming Recommendations" (p. 165).

- **Sequence of exercise.** The order in which exercises are done during a workout affects muscle fatigue. In order to minimize fatigue, larger multijoint exercises can be done first in the workout (e.g., multi-joint chest press prior to single-joint biceps curl). In addition, alternating upper body and lower body exercises can decrease fatigue. These strategies can be especially effective during the initial stages of training when early fatigue can be especially intimidating.

- **Number of sets and reps.** For older individuals, a minimum of one set of 10 to 15 repetitions should be completed for each exercise. Once a solid base is established, workouts consisting of multiple-set systems and lower repetitions can be safely completed. Gains in strength and hypertrophy are typically achieved using 8 to 12 repetitions, while muscular endurance requires 15 reps or more (figure 9.2).

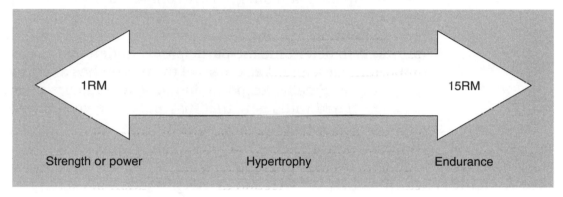

Figure 9.2 Impact of repetition selection on training effect.

- **Frequency.** Current guidelines suggest that strength training activities be completed two or more times per week.

- **Rest.** Rest periods between sets and exercises greatly influence fatigue. Shorter rest periods (±30 s) can greatly enhance muscular endurance, while longer rest periods (1-3 min) can contribute to greater recovery and greater gains in maximum strength.

Safety

Free weights are readily available and very popular. When a few safety tips are followed, they can be an effective and safe training modality. Remember to (1) load bars evenly; (2) lock dumbbells and barbells securely; (3) be aware of other equipment, such as racks and machines with extended bars, and individuals in the training area; and (4) store equipment after use.

Effective Intervention

An area that cannot be overlooked is effective intervention with participants. An instructor might design a training program that has all the proper exercises, sets, reps, and rest periods, but fails to ensure that the participant understands the why and how of the exercises.

This will affect not only the physical effectiveness of the program, but also the participant's exercise adherence. A few simple tips can make the exercise intervention more effective.

During the exercise session, engage the participant by asking about previous experience with the exercises and training. This will help you tailor your explanation and demonstration of the exercises to the individual's background and abilities. During the demonstration, describe and physically demonstrate the exercise execution, focusing on proper form and breathing. Make time for participant trials that will enable you to give feedback and encouragement. Depending on the background, adjust the amount of feedback so as to not overwhelm the participant. Maintain good eye contact, actively listen (paraphrase, question, etc.), and remember to use terminology at an appropriate level for your participant. At the end of the session, wrap up by asking questions to determine the participant's understanding and retention of the exercises, and check to see if the person has any concerns about the workout. Finally, keep in mind sensory changes (hearing, vision, etc.) associated with aging that may influence your intervention style (voice, where you stand, lighting, etc.).

The Challenge of Concurrent Training

Although concurrent training is rarely covered in textbooks, a basic understanding of this topic is critical when one is designing exercise programs. Although we typically present strength and endurance training exercise prescription principles separately, general fitness guidelines recommend the inclusion of both strength and endurance components in training. How these two modalities interact is still a question of considerable debate.

In healthy young adults, numerous studies have demonstrated that gains following concurrent strength and endurance training are comparable to those with single-mode training (Abernethy and Quigley, 1993; McCarthy et al., 2002; Sale et al., 1990). It has also been shown that short- and long-term endurance (Hickson, 1980; Marcinik et al., 1991), as well as intermediate-term anaerobic capacity (Bell et al., 1989), can be improved through the addition of strength training. These improvements occurred with little or no concomitant increase in $\dot{V}O_2$max. It is suggested that when people increase maximal strength, they can accomplish a greater total amount of work while decreasing efforts at prior submaximal workloads, thus delaying the onset of fatigue. However, some evidence exists for compromised gains in endurance (Sale et al., 1990) and strength with concurrent training (Dudley and Fleck, 1987; Hunter et al., 1987). The precise reasons for these discrepancies are unknown. Differences in program design, including scheduling, modality, frequency, volume, and intensity of the training programs, can certainly influence the outcomes observed (Kraemer et al., 2002).

Nonetheless, the majority of research in untrained subjects strongly suggests that substantial gains in strength and endurance are achieved with concurrent training regimens. In fact, these gains are often quite comparable to those with single-mode training. Although few studies addressing concurrent training in older adults have been completed, results are similar to those obtained with younger groups (Izquierdo et al., 2004; Wood et al., 2001).

In general, we must appreciate that the frequency, intensity, duration, and type of training of each modality all influence the individual's exercise response. Instructors and participants can work together in creating progressive exercise programs that are not overwhelming. Potential signs of excessive fatigue that can be monitored include decreased performance, unexpected decrease in body weight, loss of appetite, sleep disturbances, decreased desire to train, muscle tenderness, and increased colds and infections.

Programming Recommendations

Some suggestions for resistance exercises that involve both concentric and eccentric phases are provided in table 9.1. It is important to note that the initial phase of a program should involve comprehensive testing and evaluation; then the specific goals and needs of an older adult can be addressed to determine the choice of exercises. To the extent possible in order to maximize functional benefits, the recommendations should mimic activity types that are present in daily living or the sport of particular interest. However, a seated position should be used if necessary. The recommended exercise order has the largest muscle

TABLE 9.1 **Examples of Preventive Resistance Exercises to Use With Older Adults**

Exercise	Primary muscle groups
Supine dumbbell or barbell press in line with the chest, wall push-ups	Pectorals, anterior deltoid, triceps
Overhead dumbbell press	Shoulders, triceps
Side raises	Lateral head of the deltoid
Machine pull-down, bent-over dumbbell row, seated row	Back, biceps, posterior deltoid
Simultaneous barbell, dumbbell curl	Biceps
Machine-assisted dips	Chest, anterior deltoid, triceps
Machine-assisted chin-ups	Back, biceps
Bench step-ups	Entire lower body
Partial squats	Quadriceps, glutes
Standing pulley hamstring curls, supine hamstring curls	Hamstring group
Toe raises with support, free-standing toe raises	Lower compartment of the leg

Note: Timing of exercise pattern: novice—2 s for concentric movements, 3 s for the eccentric movement; advanced—2 s for the concentric movement, 4-5 s for the eccentric movement.

groups first, followed by smaller groups in descending order. Thus, this pattern would include training the legs first, followed by the back, chest, shoulders, arms, and the abdominal area last.

The preliminary phase of programming for novice strength trainers, which lasts for about 12 weeks, can involve a circuit type of program in which machines are used to allow an older person to slowly adapt to exercise before any strenuous training is initiated. Then, if the individual appears ready, free weights can be utilized as well, and the load should be increased to at least 80% of 1-repetition maximum—with the aim that failure due to fatigue occur after about six to eight repetitions. If exercise facilities are not available, other resistance methods can be used such as surgical tubing or rubber bands; even household items are adequate alternatives for the initial phase of training. Older adults should start with very light weights that will allow them to perform one set of 8 to 10 repetitions and progressively increase to three sets, using proper form (back straight, head up, abdominal muscles contracted) through a full range of motion. Emphasize controlled concentric eccentric movement to maximize the loading effect. Finally, thorough instruction in proper technique is a key factor for all age-groups in order to help them get the most out of their resistance exercise programs.

A gradual increase in the difficulty of the exercise program is important in order to avoid injury. Variations in load, repetitions, and rest periods are factors that must be taken into consideration. The training principles and acute variables are much the same regardless of training age. Taking the time to consider how these components are managed can greatly affect the success of a resistance training program. Special considerations for the frail and very old, along with those who have chronic diseases, are presented elsewhere in this book.

Examples of upper and lower body exercises using a variety of modalities are presented in tables 9.2 and 9.3. These are quite different from exercises in more advanced routines in which workouts can focus on only one or two muscle groups (split routines).

Summary

Resistance training offers many benefits to the elderly participant and is an important part of an active and healthy lifestyle. Current guidelines recommend at least two resistance training sessions per week. Nonetheless, the number of older adults participating in resistance training activities remains low. Proper design and monitoring of resistance training programs are important steps in increasing exercise adherence. Although initial strength levels can be low, elderly participants can expect significant increases in strength in the first two to three months of training.

TABLE 9.2 Examples of Upper Body Resistance Training Exercises

	Body weight exercises	Elastic band exercises	Free weight exercises
Chest			
Back			
Shoulders			

TABLE 9.3 Examples of Lower Body Resistance Training Exercises

	Body weight exercises	Elastic band exercises	Free weight exercises
Thighs			
Hamstrings			
Calves			

Questions to Consider

1. What are examples of tasks requiring muscular endurance around the home?

2. What are examples of tasks requiring muscular strength around the home?

3. List basic safety tips for using free weights.

4. List acute and chronic adaptations to resistance training.

5. How would you go about designing a basic home-based total-body routine using body weight and bands for an active 65-year-old?

6. If you were asked to design a group-based program of resistance training, what exercises and equipment would you use? Why?

7. What steps would you take to increase adherence to regular resistance training activities in older adults?

8. How would you go about promoting resistance training to older adults?

9. What signs of fatigue would you look for when monitoring a participant's progress?

chapter 10

Exercise Adherence and Safety Measures

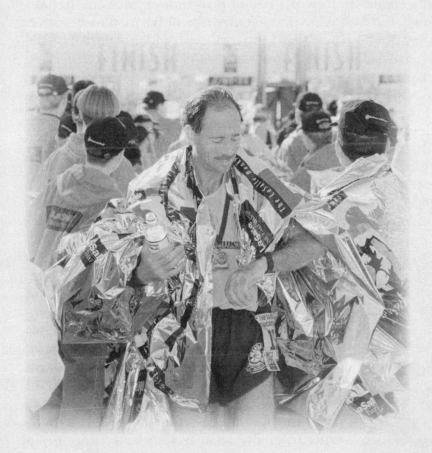

> *An activity or exercise is prescribed within the anticipated upper limit of an individual's physiological capacity, yet above the lower limit of the therapeutic threshold range, and appropriate monitoring is conducted to verify this. A thorough knowledge of signs and symptoms of distress during exercise is essential, and these need to be anticipated for each individual and taught to an older person when self-monitoring is appropriate.*
>
> Dean (1994, p. 88)

In this chapter we discuss exercise adherence, determinants of participation in physical activity, and safety with reference to elderly people. As well, we describe specific problems and needs that seniors have in relation to their exercise programs. We also discuss strategies to increase adherence such as the use of program enhancers, behavior modification, and behavior management. Safety, in particular, is a subject that cannot be neglected in work with elderly persons. We emphasize general safety precautions and contraindicated exercises and procedures.

Most people acknowledge the link between moderate physical activity and health. However, fewer have been educated as to the appropriate form, frequency, or intensity of an exercise and the inherent dangers (both physical and physiological) of inappropriate activities. This fact undoubtedly plays a role in exercise adherence and the safety factors utilized when working with older persons.

In institutional programs, an older adult's lack of mobility is often the consequence of a lack of knowledge about exercise on the part of the health care providers. How to motivate older adults to become physically active has not been part of their formal training.

Many of the principles and guidelines of training developed for younger and middle-aged populations are appropriate for older adults. Healthy older adults are capable of training at relatively heavy intensities and progressing at rates comparable to those of their younger peers. Research on exercise programs for older adults shows that a moderate intensity level is required for gains in cardiorespiratory fitness. Clearly, though, older adults may be more susceptible to joint injuries from higher-intensity programs that involve high-impact force, such as jogging. Therefore, achieving a recommended intensity is critical for adherence to exercise programs and for safe and effective exercise for older adults.

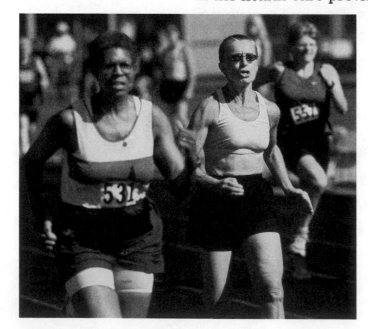

Older women running in race.

Exercise Adherence

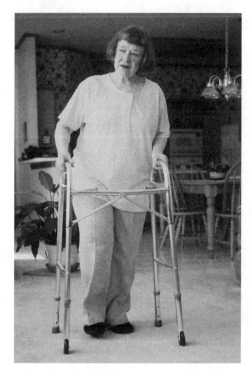

What perceived or real barriers to exercise could this woman be facing?
© Bill Crump/Brand X Pictures

At any age, many factors determine whether or not an individual adopts and adheres to regular physical activity. However, an older adult faces a growing number of perceived and real barriers. These must be overcome in order for older adults to receive the many benefits of increased physical activity. An exercise leader is able to help older adults become more active or remain physically active. Many studies have shown that the barriers to adherence are easily rectifiable and often simply related to common sense, from the senior's perspective. It is important for the leader and subject to communicate in order to eliminate potential barriers.

Psychological, physical, physiological, and clinical barriers (some investigators call these health and lifestyle barriers) affect the adherence or safety of participants, or both. Research has identified the following as barriers: muscle strength, reaction time, and psychoactive drug use (Williams and Lord, 1995); specific social support for exercise and too much initial support from exercise staff (Oka et al., 1995); lack of explanatory information and communication about the benefits and implementation of educational programs between elderly people and caregivers (Mazzeo and Tanaka, 2001); poor self-efficacy and social support throughout programs (McAuley et al., 2003; Rhodes et al., 2001); training programs that are not tailored to meet the needs of the individual (O'Grady et al., 2000); exercise-induced injuries (Kallinen and Markku, 1995); and failure of instructors to be aware of or to take into account the broad spectrum of maladies experienced by those who are elderly (Young, 1997).

Determinants of Physical Activity Participation

It is important to remember three general determinants of participation in physical activity when one is considering adherence and safety factors:

- Personal characteristics and attributes
- Environmental factors
- Characteristics of physical activity

In this chapter we discuss the first two; as the characteristics of physical activity are covered in chapters 7 and 8, we do not address those here.

Personal Characteristics and Attributes

The majority of today's seniors were raised in an era when men left the home to go to work and women stayed at home to look after the house and raise the children. As a result, women, generally, did not participate in exercise programs. In fact, until World War II, it was frowned upon for women to enter the workforce. However, because of the need for "women power" with so many of the men in the armed services, women demonstrated their ability to carry out hard physical work; and today women make up a high proportion of the workforce. During the 1970s and 1980s, women started to exercise on a regular basis and today form a very large percentage of the exercising population. Nonetheless, many older women have not been used to hard physical exercise, and it is essential for exercise leaders to be aware that an older woman may not have ever participated in a regular exercise program. Therefore, it is frequently necessary to find the ways and means to get older women involved in needed exercise.

Personality, for males and females, plays a great role; and instructors or family or friends need to have the right arguments or facts to convince older women to participate. The success rate will depend on the needs, desires, and abilities of these individuals to enjoy themselves while participating and realize the benefits of exercise programs. But it is also important for those working with older women not to set their expectations too high and thus set themselves up for disappointment.

Once participants are in a program, it is essential to observe them and to meet their physical and cognitive needs, or the attrition rate will be high.

Environmental Factors

Environmental factors can cause high attrition rates from exercise programs for elderly people. If air quality is poor, or if the site is difficult to reach (e.g., if parking facilities are inadequate or too far away), it will be difficult to retain participants or to attract new ones.

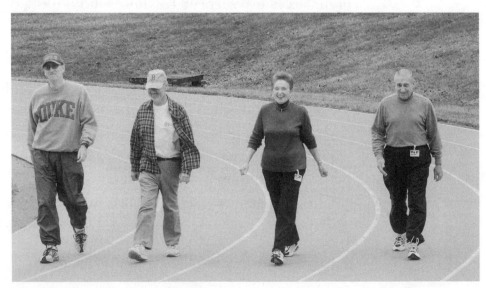

A walking class of participants 65 years and older at the CCAA at 7:00 am.

The physical environment of the exercise facility is very important. It is essential, for example, that the area be quiet, that the maladies of the clients be considered (and the instructor should be aware of these), and that any charts use font size and colors that participants can easily see. It is important to take into account accessibility, cost, attractiveness of the site; the health conditions of the site; and the health of the participants.

Strategies to Increase Adherence

A number of strategies have been used to increase adherence, not only to exercise programs, but also within the context of other behaviors such as regular and faithful prescription drug use. The following are some of the most commonly used and successful strategies for enhancing adherence.

- **Program enhancers.** In a group exercise class, program enhancers are like the spoonful of sugar that helps the medicine go down. They add variety and fun to a program. The use of equipment (e.g., balls, weights, etc.), options for activities, and especially music can greatly increase exercise adherence. If a program is interesting, participants will enjoy themselves, look forward to the class, attend regularly, and feel safe in the enviornment while participating.

- **Behavior modification.** Behavior modification involves a set of procedures that can be used to alter behavior that is deficient, inappropriate, or excessive (Watson and Tharpe, 1997). Physical inactivity is usually regarded as a deficient behavior. Planning is required in order for any type of behavior change to prove successful. Fitness leaders and exercise specialists can play an important role in exercise adoption and adherence in a pleasing and safe environment if they comply with the points already listed in this chapter. A safe, friendly, pleasing enviornment can bring about positive behavior changes.

- **Behavioral management techniques.** Increasing physical activity as a behavior change involves three stages: (1) the decision to start exercising, (2) the early stages of the behavior (*adoption*), and (3) maintenance of the new behavior (*adherence*). At each stage, different strategies are required to reinforce increased physical activity. Readers should now be able to reconsider some of the information presented in previous chapters and apply this knowledge to the three stages. The following are examples of strategies the leader and the participants can use in each of the three stages.

  - *The decision to start exercising.* When discussing the decision to start exercising with a potential participant, refer to the physiological changes that accompany aging, as well as the requirements of maintaining independence. Think about the myths of exercise—for example, "no pain, no gain." Start novice exercisers with simple exercises such as walking. And most importantly, educate individuals on the benefits of exercise and the changes to the body that can be expected.

– *Adoption.* When people move ahead to the early stages of behavior change, strategies and tactics that might be useful include putting their walking shoes by the door and marking exercise times in bold pen on their calendar. Soliciting social support from family and friends is a positive technique; and arranging for family and friends not to visit during the exercise program times is also worthwhile.

– *Adherence.* The third stage, the maintenance of the new behavior, results in an enhanced quality of life. Additional strategies that a fitness leader can use to enhance adherence are recording the practical and personal benefits that the participant is enjoying and informing the participant about ways to prevent relapse—for example, after a vacation.

Safety

Generally, older adults can safely participate in group exercise classes. As an instructor, it will be necessary for the instructor to be aware of some of the potential safety issues and to establish preventive strategies before beginning to offer a program.

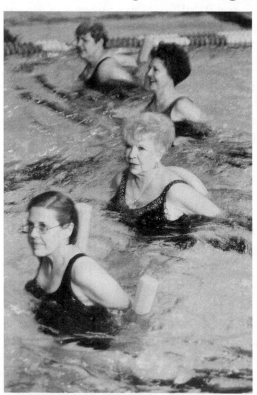

CCAA participants over the age of 80 enjoying the pool exercise program.
© Bill Crump/Brand X Pictures

• **General safety precautions.** Any fitness leader should be prepared to deal with emergency situations. It is important to be able to recognize the signs and symptoms of potential life-threatening situations and then follow an appropriate action plan. To ensure that instructors have these basic skills, one of the criteria for becoming a certified leader through the SFIC (Senior Fitness Instructor Course, offered across North America through the auspices of the Canadian Centre for Activity and Aging) is obtaining cardiopulmonary resuscitation (CPR) certification at the Heart Saver Level. In addition, the facility offering the exercise class should have a plan in place for emergency situations. A participant should stop exercising if he or she experiences

– light-headedness or dizziness,
– confusion,
– pallor,
– nausea,
– sharp leg pain,
– shortness of breath,
– chest pain, or
– musculoskeletal pain.

- **Emergency procedures.** As the saying goes, an ounce of prevention is worth a pound of cure. This certainly holds true for exercise safety of the elderly. However, in case something does go wrong during a program, the instructor should be prepared to activate an emergency plan. The steps involved in developing an emergency procedure include the following:
  - Identifying potential emergency situations
  - Regularly reviewing your facility and equipment
  - Making formal action plans for preventing, responding to, and following up on an emergency situation

- **Contraindicated exercises.** Contraindicated exercises are those that may predispose a participant to injury and should not be included in an exercise program. The contraindicated exercises listed in table 10.1 should be familiar to most fitness leaders. However, many of these exercises were thought to be quite acceptable a few years ago, and some peer leaders and participants may still be using them today. Inappropriate exercises typically involve issues of alignment, joint movement, or joint loading.

Programming Recommendations

It is undisputed that regular exercise positively affects the physiology and quality of life of older adults. However, as with younger people, the exercise must be regular and consistent. Older adults, as outlined in previous chapters, have particular problems that arise as a result of the aging process; seniors manifest the diseases and disabilities of aging, and each of these requires special consideration and treatment in relation to exercise. As a result, older adults have many problem areas that call for special safety precautions. Instructors must take the following recommendations into account when dealing with older adults:

- Be well versed in the symptoms of the various diseases of aging.
- Be certain to remove all barriers to a safe and healthy environment.
- Have a safety plan in place.
- Create an environment that is warm and friendly.
- Maintain environmental conditions, such as noise levels, that are pleasing and acceptable to older persons, in an attractive facility.
- Know the medical history of all program participants.
- Learn how to communicate with older adults to find out about their particular problems, needs, and desires.
- Keep track of attendance of seniors in your class and meet with them to ascertain why their attendance has lapsed, if this is the case.

TABLE 10.1 **Potentially Inappropriate Exercises for Elderly Participants**

Physiological factor	Exercise example	Safe alternative
Alignment issue Compression of vertebrae and blood vessels supplying the brain	Hyperextension of the neck Full neck rotations	Forward and lateral flexion Rotation in the front only Looking over each shoulder
Alignment issue Strain on lower back	Straight-leg sit-ups Lying on back and lifting straight legs up	Isometric abdominal exercises Curl-ups
Alignment issue Strain on lower back Person may pull on head/neck to complete sit-up and injure cervical vertebrae	Full sit-ups Sit-ups with feet/legs held (hip flexors do most of the work)	Isometric abdominal exercises Curl-ups
Poor alignment Strain on lower back muscles and hamstrings	Toe touches Feet shoulder-width apart and alternating toe touches (twisting) Sitting with legs stretched in front and reaching for toes	Modified hurdler's stretch
Shearing force on knee joint	Deep knee bends Duck walk	Sit to stand exercise Squat to 90° maximum
Joint loading (compression)	High-impact activities	Low impact (walking, dancing, etc.)
Issue with joint movement May injure muscles, tendons, ligaments, and joints	Bouncing while stretching	Static stretching Hold stretches for at least 15-20 s
Issue with joint movement at knee Shearing force	Hurdler's stretch	Modified hurdler's stretch Stretch for hamstrings Bring heel toward seat to stretch quads
Joint movement issue Alignment Compression of vertebrae	Rapid torso twists Lateral flexion beyond 20° Side bends with weights	Twist and hold to stretch obliques To stretch obliques and lats, reach up with one arm and bend slightly to the side

Reprinted, by permission, from Canadian Centre for Activity and Aging, 1998, *Senior fitness instructors manual* (London, Ontario, Canada: CCAA), 9.

- Be aware that older adults are more susceptible than younger people to joint injuries, and monitor each individual carefully.

- Be aware that seniors need and deserve special consideration related to sensory defects. For example, to enhance safety in a program instructors must speak clearly and precisely in a slightly louder voice than for younger people. Any visual aids must be easy to see and read (signs and charts, for example, should be printed in large type and on a matte finish). Failing to take sensory deficits into account will lead to safety and attendance problems.

- Watch for changes in behavior and learn how to react to them in a positive manner.

Summary

In this chapter we reviewed the basic assumption that exercise prescription and design for older adults are very similar to those for healthy young adults. The basic difference is one of intensity, given that most seniors have a number of maladies specific to the aging process. We reviewed the factors that determine whether or not people will participate in physical activity or in an exercise program. We also discussed strategies to increase adherence, including the use of program enhancers; behavior modification; and several behavioral management techniques, strategies, and tactics. We considered safety factors related to older adults participating in regular physical activity classes, primarily from the perspective of the instructor. General safety precautions and emergency procedures for dealing with exercising elderly persons were listed, as were contraindicated exercises, which may predispose a participant to injury.

Question to Consider

1. What factors can you identify that affect adherence to physical activity programs with aging?

2. What intervention strategies can you invoke to enhance regular participation?

3. What is the role of program enhancers in exercise adherence?

4. What pieces of equipment can be used in physical activity programs for older adults to enhance adherence and ensure safety?

5. Make a list of barriers associated with each category of the determinants of physical activity. Can you develop some strategies to address these issues?

6. Describe precautions to be taken for exercise safety, including those related to contraindicated exercises for older adults. Why should all exercise leaders be aware of the maladies of all of their participants?

7. Should the leader be more concerned with legal liability or facility and program safety? Or are the two equally important?

8. Give an example of a safety issue. How can that issue be rectified? What should be done to be certain that an unsafe situation or untoward event does not occur again?

chapter 11

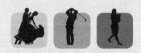

Older Athletes and Substance Abuse

Taryn-Lise Taylor, BA, MSc, MD

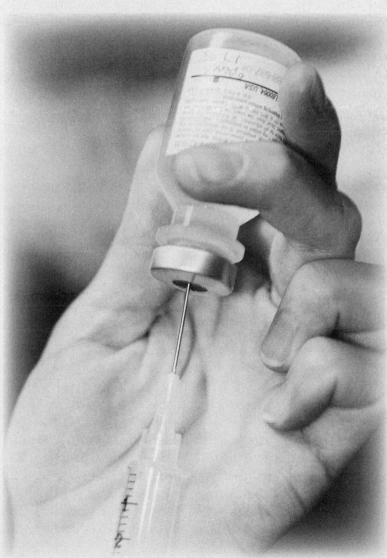

© Photodisc

>   **❝** *It is a sad commentary on human nature and society that so much effort is spent trying to detect and deter drug abuse among athletes. But a big-money, winning-is-everything mentality grips much of our social life. Since sport mirrors society, the field of competition is a stage where athletes enact social values. And if winning is everything, some athletes may try anything to win.* **❞**

> R.E. Eichner (1997, p. 70)

Chemical augmentation of athletic performance is definitely not a new concept. While the term "doping" first appeared in an English dictionary in 1879, the use of drugs has been evident throughout the history of sport. Ancient Greek Olympians ate mushrooms to win, while Aztec athletes consumed the human heart. In the late 1800s, European cyclists consumed substances such as heroin, cocaine, and ether-soaked sugar tablets. Substance use in modern-day Olympics was documented as early as 1904, when marathon runner Thomas Hicks nearly killed himself with a mixture of brandy and strychnine. Strychnine was an athlete's drug of choice well into the 20th century, until the creation of amphetamines in the 1930s. In World War II, amphetamines were introduced to U.S. troops to help keep them awake at the battlefront. However, the dangers of doping became apparent in the 1960 Rome Olympics, when Danish cyclist Knut Jensen collapsed during his race under the influence of amphetamines and later died in a hospital. In the 1967 Tour de France, British cyclist Tommy Simpson overdosed on amphetamines (Voy and Deeter, 1991).

The 1967 incident finally prompted the International Olympic Committee (IOC) to develop an official definition of doping, draw up a list of banned substances, and implement a testing policy for the 1968 Olympics (Catlin and Murray, 1996). At the 1968 Olympics in Mexico, however, seven athletes, including four medalists, had positive test results to stimulants or narcotics. Twenty years later at the 1988 Seoul Olympics, Canadian sprinter Ben Johnson was stripped of his gold medal in the 100 m and suspended for two years after testing positive for anabolic steroids. This suspension of the world's fastest man brought world attention to the use of drugs in sport. American track and field superstar Florence Griffith Joyner won three gold medals and a silver medal, setting two world records for the 100 and 200 m running events. Her victories continue to be tainted by rumors that she used human growth hormone to accomplish these feats. In the 1996 Olympics, Russian Greco-Roman wrestler Zafar Gouliev was stripped of a bronze medal for use of an amphetamine derivative; and at the 2004 Olympics in Athens, female Russian shot-putter Irina Korzhanenko tested positive for steroids after winning a gold medal, as did several weightlifters.

Unfortunately, the simple fact that testing programs are in operation does not guarantee their effectiveness. Drug screening methods are limited because of inadequate technology, and athletes (or their pharmacologists, trainers, or coaches) learn quickly how to beat the system. Sport has also developed into a significant social institution, and success in sport has become highly valued. The pressure placed on athletes to succeed has contributed to the escalation in drug taking and the number of drug-related deaths within the sporting community. For a complete list of banned substances, refer to the IOC prohibited classes of substances and prohibited methods of doping at www.usantidoping.org.

Masters Athletes

According to the 1994-1995 World Association of Veteran Athletes (WAVA) handbook, early masters athletes were mainly road runners. In 1965, track coach Bill Bowerman formed the U.S. Masters track and field team, with significant help from a lawyer named David Pain. The first masters national track and field championship was held in San Diego, California in 1968, consisting of 130 male competitors. David Pain, who was chairman of the event, arbitrarily chose the age of 40 as the starting age for masters competitors. In the United States, National Masters Championships have been held every year since 1968. The Amateur Athletic Union (AAU) adopted masters track and field in 1971, becoming its national governing body. The first International Masters meet was held in 1972 in London, England; and Toronto, Canada, hosted a major masters meet in 1975. WAVA—known today as World Masters Athletics, or WMA—was formed in 1977. The WMA is subsidized by the IAAF (International Amateur Athletics Federation) and together with 125 affiliate countries sponsors regional and world masters track and field championships that are held every two years (www.masterstrack.com).

Worldwide, roughly 50,000 older athletes refer to themselves as masters. In 1996, USA Track & Field (USATF) reported 8,189 masters members in America who listed themselves as running "track," with 3,138 competing in "field." However, many athletes compete in both. Nearly 5,800 athletes from 76 countries competed in the world meet in Durban, South Africa, in 1997, and more than 5,900 athletes from 74 nations took part in Gateshead, England, in 1999 (http://members.aol.com/trackceo). *National Masters News* is the official publication of USATF and WMA and runs a list of meets every month by U.S. region.

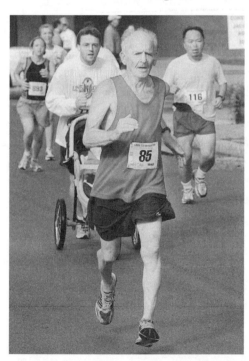

Henry Sypniewski, 85, advances to the finish line of the Linda Yalem Safety 5K Run in Amherst, New York, September 28, 2004, finishing the race with a time of 27:15. Sypniewski was a runner in high school, but for decades didn't have time to participate in the sport—until he took it up again at age 70.

© Associated Press

In masters-level sport, athletes compete in five-year age brackets: 45-49, 50-54, 55-59, and so on. WAVA has established a set of standards and formulas for comparing performances of people in different age-groups. Age grading, as it applies to masters athletics, is the process of converting actual performances to results achievable in an open age category by the application of age-related correction factors, thus allowing comparison between performances of different athletes of various ages. Age grading in masters sports helps to make the competition more equitable. The first age grading tables were developed in 1989 by WAVA; in 1994 the tables were updated, and they will continue to be updated every five years (www.ibiblio.org/drears/running/masters/agegrade.html).

In recent years, issues related to enhancement of the performance of masters athletes have received a great deal of attention. Elderly athletes must commit to a difficult training regimen in order to improve athletic performance. Modifications in training must occur in order to take into account changes associated with aging that younger athletes do not encounter, but similar pressures exist to succeed and win (Maharam et al., 1999). Doping is a real-world issue, even in masters-level athletes. There are enormous differences in how various sporting organizations regulate performance-enhancing substances. Although masters athletes are not drug tested in USATF competitions, athletes may be drug tested in WMA competitions. Therefore, it is important that athletes be familiar with any substances that may be prohibited prior to and during competition. Some prohibited substances may be permitted if a medical exemption is obtained prior to use. The international track and field community imposes the most stringent rules. The WMA antidoping program and policy are carried out in very close cooperation with the IAAF in order that attitude and measures worldwide be the same. The WMA began testing masters athletes at meets in 1995 (www.world-masters-athletics.org).

Even the healthiest masters athlete often relies on prescription medications. The Pfizer Pulse Survey (www.demko.com/cs000516.htm) showed that 64% of senior athletes take some sort of prescription medication. Most prescription medications are not on the IAAF banned list, but the ingredients in some of them are. Some athletes need to take certain medications simply to get to the meet, let alone compete.

Hormones

Hormone replacement therapy (HRT) has been shown to be beneficial to the health of some older men and women who experience a drop in hormone production. Both estrogen and testosterone can improve the quality of life of older individuals suffering from menopause or "andropause." Unfortunately, the current regulations surrounding the use of these substances in sport present a difficult dilemma for masters athletes. Human growth hormone presents a more complex dilemma, as current research is conflicting on the potential benefits versus harm associated with this substance.

Estrogen

In 1999, a 56-year-old grandmother from Phoenix, Arizona ran the 100 m dash in 13.55 s at the WAVA Championships in England. This feat was followed by running the 200 m dash in 28.34 s, a time that broke the existing age-group world record. However, sprinter Kathy Jager was required to provide a urine sample for drug testing, which is not routine at American masters meets, and tested positive for anabolic steroids. Her times were expunged and she was banned from competitions for a period of two years.

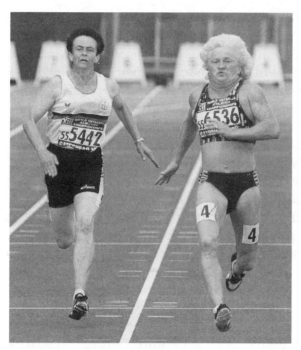

What makes Supergranny run?
© Associated Press

Jager received a letter explaining that the IAAF had found methyltestosterone metabolites (anabolic steroids) in her urine sample. She had been taking estrogen replacement to control her menopause-related hot flashes, and the formulation contained 1.25 mg per day of methyltestosterone, a synthetic testosterone. Methyltestosterone is considered a banned substance, but 1.25 mg per day is a small fraction of the amount (up to 100 mg per day) consumed by male bodybuilders. It is unclear whether or not this dose gave Jager a performance advantage, but her times have declined since she was reinstated and went off the medication. In addition, Jager stopped taking her blood pressure medication, as it too is on the IAAF's list of prohibited substances—putting her at risk for cardiovascular complications such as stroke.

During menopause, a woman's body produces less estrogen, and menstrual periods cease. This is a natural stage in a woman's life but is linked to many uncomfortable symptoms. Estrogen replacement therapy is a fact of life for many female masters athletes. Prescribed as a pill, a patch, or gel with a vaginal applicator, HRT helps to relieve distressing menopausal symptoms (hot flashes, night sweats, vaginal dryness, insomnia, difficulty concentrating). Estrogen therapy helps to prevent osteoporosis, maintain physical vitality, and reduce depression. Recent WHO research also reveals that hormone replacement therapy may reduce the risk of colorectal cancer in women.

Testosterone

The average male produces the equivalent of 100 mg of testosterone each week. Bhasin and colleagues (1996) randomly assigned 43 normal men to one of four groups: placebo with no exercise, testosterone with no exercise, placebo with exercise, and testosterone with exercise. The men received injections of 600 mg of testosterone or placebo weekly for 10 weeks. The men in the exercise groups performed standardized weightlifting exercises three times weekly. The results showed that high doses of testosterone, especially when combined with strength training, increased fat-free mass, muscle size, and strength in normal men. The IOC has banned male hormones because they offer an unfair advantage in sport.

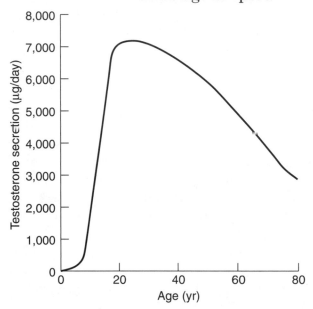

Figure 11.1   Serum testosterone secretion with age in male subjects.

Reprinted, from C. Bass, 2000, *Anti-aging medicine: Wave of the future, or wrong turn?* By permission of C. Bass. Available: www.cbass.com/Anti-Aging.htm

Serum testosterone concentrations decline with age in men (see figure 11.1). The age at which serum testosterone concentrations are significantly reduced is unclear. Some reports indicate significant decreases in serum testosterone beginning in the fifth or sixth decade of life (Vermeulen and Kaufman, 1995), whereas others indicate relatively stable serum total testosterone concentrations through the seventh decade of life (Gray et al., 1991). The average male's blood level of testosterone drops more than 40% from age 50 to 70, which can cause a decrease in male assertiveness, bone and muscle strength, and sexuality. Pharmaceutical products derived from testosterone have been used for a diverse range of indications including male infertility, athletic enhancement, libido problems, and erectile dysfunction. Thus testosterone can help improve many facets of life in men who are elderly.

However testosterone administration is also associated with a number of health risks. Massive doses of testosterone can lower high density lipoprotein (HDL) cholesterol levels, which combat the buildup of artery-clogging plaques, so in turn increase the risk of heart attack. Such doses can also intensify preexisting prostate cancer or expand an already enlarged prostate. These serious health problems need to be considered by masters athletes, as the associated risks are compounded in older individuals. Men over the age of 50 should definitely receive a blood test for prostate-specific antigen (PSA), a prostate exam, and a sonogram of the prostate before being prescribed testosterone injections; and these should be monitored during therapeutic use (Wemyss-Holden et al., 1994).

The IOC and sport governing bodies ban certain HRT drugs, and unfortunately at this time masters athletes must choose between participation in sport and the advice of a physician to use HRT to maintain health. A possible solution to this situation would be the introduction of a new drug protocol. Suggestions include permitting the administration of HRT, not to exceed normal levels, and to monitor this with blood tests. This would allow masters athletes who have difficulty participating in sport due to hormone deficiency to compete on a level playing field while instituting the necessary controls to prevent abuse (Dziepak, 2002).

Human Growth Hormone

Human growth hormone (HGH) has been traditionally prescribed for the treatment of disorders that result in HGH insufficiency. It has been used, with some success, to combat the weight loss and general wasting characteristic of AIDS and cancer. Many athletes believe that HGH has fat-burning and muscle-building properties, which enhance endurance, strength, and muscle mass, and thus use it illegally. However, studies by Yarasheski and colleagues (1992, 1993) contradict this belief and suggest no performance or strength benefit associated with the use of HGH.

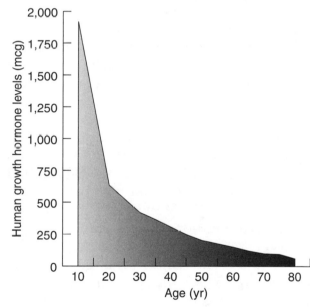

Figure 11.2 This graph shows the average decrease in human growth hormone levels (in mcg) in the body as men age. Studies indicate that human growth hormone levels decline at a rate of 15% per decade from the age of 25.

Reprinted, by permission, from DHEAUSA, 2001, "Growth Hormone." Available: http://dheause.com/AN%growth_hormone.htm.

Growth hormone has recently received a great deal of media attention in connection with its antiaging characteristics. Injections of HGH have become increasingly popular as a virtual "rejuvenator" or "fountain of youth." Over the past few years, hundreds of clinics have sprung up, providing HGH to thousands of elderly people looking for a miraculous way to reverse the aging process (muscle atrophy, thinning bones, increased body fat, loss of energy) and turn back the clock. According to IMS Health, a company that tracks drug sales in the United States, prescriptions for growth hormone more than tripled from 1997 to 2001, rising from 6000 to 21,000. The presence of HGH in a healthy adult declines at a rate of approximately 15% per decade after the age of 25 (figure 11.2). By age 60, a loss of 75% or more is not uncommon, and by age 80, HGH levels are frequently nonexistent (less than 25 mcg). This finding has encouraged researchers to determine whether HGH may be the key to the debilitating changes that occur with aging.

A six-month, randomized controlled study in healthy older men (mean age 75 years) showed slight improvements in body composition (decrease in fat mass, increase in lean mass), but no increases in strength, endurance, or cognitive function with the use of HGH (Papadakis et al., 1996). Later, in 2002, one of the largest and most carefully designed studies of HGH in healthy older people was completed. A 26-week randomized, double-blind, placebo-controlled trial was performed on 131 healthy women and men aged 65 to 88 years old. Researchers concluded that HGH can markedly transform an older person's body by increasing lean body mass and reducing fat mass. The most striking results were in the men who took both growth hormone and testosterone. These men gained almost 10 lb (4.5 kg) of lean body mass and lost a corresponding amount of fat. The increase in muscle strength and $\dot{V}O_2$max was marginal in men, and women showed no significant changes in strength or cardiovascular endurance. However, it is possible that more significant gains in strength might have occurred if the treatment had continued for a longer period of time.

The investigators caution that the gains achieved were accompanied by serious adverse side effects afflicting 24% to 46% of subjects. These included increased blood pressure, pedal edema, joint pain, and carpal tunnel syndrome (likely caused by the drug's tendency to increase water retention). There is concern that the joint pains that plagued many in the study would lead to arthritis if the drug were to be continued. In addition, half of the men who took HGH experienced an impaired ability to utilize glucose, developing either diabetes or an insulin-resistant condition. All of the adverse effects of HGH disappeared when the men and women stopped using the drug. However, adverse effects were common; so HGH intervention in elderly people should be cautious (Blackman et al., 2002).

The potential anabolic actions of HGH have made it an attractive agent for people wishing to enhance athletic ability. Human growth hormone was added to the IOC's banned list in 1989; but its use in sport is promoted by the fact that until recently, no practical method existed to detect its use in competition. Advertisements in print media and on the Internet promote the use of HGH. Many of the agents sold do not actually contain growth hormone nor do they lead to a sustained increase in concentrations of growth hormone. Several Web sites attempt to sell various oral and inhaled formulations of growth hormone; none of these have been shown to be efficacious, as the growth hormone molecule itself is too large to pass into the bloodstream and needs to be injected to be effective (Vance, 2003).

There is good evidence that chronic elevated serum concentrations of HGH may, in fact, decrease performance and cause metabolic changes that diminish the capacity for strenuous physical activity. These metabolic alterations are associated with a number of deleterious side effects such as cardiac instability, hypertension, and the development of insulin resistance and possibly type 2 diabetes. Despite the negative side effects, athletes continue to inject. The lipolytic effect of HGH causes a decrease in subcutaneous fat, which is a powerful driving force to promote abuse. The athlete perceives the resulting improvements in muscle definition almost instantly, which has a positive reinforcing effect regardless of the fact that there are no increases in strength. The embellishment of the effects of growth hormone in muscle building encourages athletes and elderly persons to expose themselves to increased risk of disease for little or uncertain benefit (Rennie, 2003).

Anabolic Steroids

Anabolic steroids (AS) are derivatives of testosterone that are effective in enhancing athletic performance. The available scientific literature explains that short-term administration of these drugs can cause strength gains of 5% to 20% and an increase in body weight of 2 to 5 kg (4.4-11 lb) attributed to an increase in lean body mass (Hartgens and Kuipers, 2004). Anabolic steroids have been widely recommended in the management of debility in association with the diseases of old age. Their action in promoting weight gain and in speeding rehabilitation makes them a tempting drug of abuse. They are often given to elderly or postoperative patients to promote muscle growth and tissue regeneration.

The trade-off, however, is the occurrence of adverse side effects that can jeopardize health. Since AS can act on several organ systems, a multitude of side effects can transpire. The frequency and severity of side effects are somewhat variable. They are influenced by several factors such as drug formulation, dosage, duration of use, and individual differences in sensitivity and response. The mechanism of action of AS may differ between compounds because of variations in the steroid molecule and affinity to androgen receptors. Serious side effects include an unhealthy cholesterol profile (increase in total cholesterol with a marked decline in HDL cholesterol), heart attack (high doses of AS increase diastolic blood pressure and cause atherosclerosis), stroke, and liver failure. Male athletes may experience prostate problems, atrophy of the testes, decrease of sperm production, and an increased frequency of erectile dysfunction. Acne is frequently reported, as well as hypertrophy of sebaceous glands and hair loss. In women, AS use results in inhibition of follicle formation and ovulation, causing irregularities of the menstrual cycle. Additional side effects specifically in women are acne, male pattern baldness, lowering of the voice, increased facial hair growth, and breast atrophy. Both genders may also suffer from various psychological side effects such as aggression, confusion, sleeping disorders, anxiety, paranoia, and hallucinations (Catlin et al., 1993).

There is some evidence that AS abuse may affect the immune system, leading to a decreased effectiveness of the body's defense system. Anabolic steroid use decreases glucose tolerance and increases insulin resistance, which in turn mimics type 2 diabetes but seems to be reversible after abstention from the drug. These are dangerous side effects for any athlete but more so for senior competitors (Cohen and Hickman, 1987).

The effects of AS are shared by the steroid precursors sold in pharmacies and health food stores. The most common of these products are androstenedione and dehydroepiandrosterone (DHEA). Androstenedione supplements are made of naturally occurring steroid hormones the body uses to make testosterone. It has been found that in young men, chronic ingestion of 100 mg or 200 mg of androstenedione three times a day caused a 40% to 50% increase in free testosterone levels; but earlier research indicates that men have to more than double their levels before supplementation can allow them to build significant muscle mass (Ballantyne et al., 2000; Rasmussen et al., 2000). Brown and colleagues (2000) investigated the effects of androstenedione ingestion in healthy 30- to 56-year-old men. The results suggested that consuming 100 mg of androstenedione three times per day does not increase serum total testosterone but does elicit increases in free testosterone, dihydrotestosterone (DHT), and estradiol. The metabolic significance of the transient increase in free testosterone is uncertain. Elevated serum concentrations of DHT (83%) can cause the prostate to enlarge, but there was no change in PSA values. However, it is possible that more prolonged supplementation may result in detectable changes in prostate function.

Levels of HDL cholesterol were reduced by 0.13 mmol/L, which corresponds to a 10% to 15% increase in the risk of atherosclerotic lesion development and heart disease. The results suggest that androstenedione is unlikely to provide the required hormonal conditions for promoting increases in muscle size and may cause undesirable health effects. In addition, there has been some speculation that athletes taking androstenedione consume doses much higher than those studied, so the magnitude of the effects is unknown. Elderly athletes should be very cautious when considering this supplement as an option, especially given the lack of evidence for its effectiveness to build muscle (Brown et al., 2000).

A Case Study in Prostate Health and Anabolic Steroid Use

The growth and development of the prostate are regulated by endogenous testosterone secretion and thus are sensitive to androgenic stimulation (Jin et al., 1996). A continuous output of testosterone is mandatory to maintain the prostate's structure and function. In an observational study, a 49-year-old male bodybuilder who was using a "cocktail" of numerous different AS volunteered to have his prostate function examined. He was studied during a 15-week period of steroid self-administration. Both objective and subjective parameters were measured, including prostatic volume (ultrasound), prostate size and consistency (digital rectal examination), urine flow rate, PSA level (a blood marker for enlarged prostate and prostate cancer), and bladder outflow obstruction (symptom rating). The subject noted an increase in nocturnal urinary frequency, libido, and aggression. Results also showed that during the period of steroid use, prostatic volume increased significantly and urine flow decreased. Four weeks after steroid administration ceased, these parameters approached, but did not reach, presteroid use levels. Any effects of AS are shared by the steroid precursors such as androstenedione and DHEA. This is especially important information that must be considered by elderly male athletes thinking about AS use (Wemyss-Holden et al., 1994; Prostate Health and OTC Medications, www.uspharmacist.com).

Analgesics and Anti-Inflammatories

An analgesic (colloquially known as a painkiller) is any member of the diverse group of drugs used to relieve pain. Analgesic drugs act in various ways on the peripheral and central nervous systems. Nonsteroidal anti-inflammatory drugs (NSAIDs) reduce fever and inflammation as well as relieve pain. Narcotic analgesics depress the central nervous system and alter the perception of pain and are often used to alleviate pain not relieved by the NSAIDs. Pain relief is a significant part of arthritis treatment that is common after the age of 50.

Narcotic Analgesics

Prescription painkillers are the opioid most commonly misused by athletes (Nativ and Puffer, 1991). Athletes who use narcotic analgesics (e.g., codeine, morphine, fentanyl, hydromorphone, and meperidine) can experience feelings of euphoria or psychological stimulation leading to false feelings of invincibility. Narcotic analgesics increase the pain threshold, and as a result an athlete may fail to recognize injury and suffer more serious injury. Athletes often use these drugs to mask injury in order to continue to participate in their sports, despite musculoskeletal injuries. Narcotic analgesics produce physical and psychological dependence. Adverse effects include drowsiness, mental clouding, nausea, vomiting, dizziness, constipation, and an inability to urinate. High doses of opioids can lead to respiratory depression, apnea, circulatory depression, hypotension or low blood pressure, muscle rigidity, coma, shock, and cardiac arrest. These are serious side effects that may be amplified in elderly persons, as lower doses are required to produce an effect and this may be difficult to calculate.

NSAIDs

Pain and inflammation are probably the most common ailments of athletes due to strains, sprains, and other minor injuries. Ibuprofen (including Advil and Motrin), along with other NSAIDs such as naprosyn (Aleve) and aspirin, is generally considered effective for mild to moderate pain and inflammation (see table 11.1). Degenerative joint disease and osteoarthritsis are common ailments, affecting persons as they age, and may result in abuse of NSAIDs in masters athletes.

Although NSAIDs are available without prescription, taking them can be potentially harmful. The widespread use of NSAIDs has led to the recognition of numerous associated adverse effects that limit their use (see figure 11.3). Many of the toxic effects of NSAIDs are related to the inhibition of prostaglandin (PG) synthesis and of cyclooxygenase (COX), which are the main mechanisms of action. The most important

TABLE 11.1 **NSAIDs and COX-2 Inhibitors**

Traditional NSAIDS	Trade names
Acetylsalicylic acid (ASA)	Aspirin
Diclofenac	Voltaren
Ibuprofen	Advil, Motrin
Naproxen	Naprosyn, Anaprox
Celecoxib	Celebrex
Lumiracoxib	Prexige
Meloxicam	Mobicox

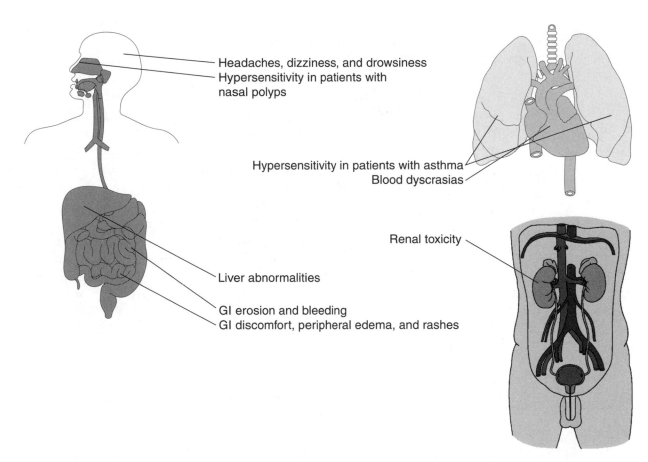

Headaches, dizziness, and drowsiness
Hypersensitivity in patients with nasal polyps

Hypersensitivity in patients with asthma
Blood dyscrasias

Liver abnormalities

GI erosion and bleeding
GI discomfort, peripheral edema, and rashes

Renal toxicity

Figure 11.3 Adverse effects of nonsteroidal anti-inflammatory drugs.
Reprinted by permission from www.ama-cmeonline.com/.../04pharm/06_01.htm.

complications include gastrointestinal toxicity (dyspepsia, peptic ulcer disease, and GI bleeding), acute renal failure due to renal vasoconstriction (PG maintains blood flow), and modest worsening of underlying hypertension or congestive heart failure. Dehydration increases the risk of kidney problems, which is an issue especially for endurance athletes. COX-2 inhibitors (Celebrex, Prexige, Mobicox) are a class of

NSAIDs that are less problematic for gastrointestinal bleeding but are still potentially dangerous when it comes to the kidneys and cardiovascular system (Ruscin and Page, 2002). NSAIDS mask pain and do not cure injury. An athlete may chose to abuse these medications to complete training; but if the body's message to cease a damaging activity is ignored, there is risk of further injury.

Hypertension Medications

It is known that physical activity is an effective way to lower high blood pressure (BP). Hernelahti and colleagues (1998) compared the prevalence of hypertension in two groups of middle-aged men. One group engaged in vigorous endurance training and were top-level masters orienteering runners, and the control group were considered representative of the general population born after 1925, who had been classified as healthy when young adults. The prevalence of hypertension was more than three times higher in the control group (27.8%) than in the exercise group (8.7%), and the difference remained significant after body mass index was adjusted for. The conclusion was that long-term intense endurance exercise is associated with a decreased prevalence of hypertension. Masters athletes are usually thought to be free of cardiovascular disease and hypertension because of their apparently high level of fitness. Hypertension is a problem in 20% to 25% of adults 30 to 60 years of age (Gifford et al., 1989). Older athletes and other physically active individuals should be screened for hypertension and given appropriate therapy if required to reduce the risk of morbidity and mortality associated with cardiovascular disease. Recommendations on exercise and sport participation for patients with hypertension are provided in table 11.2.

In older athletes it is important to focus on behaviors that may affect blood pressure, such as a high intake of sodium and saturated fats and the use of alcohol and drugs (e.g., stimulants taken before competition, AS). Many over-the-counter medications, including NSAIDs, caffeine, diet pills, and decongestants (ephedrine), can also cause blood pressure to rise (see "Risk Factors for Hypertension . . ." [p. 193] and Joint National Committee on Prevention, Detection, Evaluation, and Treatment of High Blood Pressure, 1997; Julius and Nesbitt, 1996). Athletes should also be cautious when using herbs and dietary supplements purported to increase energy or control weight. These supplements are not regulated and often contain "natural" substances that act as stimulants, such as ephedra, guanara, and ma huang, which can elevate blood pressure (Nieldfeldt, 2002).

It is important for athletes to monitor medication effects, because some antihypertensive drugs may have an adverse influence on exercise tolerance (figure 11.4). A high-performance athlete may experience problems that would not come into play for less active individuals. NSAIDs may

TABLE 11.2 **Exercise and Sport Participation in Athletes and Other Physically Active Persons With Hypertension**

Exercise: The recommended mode, frequency, duration, and intensity of exercise are generally the same as those for persons without hypertension.
Sport participation: Blood pressure should be controlled before resumption of participation in vigorous sports, because both dynamic and isometric exercise can cause remarkable increases in blood pressure.

Recommendations on exercise restrictions

High-normal blood pressure	No restrictions
Controlled mild to moderate hypertension (<140/90 mmHg)	No restrictions on dynamic exercise; possible limit on isometric training or sports in some patients
Uncontrolled hypertension (>140/90 mmHg)	Limited to low-intensity dynamic exercise; avoid isometric sports
Controlled hypertension with end-organ damage	Limited to low-intensity dynamic exercise; avoid isometric sports
Severe hypertension with no end-organ involvement	Limited to low-intensity dynamic exercise, with participation only if blood pressure is under adequate control
Secondary hypertension of renal origin	Limited to low-intensity dynamic exercise; avoid "collision" sports that could lead to kidney damage

Table 2 from "Managing Hypertension in Athletes and Physically Active Patients" [Mark Nieldfeldt, MD-author: *American Family Physician*, vol. 66(3): 445-452; August 1, 2002].

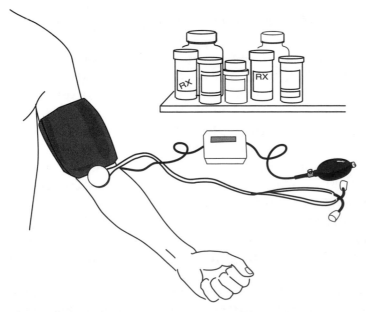

Figure 11.4 Blood pressure can be affected if people use or stop the use of certain drugs and medications.

Adapted from http://health.allrefer.com/pictures-images/drug-induced-hypertension.html.

decrease the action of antihypertensive medications, including diuretics, beta-blockers, and angiotensin converting enzyme inhibitors, which is important for athletes taking any of these medications (Fuentes and Rosenberg, 1999). Athletes also need to be aware that the U.S. Olympic Committee (USOC) has banned the use of some antihypertensive medications. However, the more important issue for masters athletes is the danger of avoiding treatment of high BP for the purpose of competition (IOC prohibited classes of substances and prohibited methods of doping, from www.usantidoping.org; USADA guide to prohibited classes of substances and prohibited methods of doping, from www.usantidoping.org).

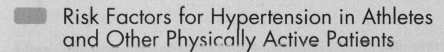

Risk Factors for Hypertension in Athletes and Other Physically Active Patients

- High sodium intake
- Excessive alcohol consumption (binge drinking)
- Illicit drug use (e.g., cocaine)
- Anabolic steroid use
- Stimulant use (e.g., in supplements taken to enhance energy or control weight)
- High stress levels
- Male gender
- Race (blacks affected more often than whites by about a 2-to-1 ratio; Asians affected the least)
- Family history of hypertension or cardiac disease in men over 55 years of age and women over 65 years of age
- Diabetes mellitus or glucose intolerance
- Smoking or chewing tobacco
- Obesity

From "Managing Hypertension in Athletes and Physically Active Patients" [Mark Nieldfeldt, MD-author: *American Family Physician*, vol. 66(3): 445-452; August 1, 2002].

- **Diuretics.** Both thiazide (e.g., hydrochlorothiazide) and loop diuretics (e.g., furosamide) decrease plasma volume, cardiac output, and vascular resistance. Loop diuretics are inappropriate for use in the treatment of hypertension in athletes. The thiazide diuretics have less pronounced effects, are inexpensive, and may be used as first-line treatment for hypertension in casually active patients. However, diuretic therapy is less desirable in high-intensity or endurance athletes because of the risk of dehydration or hypokalemia (Nieldfeldt, 2002). These side effects can lead to syncope, muscle cramps, and arrhythmias in patients who are exercising intensely or competing in warm weather. Sport regulatory bodies have banned the use of all diuretics because they are dangerous when used by athletes for the purpose of making a weight class. Diuretics cause excretion enhancement for the purpose of losing weight rapidly prior to competitions in which weight limits are set (boxing, wrestling, weightlifting, judo, lightweight rowing). They are often used in combination with other dehydration techniques which can be extremely dangerous in those who are elderly. Diuretics can be abused in an attempt to "dilute" the urine and make detection of other drugs more difficult (Chick et al., 1988).

- **Angiotensin converting enzyme (ACE) inhibitors.** ACE inhibitors (e.g., ramipril, enalapril, captopril) are excellent choices for treating mild to moderate hypertension. These agents block the conversion of angiotensin I to angiotensin II, which is a potent vasoconstrictor and a source of sodium retention. Reducing angiotensin II allows blood vessels to relax and dilate, which in turn lowers blood pressure. ACE inhibitors are associated with a slight decrease in heart rate, an increase in stroke volume, and a decrease in total peripheral resistance (Gifford, 1997). In exercise, ACE inhibitors have no major effects on energy metabolism and cause no impairment of maximum oxygen uptake. In general, these drugs have no deleterious effects on training or competition (Chick et al., 1988). An adequate cool-down period is recommended for athletes taking ACE inhibitors because there have been reports of postural hypotension after intense exercise. ACE inhibitors are often the first-line agents for the treatment of high blood pressure in physically active patients, especially those with diabetes. A dry cough is experienced in a small percentage of patients, which is an indication to stop the medication.

- **Calcium channel blockers.** Calcium channel blockers are generally well tolerated and effective in physically active patients. These drugs reduce the calcium concentration in vascular smooth muscle causing vasodilation, which results in decreased systemic vascular resistance and decreased blood pressure (Gifford, 1997). Amlodipine and nifedipine can cause reflex tachycardia, palpitations, flushing, fluid retention (pedal edema), and headaches, which may affect adherence to the prescribed medication regimen. Verapamil and diltiazem can cause minor impairment of maximal heart rate, lower limb edema, severe dizziness or fainting, and difficulty urinating, which can also affect compliance (Joint National Committee on Prevention, Detection, Evaluation, and Treatment of High Blood Pressure, 1997). Although there is a potential for early onset of the lactate threshold, calcium channel blockers have no deleterious effects on energy metabolism during exercise, and maximum oxygen uptake is typically preserved (Chick et al., 1988).

- **Beta-blockers.** Beta-blockers (e.g., metoprolol, atenolol) significantly decrease heart rate and contractility while impairing cardiac output and maximum oxygen uptake, particularly in athletes. These drugs inhibit lipolysis and glycogenolysis, which can cause hypoglycemia after intense exercise. In addition, athletes who take beta-blockers perceive greater exertion during exercise and often stop taking the drug because they feel it impairs their performance, which in turn puts them at high risk for a cardiac event (Chick et al., 1988). However, beta-blockers are often abused due to their anxiolytic and antitremor effects. As a result the USOC has banned the use of beta-blockers in athletes participating in precision events such as archery, shooting, diving, and ice skating (IOC prohibited classes of substances and prohibited methods of doping, from www.usantidoping.org; USADA guide to prohibited classes of substances and prohibited methods of doping, from www.usantidoping.org).

Other Medications

A variety of other medications that were originally developed to treat medical conditions were later used to enhance athletic performance. Erythropoietin is used legitimately to treat certain types of anemia. Acetazolamide (Diamox) is used in the treatment of glaucoma. Beta-2 agonists such as Ventolin provide crucial lifesaving management of asthma. However, the mechanisms of action of these drugs have been monopolized by athletes to maximize their abilities.

Erythropoietin

Erythropoietin (EPO) is a favorite drug of abuse for endurance athletes such as long-distance cyclists, cross-country skiers, and marathon runners. Recombinant EPO has been available since 1985. It is a form of modern-day blood doping (no transfusion required) that enhances the oxygen-carrying capacity of the blood, which is why it is banned by most sporting organizations, including USATF and the IOC.

Erythropoietin is a protein produced primarily in the kidneys that stimulates the bone marrow and regulates the production of red blood cells. Natural EPO production may be increased due to low oxygen pressures or anemia, as well as strenuous training and transition from sea level to high altitude. Maximal cardiovascular performance decreases with age, as evidenced by the decline in maximal oxygen consumption ($\dot{V}O_2$max) of 8% to 10% per decade after the age of 25 (Heath et al.,

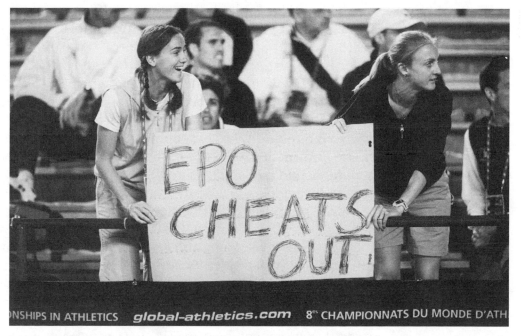

British distance runners Hayley Tullett and Paula Radcliff protest lack of action on positive erythropoietin tests at the 2001 Track & Field World Championships in Edmonton, Canada.
© Victah Sailor

1981; Ogawa et al., 1992). Studies in healthy athletes have shown that several weeks of EPO injections lead to improvements in $\dot{V}O_2$max of up to 8%. This can produce an enormous boost to someone training for any type of endurance event (Ruscin and Page, 2002).

Erythropoietin is believed to enhance the activity of platelets, which are responsible for forming blood clots. This puts any athlete at increased risk for thrombosis, heart attack, or stroke, but elderly athletes more so. A cerebrovascular accident (especially with dehydrating endurance exercise) is a serious side effect and may be fatal. The risk of thrombosis has been implicated in a number of deaths among cyclists. Erythropoietin has been shown to increase blood pressure and heart rate even during submaximal exercise. Athletes who have abused EPO have also experienced documented iron overload, which may eventually produce damage in the heart, lungs, liver, and kidneys (Ruscin and Page, 2002). Masters athletes should be cautioned to avoid EPO abuse since such abuse amplifies the protential risks.

Acetazolamide (Diamox)

Acetazolamide is classified as a carbonic anhydrase inhibitor, which is effective therapy for glaucoma, convulsive disorders (e.g., epilepsy), and in the promotion of diuresis in instances of abnormal fluid retention (e.g., cardiac edema). Acetazolamide has become popular among high-altitude athletes because it can help prevent some of the symptoms associated with altitude sickness, such as headache, dizziness, and nausea.

Adverse reactions common to all sulfonamide derivatives, including acetazolamide, may also occur, including fever, rash, fulminant hepatic necrosis, renal calculus (kidney stones), bone marrow depression, blood dyscrasias, anaphylaxis, and death. One in 15,000 patients per year taking acetazolamide will develop aplastic anemia, which is a potentially fatal suppression of the bone marrow. It usually occurs in the first six months of therapy and has been reported most often in elderly people (www.vh.org/adult/patient/ophthalmology/iih/diamox.html). Acetazolamide treatment may cause dangerous electrolyte imbalances, including hyponatremia (low sodium) and hypokalemia (low potassium), as well as metabolic acidosis. Particular caution is recommended in athletes with impaired renal function (including elderly patients or athletes, patients with diabetes mellitus, and patients with lung disease).

Caution is advised for athletes receiving concomitant salicylate (aspirin) and acetazolamide, as severe toxicity has been reported. Studies showed that the renal clearance of acetazolamide was significantly reduced with chronic aspirin use. Salicylate appears to inhibit renal secretion of the acetazolamide and may produce serious metabolic acidosis (www.medsafe.govt.nz/Profs/Datasheet/d/Diamoxtabinj.htm).

Beta-2 Agonists

Beta-2 agonists act by relaxing muscles in the airways to improve breathing and reduce bronchospasm (wheezing, shortness of breath) associated with reversible obstructive airway disease such as asthma. Beta-2 agonists (e.g., albuterol/Ventolin, salmeterol) are potentially anabolic, which is why their systemic use is banned in sport. They are legal only in the inhaled form for exercise-induced asthma with proper documentation and exemption forms. In a three-week study of a slow-release oral form of albuterol, voluntary strength of young men appeared to increase significantly (Martineau et al., 1992). However, in two other studies, long-acting inhaled salmeterol had no ergogenic effect on maximal or endurance cycling in asthmatic men, or on anaerobic cycling or peak leg torque in nonasthmatic men (Robertson et al., 1994; Morton et al., 1996). Whether the legal inhaled form of albuterol is ergogenic remains controversial. The weight of the evidence suggests that single doses of albuterol are not ergogenic for asthmatic or nonasthmatic athletes, but further study is required.

Certain masters athletes may be afflicted with chronic obstructive pulmonary disease (COPD), emphysema, or asthma, all requiring the use of a beta-2 agonist. Although use may be approved for these athletes, the potential for abuse still exists.

Beta-2 agonists, like other sympathomimetic agents, can cause adverse reactions such as tremors, flushing, restlessness, sweating, and anxiety, as well as important cardiovascular side effects such as increased heart rate, palpitations, hypertension, and angina or chest pain. If used in excess, beta-2 agonists may precipitate or mask a potential life-threatening cardiac event, especially in senior athletes.

Dietary Supplementation and Ergogenics

The use of nutritional products in attempts to increase athletic performance has become so widespread that it is important to provide a review of the latest evidence. Ergogenic aids are substances, strategies, or treatments that are theoretically designed to improve physical performance above and beyond the effects of normal training. Some ergogenic aids are used during training to enhance the effect on performance over time, while others are used just prior to or during the event to provide an immediate competitive edge. Caution is advised with the use of any nutritional ergogenic in an attempt to enhance sport performance, and individuals should consult a sport nutrition expert or physician before commencing such use.

Vitamin Supplementation

Nutritional needs of the older athlete are complex and must be viewed in relation to the basic physiologic requirements of aging and exercise as well as the reduction of chronic disease risk factors (for more information on this topic, see chapters 5 and 6). The elderly athlete has certain elevated nutritional needs compared to younger athletes, but these must be balanced with the promotion of weight management. The current dietary recommendations for elderly people include the following for macronutrients: 60% to 65% carbohydrate, 10% to 20% protein, and <30% fat. Recent dietary recommendations promote reducing fat in the diet and increasing fiber. It appears that greater amounts of protein are required with aging in order to maintain lean body mass. Protein shakes can help meet the higher demands, and most meal replacement drinks are well-balanced liquid meals with an ample supply of vitamins and minerals, varying amounts of carbohydrate and fat, and a increased protein content. Masters athletes can choose from a multitude of protein-packed liquid meals, some having up to 40 g of protein per serving (Maharam et al., 1999).

When one is making nutrition recommendations to the exercising elderly population, research suggests that four important areas should be taken into consideration:

- The changing needs that occur with age
- The changing needs that occur with exercise
- The presence of chronic illness or disease
- The level of competition

It has been reported that the nutrients for which food consumption is often inadequate and that have the largest impact on the exercising elderly population include vitamin B_6, vitamin B_{12}, calcium, and vitamin D. When adequate dietary intakes cannot be obtained, supplementation with a multivitamin is recommended (see table 11.3 and Sacheck and Roubenoff, 1999).

Adequate fluid replacement to avoid the dangers of dehydration is essential for all athletes. There is evidence for the effectiveness of 4% to 10% carbohydrate-containing sport drinks for older athletes competing in high-intensity endurance exercise. Many commercial sport drinks exist in an assortment of flavors, containing varying ingredients and electrolyte quantities. Consulting a registered dietitian may be helpful and provide guidance for many masters athletes (Rock, 1991).

Caffeine

Caffeine is the most frequently consumed drug in the world, and athletes often use it as an ergogenic aid. A familiar substance in the diet of most athletes, caffeine appears in energy drinks, sport gels, and diet

TABLE 11.3 **U.S. Government Guidelines for Vitamin and Mineral Intake for Adults Aged 51 Years and Older**

Micronutrient	Males	Females
Retinol/Vit A (mcg/RE/day)	1,000	800
Cholecalciferol/Vit D3 (mcg/day)	5	5
Tocopherol/Vit E (mg/TE/day)	10	8
Phylloquinone/Vit K (mcg/day)	80	65
Ascorbic acid/Vit C (mg/day)	60	60
Thiamin/Vit B1 (mg/day)	1.2	1.0
Riboflavin/Vit B2 (mg/day)	1.4	1.2
Nicotinic acid/Vit B3 (mg/day)	1.5	1.3
Pyridoxine/Vit B6 (mg/day)	2.0	1.6
Folic acid (mg/day)	200	180
Cyanocobalamin/Vit B12 (mg/day)	2.0	2.0
Calcium (mg/day)	800	800
Phosphorus (mg/day)	800	800
Magnesium (mg/day)	350	280
Iron (mg/day)	10	10
Zinc (mg/day)	15	12
Iodide (mg/day)	150	150
Selenium (mg/day)	70	55

RE = retinol equivalents; TE = tocopherol equivalents.

Reprinted, by permission, from L.G. Maharam et al., 1999, "Masters Athletes: Factors Affecting Performance," *Sports Medicine* 28: 273-285.

aids. Caffeine was recently removed from the World Antidoping Agency (WADA) 2007 list of prohibited substances.

Recent research suggests that caffeine can enhance performance of a 20 min swim, a 100 m swim trial, a 1,500 m treadmill run, and brief bursts of all out cycling (Graham and Spriet, 1996). The mechanism by which caffeine elicits its ergogenic effects are unknown, but the popular theory is that it increases plasma free fatty acid levels and muscle triglyceride use to enhance fat oxidation while sparing muscle glycogen use early in exercise. Another study examined the effects of a high caffeine dose on endurance performance, and the results indicated that caffeine ingestion before exercise decreased muscle glycogenolysis by approximately 55% over the first 15 min of exercise (Spriet et al., 1992). This effect may account for the prolonged time to exhaustion with caffeine ingestion, but it is an incomplete explanation.

There is debate about whether the effects are a direct result of caffeine itself or its metabolites (e.g., dimethylxanthines). Caffeine may act by stimulating epinephrine release, or possibly influence neurotransmitter function (e.g., dopamine or norepinephrine). Caffeine improves concentration, enhances alertness or mental awareness, and reduces the perception of fatigue, such that time to exhaustion in endurance activities is increased (Schwenk and Costley, 2002). Caffeine is a relatively safe ergogenic aid and has no known negative performance effects, nor does it cause significant dehydration or electrolyte imbalance during exercise (Paluska, 2003). Routine caffeine consumption may cause tolerance or dependence, and abrupt discontinuation produces irritability, mood shifts, headache, drowsiness, or fatigue. Caffeine does increase an athlete's heart rate, and there have been instances in which older athletes have suffered heart attacks from abuse of this drug. Elderly athletes need to be cautious when introducing any type of sympathomimetic agent into their training regime, especially if there is a history of heart disease (Eichner, 1997).

Creatine

Creatine supplementation has become tremendously popular, in recent years, as athletes take it to "bulk up" their muscles. Creatine supplementation is a legal practice and was first used by British sprinters and hurdlers in the 1992 Olympics. Creatine has been claimed to increase muscle strength and delay fatigue, allowing athletes to train harder and achieve muscle gains beyond normal capacities. Creatine monohydrate plays a role in cellular energy metabolism (figure 11.5) and potentially has a role in protein metabolism. People ingest roughly 1 g of creatine per day naturally from eating a regular, mixed diet. Muscles take up the majority of the creatine, where it is converted to phosphocreatine (PCr), which is necessary for adenosine triphosphate (ATP) production. Creatine monohydrate supplementation increases PCr levels in muscle, especially when accompanied by exercise or carbohydrate intake (see figure 11.6, and Green et al., 1996). During brief, intense, anaerobic

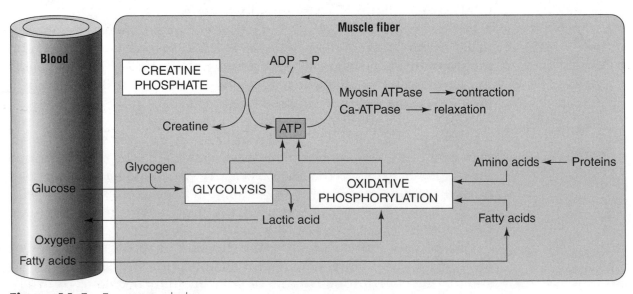

Figure 11.5 Energy metabolism.

From A.S. Vander, J.H. Sherman, and D.S. Luciano, 1998, *Human physiology: Mechanisms of body function*, 7th ed. (New York: McGraw-Hill Companies), 313. Adapted by permission of The McGraw-Hill Companies.

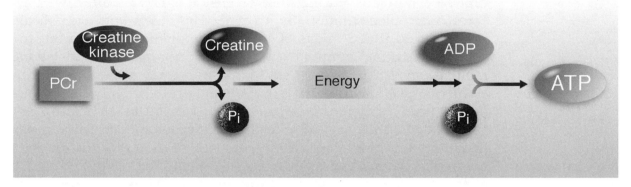

Figure 11.6 The production of energy in the body.

Reprinted, by permission, from J. Wilmore and D. Costill, 2003, *Physiology of sport and exercise*, 3rd ed. (Champaign, IL: Human Kinetics), 123

actions, creatine phosphate regenerates ATP to provide the energy necessary for muscle contraction. The aim of supplemental creatine is to increase resting levels of creatine phosphate so as to regenerate more ATP and sustain a high-power output, thus delaying fatigue and improving performance. Creatine stores vary greatly among individuals; and apart from diet, the reasons are unclear. Athletes with low stores may be most apt to benefit from supplementation (Gaie, 1996). Creatine supplementation does not benefit aerobic performance, such as long-distance running; and perhaps because of the associated weight gain, it may actually inhibit distance running times (Balsom et al., 1993).

Several studies show that creatine supplementation significantly enhances the ability to produce higher muscular force or power output (or both) during short bouts of maximal exercise in healthy young adults. This translates into improvements in exercise performance in events that require explosive, high-energy output of a repeated nature such as weightlifting, sprinting, football, and rowing (Terjung et al., 2000). Most controlled studies have shown that 20 g per day of creatine monohydrate, taken for five to six days by sedentary or moderately active people, is sufficient to initiate improvements in performance and delay muscle fatigue during short-duration, high-intensity exercise (Toler, 1997; Greenhaff, 1997; Greenhaff et al., 1993).

One of the most debilitating symptoms of aging is a loss of muscle strength and consequently independence. One cause of this muscle degeneration is a reduced level of creatine in aging muscles. For reasons that are unknown, muscular PCr levels decline with age after the fifth decade. Creatine monohydrate supplementation has been shown to increase skeletal muscle PCr concentration, increase fat-free mass, and enhance high-intensity exercise performance in young healthy individuals.

Very few studies employing short-term creatine supplementation have involved older individuals. In one study, four subjects (mean age of 58 years) exhibited increased muscle PCr concentrations and improved time to exhaustion during knee extension exercises after five days of creatine supplementation (Smith et al., 1998). Rawson and colleagues (1999) found that 30 days of creatine supplementation in 60- to 82-year-old men had minimal effect on performance and showed either no or a small (0.5 kg, or 1 lb) increase in body mass. Furthermore, eight weeks of creatine ingestion demonstrated no changes in lower limb volume, body mass, or percentage body fat in 32 healthy elderly subjects who took part in an eight-week resistance training program (Bermon et al., 1998). Creatine supplementation did not induce any additional strength gains or resistance to fatigue compared to values in the group with resistance training alone. Thus, the weight of the data reported, to date, suggests that older subjects do not respond to creatine supplementation to the same extent as young subjects. Elderly people appear to gain only minimal, if any, exercise performance benefits from creatine supplementation. Tarnopolsky (2000), one of the leading researchers in creatine supplementation in the elderly population, states that future studies will be required to address the potential for creatine monohydrate supplementation to attenuate age-related muscle atrophy and strength loss.

Supplementing creatine in the correct dosage and duration can aid in improving anaerobic performance in masters athletes. In the loading method, 20 g per day of creatine is taken for five to six days. To maintain muscle creatine levels after this loading period, 2 to 10 g per day is effective (Vandenberghe et al., 1997). In another method, 3 g per day of creatine monohydrate is taken over an extended *training* period of at least four weeks, during which muscle creatine levels rise more slowly, eventually reaching levels similar to those achieved with the loading method (Hultman et al., 1996).

Creatine is available commercially but is classified as a nutritional supplement, so purity and safety are not assured. As with any nutraceutical preparation, it is not subject to a certification process such as that conducted by the Food and Drug Administration (FDA). Little is known about the long-term side effects of creatine, but no consistent toxicity has been reported (Poortmans and Francaux, 2000). Some observers believe high doses of creatine promote dehydration and possibly muscle cramping. Creatine is metabolized in the kidneys and degraded to creatinine and eliminated in the urine. Uncertainty remains about the potential long-term effects on the kidneys. It is recommended that any elderly person who elects to take creatine have his or her renal function measured periodically. People who currently suffer from renal disease should not start taking creatine (Gaie, 1996; http://healthlink.mcw.edu/article/969991656.html).

Glucosamine and Chondroitin

Glucosamine sulfate and chondroitin sulfate do not tend to be abused in the traditional sense, but many elderly athletes with arthritis take these over-the-counter supplements and should be aware of the associated risks. Dietary supplements do not fall under the same rigorous and strict standards that traditional medications do and are not tested or analyzed by the FDA before they are sold to consumers. This means that consumers cannot be sure they are getting what they pay for. In fact, a recent study by ConsumerLab.com showed that almost half of the glucosamine/chondroitin supplements tested did not contain the labeled amounts of ingredients (http://orthoinfo.aaos. org). Masters athletes should ask their health care provider and their pharmacist for suggestions on which brand they believe to have the highest-quality product to ensure they do not consume substances from the banned list.

Glucosamine sulfate and chondroitin sulfate are naturally occurring substances found in the connective tissues of the body, including the hyaline cartilage that covers the ends of bones in the joints.

The primary role of glucosamine sulfate in ceasing or reversing joint degeneration appears to be related to its ability to function as the primary building block for glycosaminoglycans and the hyaluronic acid backbone needed for the formation of proteoglycans found in joints. Proteoglycans are large molecules in cartilage that give it viscoelastic (buffering) properties. There is no direct evidence that such repair or protection occurs in vivo, or that the use of glucosamine sulfate changes articular cartilage either structurally or functionally. Several placebo-controlled studies showed that, irrespective of any structural or biochemical change in articular cartilage, oral glucosamine sulfate supplementation results in substantial functional improvement in patients with osteoarthritis (Leffler et al., 1999). Glucosamine sulfate has also been shown to have unique anti-inflammatory effects.

Chondroitin sulfate is also associated with the proteoglycans found naturally in articular cartilage and associated structures that give cartilage elasticity and resiliency. The proposed mechanism of action is the stimulation of chondrocytes to replace or repair damaged proteoglycans in the joint matrix. Past studies show that some people with mild to moderate osteoarthritis taking either glucosamine or chondroitin sulfate reported pain relief at a level similar to that with NSAIDs, such as aspirin and ibuprofen. The difference is that NSAIDs carry an increased risk of side effects while the joint supplements have few side effects, and thus their use would be preferred if the effects of pain reduction were indeed the same (Muller-Fassbender et al., 1994). Some research indicates that the supplements might also slow cartilage damage in people with osteoarthritis (Morreale et al., 1996). Chondroitin sulfate has been studied much less extensively than glucosamine, but early results show that it also seems to work as an anti-inflammatory and reduces pain.

The combined use of glucosamine sulfate and chondroitin sulfate in the treatment of degenerative joint disease has become an extremely popular supplementation protocol in arthritic conditions of the joints. Although glucosamine and chondroitin are often administered together, no information is available to demonstrate that the combination produces better results than glucosamine alone (Kelly, 1998). Supplementation of both glucosamine and chondroitin is recommended in what are essentially megadoses compared with their natural occurrence, roughly 1,500 mg/day for glucosamine and 1,200 mg/day for chondroitin. Many over-the-counter preparations combine the two, despite a lack of evidence of enhanced benefit, that is, 500 mg glucosamine and 400 mg chondroitin to be taken three times daily. Oral supplementation is well tolerated with infrequent, mild side effects reported (Schwenk and Costley, 2002).

This is not likely to be a drug of abuse in elderly athletes and may in fact be a safe and effective way to avert osteoarthritic pain and suffering that may prevent an athlete from competing.

Summary

Every health professional working with older competitive athletes should, at a minimum, be familiar with the following facts:

- Drug use is a major problem facing sports today.
- Taking performance-enhancing drugs, or "doping," has a long history in sport.
- The elderly athlete has certain elevated nutritional needs over younger athletes.
- Estrogen in women may prevent osteoporosis, maintain physical vitality, treat postmenopausal symptoms, and reduce depression; but certain HRT drugs are banned.
- High doses of testosterone, especially when combined with strength training, increase fat-free mass, muscle size, and strength in men.
- Performance-enhancing drugs can have a deleterious effect on the prostate.
- Anabolic steroids can cause an unhealthy cholesterol profile, heart attack, stroke, liver failure, and type 2 diabetes.
- HGH can cause hypertension, pedal edema, carpal tunnel syndrome, and a prediabetic condition.
- Deaths have occurred with amphetamine use when people undertook maximal physical activity.
- Beta-2 agonists are legal only in inhaled form, for exercise-induced asthma.

- Caffeine causes increased alertness, shortened reaction time, and improved concentration.
- Older athletes do not respond to creatine supplementation to the same extent as young athletes.
- Erythropoietin has allegedly become widespread among people engaged in endurance sports.
- Prescription painkillers are the most common opioid misused by athletes.
- NSAIDs can cause gastrointestinal toxicity, renal failure, and modest worsening of underlying hypertension or congestive heart failure.
- Glucosamine and chondroitin may be safe and effective drugs for avoiding osteoarthritic pain.
- Acetazolamide has become popular among high-altitude athletes for preventing altitude sickness.
- Master athletes should be screened for hypertension and given appropriate therapy, keeping in mind that sports regulatory bodies have banned the use of many antihypertensives.

But these facts must also be put into the larger context of the potential abuse of performance-enhancing drugs by older athletes and the problem of unintentionally gaining advantage over competitors through the use of medications necessary for conditions that have developed with age.

Since the beginning of athletic competition, athletes have abused performance-enhancing drugs. The growing problem of doping in amateur sport is fast becoming a public health issue. Although today's athletes face being stripped of their medals or banned from their sports if they are caught doping, the "win at all costs" mentality drives them to continue to risk all for victory. Use of drugs is contrary to the rules and ethical principles of athletic competition. It is doleful and frustrating that these individuals reject the standards of fair play and safe, healthy training habits.

Many performance-enhancing drugs are potentially hazardous, and it is important for athletes to understand the full extent of the dangers. Without question, health risks are involved in the self-administration of any prescription medicine, particularly in the absence of a physician's advice with respect to dosages and duration of use. Further, without regular monitoring by a doctor, some side effects may go unnoticed or untreated until it is too late. However, for masters athletes it is also dangerous to avoid taking prescription medication for the purpose of competition. When the ultimate goal of the athlete is to win at any cost, those costs may be greater than the athlete realizes. Where to draw the line between performance-enhancing drugs and life-enhancing medications has been an ongoing battle in the world of masters athletics. The current controversy is this: Should there be a move to modify the list of prohibited substances, or should the zero-tolerance system be maintained? It is becoming popular opinion that, although most favor the testing of masters athletes, the list of prohibited substances must be rewritten to take into account the health differences that exist in the aging athlete.

There are multiple factors influencing elderly athletes to abuse drugs. It is important to educate athletes on the health risks associated with drug use and to establish effective and appropriate policy, rules, and guidelines that target the prevention and reduction of substance use among athletes. Programs are in place to address and deter use through testing and discipline. Though many programs have instituted drug screening, they are often too narrow to catch many drugs or are unable to keep up with innovations in performance-enhancing drugs. Community attitudes and expectations of success compound the problem.

Collaboration is needed between the sporting community and governing bodies in order to standardize antidoping policies and practices at an international level so athletes stop viewing drugs as essential for success.

Questions to Consider

1. Discuss some reasons why elderly athletes would take drugs to enhance performance.

2. Describe some of the benefits of hormone replacement therapy in elderly men and women.

3. Describe some of the side effects of taking anabolic steroids.

4. What would be your recommendation to an elderly athlete interested in taking human growth hormone to enhance performance?

5. List the important risk factors for hypertension in physically active elderly athletes.

6. Discuss the dangers associated with masters athletes stopping the use of certain medications for the purpose of competition, and possible solutions.

7. Which nutrients are often found to be inadequate in the diet and have the largest impact on the exercising elderly population?

8. Discuss the use of nutraceuticals in the elderly athlete.

9. Do you think masters athletes gain an unfair advantage if they are using drugs to improve their performance?

10. What do you feel would be a suitable punishment for masters athletes caught taking drugs?

appendix a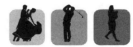

Web Resources

*Canada's Physical Activity Guide to Healthy Active Living
for Older Adults*
www.paguide.com

Canadian Society for Exercise Physiology
www.csep.ca

Health Canada
www.hc-sc.gc.ca

*International Curriculum Guidelines for Preparing Physical Activity
Instructors of Older Adults*
www.ISAPA.org

My Pyramid
www.mypyramid.gov

National Institute of Aging
www.nia.nih.gov

Using the Food Guide
www.hc-sc.gc.ca/nutrition

appendix b

Forms

Appendix B contains several internationally recognized and accepted tests to screen, assess, and test elderly subjects. Some of the tests are difficult to locate, as they are published in manuals produced by local organizations and associations. PAR-Q and You, the Three-Day Nutritional Assessment, and Determine Your Nutritional Health may be filled out by clients who do not need assistance to do so. The other forms should be filled out by the fitness or medical professional as they interview the client or patient or review that individual's results on other tests. The instructions on the forms are self-explanatory. The forms will be useful not only for fitness professionals, but also for students carrying out research projects for classes.

The Par-Q & You and the PARmed-X forms are widely recognized in the fitness field. The Health History and Activity Questionnaire and the Three-Day Nutritional Assessment form were both developed at the Canadian Centre for Activity and Aging (CCAA). The latter is jointly owned by Dr. Shanthi Jacob-Johnson. The Client Report Form was produced by A.W. Taylor and M. Johnson in conjunction with staff members at the CCAA. It is a useful format for compiling and interpreting the results of several tests as well as for developing individualized physical activity and nutrition recommendations based on those results. The Determine Your Nutritional Health form may be given to clients or patients whose nutritional status is questionable. This form is a self-assessment that may alert older persons (or enable them to accept it) when they should seek help regarding their nutritional circumstances and conditions. Although the results of the Yale Physical Activity Survey for Older Adults and the Timed Up and Go Test are required to complete the Client Report Form, we have included space for these results in the Client Report Form, but we have not included those actual forms in this appendix because they have been widely published elsewhere and are easily available to health professions. We strongly suggest using these tests: there are good reasons why they are the two most used activity surveys in North America.

All the forms in this appendix may be photocopied by readers for use with their clients, patients, or research subjects. They are as follows:

- Health History and Activity Questionnaire
- Medical Clearance by Personal Physician
- Three-Day Nutritional Assessment
- Client Report Form
- Daily Food Diaries
- Determine Your Nutritional Health
- Physical Activities Readiness Questionnaire (PAR-Q & You)
- Physical Activity Readiness Medical Examination (PARmed-X)

Health History and Activity Questionnaire

1. Date _____

   Name: _____

   Address: _____ City: _____ State: _____ Zip: _____

   Home phone #: _____ Sex: Male _____ Female _____

   Age: _____ Date of birth: _____ Height: _____ Weight: _____

   Highest level of education completed: _____ Ethnicity: _____

   Whom to contact in case of emergency: _____ Phone #: _____

   Name of your physician: _____ Phone #: _____

2. Have you ever been diagnosed as having any of the following symptoms or conditions?

	Yes (✓)	Year it began (approximate)
Heart attack		
Transient ischemic attack		
Angina (chest pain)		
Stroke		
Peripheral vascular disease		
Heart surgery		
High blood pressure		
High cholesterol		
Diabetes		
Respiratory disease		
Osteoporosis		
Joint replacement (site: _____)		
Cancer (type: _____)		
Cognitive disorder (type: _____)		
Neuropathies (problems with sensations)		

	Yes (✓)	Year it began (approximate)
Parkinson's disease		
Multiple sclerosis		
Polio or postpolio syndrome		
Epilepsy or seizures		
Other neurological conditions		
Rheumatoid arthritis		
Other arthritic conditions		
Visual or depth perception problems		
Inner ear problems or recurrent ear infections		
Cerebellar problems (ataxia)		
Other movement disorders		
Chemical dependency (alcohol or drugs)		
Depression		

   Please describe any other health concerns:

   _____

   _____

3. Do you currently have a medical condition that might limit your physical performance?

   Yes ___ No ___ If YES, please describe the condition(s): _____

   _____

4. Do you have a pacemaker?

   Yes ___ No ___ Does it automatically resuscitate?

From A.W. Taylor and M.J. Johnson, 2008, *Physiology of Exercise and Healthy Aging* (Champaign, IL: Human Kinetics). Reprinted, by permission, from the CCAA (Canadian Centre for Activity and Aging).

5. Do you currently suffer any of the following symptoms in your legs or feet?

Yes (✓)

Numbness ____

Tingling ____

Arthritis ____

Swelling ____

6. Do you currently have any medical conditions for which you see a physician regularly?

Yes ___ No ___ If YES, please describe the condition(s): _____

_____

_____

7. Have you required emergency medical care or hospitalization in the last **three years?**

Yes ___ No ___ If YES, please state when this occurred and briefly explain why:

_____

_____

8. In general, how depressed have you felt within the past four weeks?

Not at all ___ Slightly ___ Moderately ___ Quite a bit ___ Extremely ___

9. Do you require eyeglasses? Yes ___ No ___

10. Do you require hearing aids? Yes ___ No ___

11. Do you use an assistive device for walking? Yes ___ No ___ Sometimes ___ Type: _____

_____

12. How would you describe your health?

Excellent ____ Very good ____ Good ____ Fair ____ Poor ____

13. Have you had a close relative who had a heart attack before age 55 (father or brother) or before age 65 (mother or sister)?

Yes ___ No ___ If YES, who and at what age: _____

_____

14. List the prescription medications that you currently take (by exact name or by type):

Type of medication

_____

_____

_____

_____

_____

For what condition

_____

_____

_____

_____

From A.W. Taylor and M.J. Johnson, 2008, *Physiology of Exercise and Healthy Aging* (Champaign, IL: Human Kinetics). Reprinted, by permission, from the CCAA (Canadian Centre for Activity and Aging).

15. Do you currently smoke cigarettes? Yes ___ No ___

Number smoked on an average day: _____

If NO, have you ever smoked? Yes ___ No ___ How many years? _____

How many years since you stopped? _____

Number formerly smoked an average day: _____

16. In the past four weeks, to what extent did health problems limit your everyday physical activities (such as walking and household chores)?

Not at all ___ Slightly ___ Moderately ___ Quite a bit ___ Extremely ___

17. How many times have you fallen **within the past year?** _____

Did you require medical treatment? Yes ___ No ___

If you have fallen once or more in the past year, please list the approximate date of the fall, the medical treatment required, and the reason you fell **in each case** (e.g., uneven surface, going down stairs): _____

_____

18. Have you ever had any condition or suffered any injury that has affected your balance or ability to walk without assistance?

Yes ___ No ___ If YES, please list when this occurred and briefly explain the condition or injury:

_____

_____

19. Are you **worried** about falling? (Circle approximate number.)

1	2	3 4	5	6 7
Not at all	A little	Moderately	Very	Extremely

20. In general, do you currently require household or nursing assistance to carry out daily activities? Yes ___ No ___ If YES, please check the reasons:

a. Health problems ___

b. Chronic pain ___

c. Lack of strength or endurance ___

d. Lack of flexibility or balance ___

e. Other reasons: _____

21. In a typical week, how often do you leave your house (to run errands or go to work, meetings, classes, church, social functions, etc.)?

_____ less than once a week   _____ 3-4 times a week

_____ 1-2 times a week   _____ almost every day

22. Please indicate your ability to do each of the following. (Circle appropriate response.)*

	Can do	Can do with difficulty or with help	Cannot do
a. Take care of own personal needs, such as dressing yourself	2	1	0
b. Bathe yourself, using tub or shower	2	1	0
c. Climb up and down a flight of stairs (e.g., to a second story in a house)	2	1	0
d. Walk outside one or two blocks	2	1	0
e. Do light household activities, such as cooking, dusting, washing dishes, sweeping a walkway	2	1	0
f. Do own shopping for groceries or clothes	2	1	0
g. Walk 1/2 mile (6-7 blocks, 0.8 kilometers)	2	1	0
h. Walk 1 mile (12-14 blocks, 1.6 kilometers)	2	1	0
i. Lift and carry 10 pounds (4.5 kilograms, a full bag of groceries)	2	1	0
j. Lift and carry 25 pounds (11.3 kilograms, a medium to large suitcase)	2	1	0
k. Do most heavy household chores, such as scrubbing floors, vacuuming, raking leaves	2	1	0
l. Do *strenuous* activities, such as hiking, digging in garden, moving heavy objects, bicycling, aerobic dance exercises, strenuous calisthenics.	2	1	0

*Composite Physical Function Scale (Rikli and Jones, 1998).

23. Do you currently participate in regular physical activity (such as walking, jogging, sports, exercise classes, housework, yard work) that is strenuous enough to cause a noticeable increase in breathing, heart rate, or perspiration? Yes ___ No ___ If YES, how many days per week? (Circle appropriate number.)   1   2   3   4   5   6   7

24. Do you go for walks on a regular basis? Yes ___ No ___ If YES, how many times per week on average? _____

How many minutes at a time usually? _____

How far do you usually walk? _____

25. When you go for walks (if you do), which of the following best describes your usual pace:

Strolling (easy pace, takes 30 minutes or more to walk a mile [1.6 kilometers]) _____

Average or normal (can walk a mile [1.6 kilometers] in 20-30 minutes) _____

Fairly brisk (fast pace, can walk a mile [1.6 kilometers] in 15-20 minutes) _____

Do not go for walks on a regular basis _____

26. Please list all other types of exercise activities (other than walking) that you usually do each week. Include activities such as exercise, light or heavy housework or yard work, and so on. Think through the past week (or a typical week in the past month); list **only** your **regular** physical activities.

Activity	Number of days per week	Number of minutes or hours per day

27. What is your current occupational status?

Working _____   Semi-retired _____   Retired/Not working _____

From A.W. Taylor and M.J. Johnson, 2008, *Physiology of Exercise and Healthy Aging* (Champaign, IL: Human Kinetics). Reprinted, by permission, from the CCAA (Canadian Centre for Activity and Aging).

28. What have been your major occupations? How long were you in each occupation? How would you describe the physical demands of these jobs?

Occupations	From (age)	To (age)	Mostly sedentary	Light exercise	Moderate exercise	Heavy labor

29. In general, how would you rate the quality of your life? (Circle appropriate number.)

1	2	3 4	5	6	7
Very low	Low	Moderate		High	Very high

30. Did you require assistance in completing this form?

None (or very little) _____   Needed quite a bit of help _____

Reason: _____

Thank you!

From A.W. Taylor and M.J. Johnson, 2008, *Physiology of Exercise and Healthy Aging* (Champaign, IL: Human Kinetics). Reprinted, by permission, from the CCAA (Canadian Centre for Activity and Aging).

Medical Clearance by Personal Physician

Your patient, _____, has expressed an interest in participating in one of the programs offered by _____. We would appreciate your medical opinion and recommendations concerning this individual's participation in exercise. If you feel that this person might benefit from participation in the program, we would also greatly appreciate your endorsement of his or her participation.

Assessments: The program participants are required to complete a medical and activity questionnaire, followed by a series of functional fitness assessments. This is done to identify weaknesses in physical parameters associated with activities of daily living and to more effectively prescribe appropriate exercise.

Physical Parameters	Assessments	Approval	
Cardiovascular	Two-minute step-in-place	Yes	No
	Six-minute walk	Yes	No
Muscular strength and endurance	30-second chair stand	Yes	No
	30-second arm curl	Yes	No
Flexibility	Chair sit-and-reach	Yes	No
	Back scratch	Yes	No
Balance and gait	8-foot (2.4-meter) up-and-go	Yes	No
	50-foot (15.2-meter walking speed)	Yes	No

Exercise program description:

_____

_____

_____

_____

_____

_____

Exercise class approval: Yes ___ No ___

Please list any modifications or comments for testing and exercise class: _____

_____

Patient's last blood pressure reading: ____/____

Please indicate by your signature below that your patient is medically cleared to participate in the specific testing and training described. Please call _____ at _____ if you have any questions concerning the program.

Signature of physician	Print name of physician	Date

Physician's phone #: _____

From A.W. Taylor and M.J. Johnson, 2008, *Physiology of Exercise and Healthy Aging* (Champaign, IL: Human Kinetics). Client Report

Client Report

Kinesiologist: _____ Date: _____

General Client Information

Client name: _____

Date of birth: _____ (month/day/year)

Height (cm): _____ Weight (kg): _____

Dominant leg: __ Right __ Left

Ambulatory aid: __ Yes __ No Description: _____

Notes:

Medical History

Has the client had:	Yes (✓)	No (✓)
Arthritis		
Asthma or hay fever		
Cancer		
Chronic lung disease		
Convulsions		
Diabetes		
Heart disease		
High blood pressure		
Kidney disease		
Nervous or mental disease		
Rheumatic fever		
Stomach or intestinal trouble		
Thyroid disorder		
Tuberculosis		
A learning disability		
Does the client's medical history include:	**Yes (✓)**	**No (✓)**
Back problems		
Eye defect		
Hearing defect		
Reason for limited physical activity		
Add details pertaining to any "YES" answers:		

From A.W. Taylor and M.J. Johnson, 2008, *Physiology of Exercise and Healthy Aging* (Champaign, IL: Human Kinetics).

Fall History

Has the client ever fallen?   Yes ___   No ___

When did the falls occur (month/year)?   1. _____   Cause: _____

2. _____   Cause: _____

3. _____   Cause: _____

Injuries from falls: _____

_____

_____

_____

Fracture History

Has the client had a recent fracture?   Yes ___   No ___

Record age for fractures of hip, knee, ankle, vertebrae, ribs, or other:

Hip: L _____   Knee: L _____   Ankle: L _____

R _____   R _____   R _____

Vertebrae: Level _____   Ribs: _____

Other: _____

Notes:

Medications

List all medications, vitamins, minerals, over-the-counter products, health food store preparations, and prescribed medicines that the client is currently taking:

Name   *Dosage*   *Year started*

1. _____   _____   _____

2. _____   _____   _____

3. _____   _____   _____

4. _____   _____   _____

5. _____   _____   _____

Notes and/or additional medications:

From A.W. Taylor and M.J. Johnson, 2008, *Physiology of Exercise and Healthy Aging* (Champaign, IL: Human Kinetics).

Yale Physical Activity Survey for Older Adults Results

Activity checklist   *Expenditure (total hours/wk × intensity code)*

Work   _____

Yard work   _____

Caretaking   _____

Exercise   _____

Recreational activities   _____

Sum: _____

Activity dimensions:

Vigorous activity index score   _____

Leisurely walking index score   _____

Moving index score   _____

Standing index score   _____

Sitting index score   _____

Sum of activity dimensions: _____

Seasonal adjustment score: _____

Notes:

Timed Up & Go Results

Chair seat height (cm): _____   Trial #1 (s): _____

Gait aid (specify): _____   Trial #2 (s): _____

Floor surface: _____   Trial #3 (s): _____

                                        Average (s): _____

Group 1 (0-9 s)   __

Group 2 (10-19 s)   __

Group 3 (20-29 s)   __

Notes:

From A.W. Taylor and M.J. Johnson, 2008, *Physiology of Exercise and Healthy Aging* (Champaign, IL: Human Kinetics).

Three-Day Nutritional Assessment Results

Daily food group servings

	Day 1	Day 2	Day 3	Average
Grain products	____	____	____	____
Vegetables and fruit	____	____	____	____
Milk products	____	____	____	____
Meat and alternatives	____	____	____	____

Notes:

General Health

Observations:

Recommendations:

Mobility

Observations:

Recommendations:

Physical Activity

Observations:

Recommendations:

From A.W. Taylor and M.J. Johnson, 2008, *Physiology of Exercise and Healthy Aging* (Champaign, IL: Human Kinetics). Meal Diary

Nutrition

Observations:

Recommendations:

Exercise Prescription

Aerobic

Recommendations:

Considerations:

Strength

Recommendations:

Considerations:

Flexibility

Recommendations:

Considerations:

Concluding Remarks (up to four pages):

From A.W. Taylor and M.J. Johnson, 2008, *Physiology of Exercise and Healthy Aging* (Champaign, IL: Human Kinetics). Meal Diary

Meal Diary

Food Record Instructions

1. Use the record sheets to track two weekdays and one weekend day. This gives us a better idea of the overall diet.

2. This record is used to get an accurate representation of your usual daily intake. It is very important that you do not alter what you eat in order to change the outcome in any way. Please try to weigh and record every item that you consume (this includes all beverages, condiments, vitamins, etc.).

3. Be sure to weigh and record all items taken in; this means any snacks, however small, also any condiments or toppings added to items. Often these items are consumed unpredictably, so remember that it is vital that the scale and food record are with you at all times.

4. It is important to assess the serving sizes as accurately as possible, thus, whenever it is feasible, measure the item after it has been cooked. Always weigh food items immediately prior to consumption. If possible, also record information from food packages (brand names).

5. If items are to be cooked, be sure to describe the cooking method, for example, barbequed chicken, fried fish, braised beef. The "notes" column may also be useful for this.

6. All beverages should also be included; this includes water, coffee, tea, etc. Be sure to record any cream, milk, or sugar added to coffee or tea.

From A.W. Taylor and M.J. Johnson, 2008, *Physiology of Exercise and Healthy Aging* (Champaign, IL: Human Kinetics) Reprinted, by permission, from Canadian Centre for Activity and Aging, 1998.

Food Diary

Day One

Meal	Food item	Amount
Breakfast		
Snack		
Lunch		
Snack		
Dinner		
Snack		

Day Two

Meal	Food item	Amount
Breakfast		
Snack		
Lunch		
Snack		
Dinner		
Snack		

From A.W. Taylor and M.J. Johnson, 2008, *Physiology of Exercise and Healthy Aging* (Champaign, IL: Human Kinetics).

Day Three

Meal	Food item	Amount
Breakfast		
Snack		
Lunch		
Snack		
Dinner		
Snack		

From A.W. Taylor and M.J. Johnson, 2008, *Physiology of Exercise and Healthy Aging* (Champaign, IL: Human Kinetics).

The Warning Signs of poor nutritional health are often overlooked. Use this Checklist to find out if you or someone you know is at nutritional risk.

Read the statements below. Circle the number in the "yes" column for those that apply to you or someone you know. For each "yes" answer, score the number in the box. Total your nutritional score.

DETERMINE YOUR NUTRITIONAL HEALTH

	YES
I have an illness or condition that made me change the kind and/or amount of food I eat.	2
I eat fewer than 2 meals per day.	3
I eat few fruits or vegetables or milk products.	2
I have 3 or more drinks of beer, liquor or wine almost every day.	2
I have tooth or mouth problems that make it hard for me to eat.	2
I don't always have enough money to buy the food I need.	4
I eat alone most of the time.	1
I take 3 or more different prescribed or over-the-counter drugs a day.	1
Without wanting to, I have lost or gained 10 pounds in the last 6 months.	2
I am not always physically able to shop, cook and/or feed myself.	2
	TOTAL

Total Your Nutritional Score. If it's –

0-2   **Good!** Recheck your nutritional score in 6 months.

3-5   **You are at moderate nutritional risk.** See what can be done to improve your eating habits and lifestyle. Your office on aging, senior nutrition program, senior citizens center or health department can help. Recheck your nutritional score in 3 months.

6 or more   **You are at high nutritional risk.** Bring this Checklist the next time you see your doctor, dietitian or other qualified health or social service professional. Talk with them about any problems you may have. Ask for help to improve your nutritional health.

Remember that Warning Signs suggest risk, but do not represent a diagnosis of any condition. Turn the page to learn more about the Warnings Signs of poor nutritional health.

These materials are developed and distributed by the Nutrition Screening Initiative, a project of:

 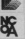 AMERICAN ACADEMY
OF FAMILY PHYSICIANS

THE AMERICAN
DIETETIC ASSOCIATION

THE NATIONAL COUNCIL
ON THE AGING, INC.

 The Nutrition Screening Initiative • 1010 Wisconsin Avenue, NW • Suite 800 • Washington, DC 20007
The Nutrition Screening Initiative is funded in part by a grant from Ross Products Division of Abbott Laboratories, Inc.

From A.W. Taylor and M.J. Johnson, 2008, *Physiology of Exercise and Healthy Aging* (Champaign, IL: Human Kinetics). Reprinted, by permission, from Nutrition Screening Initiative.

Disease

Any disease, illness or chronic condition which causes you to change the way you eat, or makes it hard for you to eat, puts your nutritional health at risk. Four out of five adults have chronic diseases that are affected by diet. Confusion or memory loss that keeps getting worse is estimated to affect one out of five or more of older adults. This can make it hard to remember what, when or if you've eaten. Feeling sad or depressed, which happens to about one in eight older adults, can cause big changes in appetite, digestion, energy level, weight and well-being.

Eating Poorly

Eating too little and eating too much both lead to poor health. Eating the same foods day after day or not eating fruit, vegetables, and milk products daily will also cause poor nutritional health. One in five adults skip meals daily. Only 13% of adults eat the minimum amount of fruit and vegetables needed. One in four older adults drink too much alcohol. Many health problems become worse if you drink more than one or two alcoholic beverages per day.

Tooth Loss/Mouth Pain

A healthy mouth, teeth and gums are needed to eat. Missing, loose or rotten teeth or dentures which don't fit well, or cause mouth sores, make it hard to eat.

Economic Hardship

As many as 40% of older Americans have incomes of less than $6,000 per year. Having less -- or choosing to spend less -- than $25-30 per week for food makes it very hard to get the foods you need to stay healthy.

Reduced Social Contact

One-third of all older people live alone. Being with people daily has a positive effect on morale, well-being and eating.

Multiple Medicines

Many older Americans must take medicines for health problems. Almost half of older Americans take multiple medicines daily. Growing old may change the way we respond to drugs. The more medicines you take, the greater the chance for side effects such as increased or decreased appetite, change in taste, constipation, weakness, drowsiness, diarrhea, nausea, and others. Vitamins or minerals, when taken in large doses, act like drugs and can cause harm. Alert your doctor to everything you take.

Involuntary Weight Loss/Gain

Losing or gaining a lot of weight when you are not trying to do so is an important warning sign that must not be ignored. Being overweight or underweight also increases your chance of poor health.

Needs Assistance in Self Care

Although most older people are able to eat, one of every five have trouble walking, shopping, buying and cooking food, especially as they get older.

Elder Years Above Age 80

Most older people lead full and productive lives. But as age increases, risk of frailty and health problems increase. Checking your nutritional health regularly makes good sense.

The Nutrition Screening Initiative • 1010 Wisconsin Avenue, NW • Suite 800 • Washington, DC 20007
The Nutrition Screening Initiative is funded in part by a grant from Ross Products Division of Abbott Laboratories, Inc.

Physical Activity Readiness
Questionnaire - PAR-Q
(revised 2002)

PAR-Q & YOU

(A Questionnaire for People Aged 15 to 69)

Regular physical activity is fun and healthy, and increasingly more people are starting to become more active every day. Being more active is very safe for most people. However, some people should check with their doctor before they start becoming much more physically active.

If you are planning to become much more physically active than you are now, start by answering the seven questions in the box below. If you are between the ages of 15 and 69, the PAR-Q will tell you if you should check with your doctor before you start. If you are over 69 years of age, and you are not used to being very active, check with your doctor.

Common sense is your best guide when you answer these questions. Please read the questions carefully and answer each one honestly: check YES or NO.

YES	NO		
☐	☐	1.	Has your doctor ever said that you have a heart condition <u>and</u> that you should only do physical activity recommended by a doctor?
☐	☐	2.	Do you feel pain in your chest when you do physical activity?
☐	☐	3.	In the past month, have you had chest pain when you were not doing physical activity?
☐	☐	4.	Do you lose your balance because of dizziness or do you ever lose consciousness?
☐	☐	5.	Do you have a bone or joint problem (for example, back, knee or hip) that could be made worse by a change in your physical activity?
☐	☐	6.	Is your doctor currently prescribing drugs (for example, water pills) for your blood pressure or heart condition?
☐	☐	7.	Do you know of <u>any other reason</u> why you should not do physical activity?

If you answered

YES to one or more questions

Talk with your doctor by phone or in person BEFORE you start becoming much more physically active or BEFORE you have a fitness appraisal. Tell your doctor about the PAR-Q and which questions you answered YES.

- You may be able to do any activity you want — as long as you start slowly and build up gradually. Or, you may need to restrict your activities to those which are safe for you. Talk with your doctor about the kinds of activities you wish to participate in and follow his/her advice.
- Find out which community programs are safe and helpful for you.

NO to all questions

If you answered NO honestly to <u>all</u> PAR-Q questions, you can be reasonably sure that you can:

- start becoming much more physically active — begin slowly and build up gradually. This is the safest and easiest way to go.
- take part in a fitness appraisal — this is an excellent way to determine your basic fitness so that you can plan the best way for you to live actively. It is also highly recommended that you have your blood pressure evaluated. If your reading is over 144/94, talk with your doctor before you start becoming much more physically active.

→

DELAY BECOMING MUCH MORE ACTIVE:

- if you are not feeling well because of a temporary illness such as a cold or a fever — wait until you feel better; or
- if you are or may be pregnant — talk to your doctor before you start becoming more active.

PLEASE NOTE: If your health changes so that you then answer YES to any of the above questions, tell your fitness or health professional. Ask whether you should change your physical activity plan.

<u>Informed Use of the PAR-Q</u>: The Canadian Society for Exercise Physiology, Health Canada, and their agents assume no liability for persons who undertake physical activity, and if in doubt after completing this questionnaire, consult your doctor prior to physical activity.

No changes permitted. You are encouraged to photocopy the PAR-Q but only if you use the entire form.

NOTE: If the PAR-Q is being given to a person before he or she participates in a physical activity program or a fitness appraisal, this section may be used for legal or administrative purposes.

"I have read, understood and completed this questionnaire. Any questions I had were answered to my full satisfaction."

NAME _____

SIGNATURE _____ DATE _____

SIGNATURE OF PARENT _____ WITNESS _____
or GUARDIAN (for participants under the age of majority)

Note: This physical activity clearance is valid for a maximum of 12 months from the date it is completed and becomes invalid if your condition changes so that you would answer YES to any of the seven questions.

© Canadian Society for Exercise Physiology

Supported by: Health Canada   Santé Canada

continued on other side...

From A.W. Taylor and M.J. Johnson, 2008, *Physiology of Exercise and Healthy Aging* (Champaign, IL: Human Kinetics). Source: Physical Activity Readiness Medical Examination (PAR-Q). © 2002. Reprinted with permission from the Canadian Society for Exercise Physiology. www.csep.ca/forms.asp.

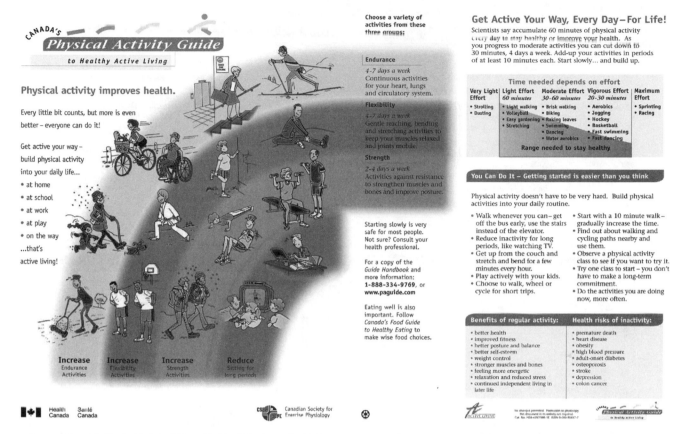

Source: *Canada's Physical Activity Guide to Healthy Active Living*, Health Canada, 1998 http://www.hc-sc.gc.ca/hppb/paguide/pdf/guideEng.pdf
© Reproduced with permission from the Minister of Public Works and Government Services Canada, 2002.

FITNESS AND HEALTH PROFESSIONALS MAY BE INTERESTED IN THE INFORMATION BELOW:

The following companion forms are available for doctors' use by contacting the Canadian Society for Exercise Physiology (address below):

The **Physical Activity Readiness Medical Examination (PARmed-X)** – to be used by doctors with people who answer YES to one or more questions on the PAR-Q.

The **Physical Activity Readiness Medical Examination for Pregnancy (PARmed-X for Pregnancy)** – to be used by doctors with pregnant patients who wish to become more active.

References:

Arraix, G.A., Wigle, D.T., Mao, Y. (1992). Risk Assessment of Physical Activity and Physical Fitness in the Canada Health Survey Follow-Up Study. **J. Clin. Epidemiol.** 45:4 419-428.

Mottola, M., Wolfe, L.A. (1994). Active Living and Pregnancy, In: A. Quinney, L. Gauvin, T. Wall (eds.), **Toward Active Living: Proceedings of the International Conference on Physical Activity, Fitness and Health**. Champaign, IL: Human Kinetics.

PAR-Q Validation Report, British Columbia Ministry of Health, 1978.

Thomas, S., Reading, J., Shephard, R.J. (1992). Revision of the Physical Activity Readiness Questionnaire (PAR-Q). **Can. J. Spt. Sci.** 17:4 338-345.

To order multiple printed copies of the PAR-Q, please contact the:

Canadian Society for Exercise Physiology
202-185 Somerset Street West
Ottawa, ON K2P 0J2
Tel. 1-877-651-3755 • FAX (613) 234-3565
Online: www.csep.ca

 © Canadian Society for Exercise Physiology

Supported by: Health Canada Santé Canada

The original PAR-Q was developed by the British Columbia Ministry of Health. It has been revised by an Expert Advisory Committee of the Canadian Society for Exercise Physiology chaired by Dr. N. Gledhill (2002).

Disponible en français sous le titre «Questionnaire sur l'aptitude à l'activité physique - Q-AAP (revisé 2002)».

From A.W. Taylor and M.J. Johnson, 2008, *Physiology of Exercise and Healthy Aging* (Champaign, IL: Human Kinetics). Source: Physical Activity Readiness Medical Examination (PAR-Q). © 2002. Reprinted with permission from the Canadian Society for Exercise Physiology. www.csep.ca/forms.asp.

PARmed-X

PHYSICAL ACTIVITY READINESS MEDICAL EXAMINATION

The PARmed-X is a physical activity-specific checklist to be used by a physician with patients who have had positive responses to the Physical Activity Readiness Questionnaire (PAR-Q). In addition, the Conveyance/Referral Form in the PARmed-X can be used to convey clearance for physical activity participation, or to make a referral to a medically-supervised exercise program.

Regular physical activity is fun and healthy, and increasingly more people are starting to become more active every day. Being more active is very safe for most people. The PAR-Q by itself provides adequate screening for the majority of people. However, some individuals may require a medical evaluation and specific advice (exercise prescription) due to one or more positive responses to the PAR-Q.

Following the participant's evaluation by a physician, a physical activity plan should be devised in consultation with a physical activity professional (CSEP-Professional Fitness & Lifestyle Consultant or CSEP-Exercise Therapist™). To assist in this, the following instructions are provided:

PAGE 1: • Sections A, B, C, and D should be completed by the participant BEFORE the examination by the physician. The bottom section is to be completed by the examining physician.

PAGES 2 & 3: • A checklist of medical conditions requiring special consideration and management.

PAGE 4: • Physical Activity & Lifestyle Advice for people who do not require specific instructions or prescribed exercise.

• Physical Activity Readiness Conveyance/Referral Form — an optional tear-off tab for the physician to convey clearance for physical activity participation, or to make a referral to a medically-supervised exercise program.

This section to be completed by the participant

A PERSONAL INFORMATION:

NAME _____

ADDRESS _____

_____

TELEPHONE _____

BIRTHDATE _____ GENDER _____

MEDICAL No. _____

B PAR-Q: Please indicate the PAR-Q questions to which you answered YES

- ❏ Q 1 Heart condition
- ❏ Q 2 Chest pain during activity
- ❏ Q 3 Chest pain at rest
- ❏ Q 4 Loss of balance, dizziness
- ❏ Q 5 Bone or joint problem
- ❏ Q 6 Blood pressure or heart drugs
- ❏ Q 7 Other reason:

_____

C RISK FACTORS FOR CARDIOVASCULAR DISEASE:
Check all that apply

- ❏ Less than 30 minutes of moderate physical activity most days of the week.
- ❏ Currently smoker (tobacco smoking 1 or more times per week).
- ❏ High blood pressure reported by physician after repeated measurements.
- ❏ High cholesterol level reported by physician.
- ❏ Excessive accumulation of fat around waist.
- ❏ Family history of heart disease.

Please note: Many of these risk factors are modifiable. Please refer to page 4 and discuss with your physician.

D PHYSICAL ACTIVITY INTENTIONS:

What physical activity do you intend to do?

_____

_____

_____

This section to be completed by the examining physician

Physical Exam:

Ht	Wt	BP i) /
		BP ii) /

Conditions limiting physical activity:

- ❏ Cardiovascular
- ❏ Musculoskeletal
- ❏ Respiratory
- ❏ Abdominal
- ❏ Other

Tests required:

- ❏ ECG
- ❏ Blood
- ❏ Exercise Test
- ❏ Urinalysis
- ❏ X-Ray
- ❏ Other

Physical Activity Readiness Conveyance/Referral:

Based upon a current review of health status, I recommend:

- ❏ No physical activity
- ❏ Only a medically-supervised exercise program until further medical clearance
- ❏ Progressive physical activity:
  - ❏ with avoidance of: _____
  - ❏ with inclusion of: _____
  - ❏ under the supervision of a CSEP-Professional Fitness & Lifestyle Consultant or CSEP-Exercise Therapist™
- ❏ Unrestricted physical activity—start slowly and build up gradually

Further Information:
- ❏ Attached
- ❏ To be forwarded
- ❏ Available on request

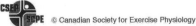

© Canadian Society for Exercise Physiology

Supported by: Health Canada   Santé Canada

1

PARmed-X
PHYSICAL ACTIVITY READINESS MEDICAL EXAMINATION

Following is a checklist of medical conditions for which a degree of precaution and/or special advice should be considered for those who answered "YES" to one or more questions on the PAR-Q, and people over the age of 69. Conditions are grouped by system. Three categories of precautions are provided. Comments under Advice are general, since details and alternatives require clinical judgement in each individual instance.

	Absolute Contraindications	Relative Contraindications	Special Prescriptive Conditions	ADVICE
	Permanent restriction or temporary restriction until condition is treated, stable, and/or past acute phase.	Highly variable. Value of exercise testing and/or program may exceed risk. Activity may be restricted. Desirable to maximize control of condition. Direct or indirect medical supervision of exercise program may be desirable.	Individualized prescriptive advice generally appropriate: • limitations imposed; and/or • special exercises prescribed. May require medical monitoring and/or initial supervision in exercise program.	

Cardiovascular	❑ aortic aneurysm (dissecting)
	❑ aortic stenosis (severe)
	❑ congestive heart failure
	❑ crescendo angina
	❑ myocardial infarction (acute)
	❑ myocarditis (active or recent)
	❑ pulmonary or systemic embolism—acute
	❑ thrombophlebitis
	❑ ventricular tachycardia and other dangerous dysrhythmias (e.g., multi-focal ventricular activity)
		❑ aortic stenosis (moderate)
		❑ subaortic stenosis (severe)
		❑ marked cardiac enlargement
		❑ supraventricular dysrhythmias (uncontrolled or high rate)
		❑ ventricular ectopic activity (repetitive or frequent)
		❑ ventricular aneurysm
		❑ hypertension—untreated or uncontrolled severe (systemic or pulmonary)
		❑ hypertrophic cardiomyopathy
		❑ compensated congestive heart failure
			❑ aortic (or pulmonary) stenosis—mild angina pectoris and other manifestations of coronary insufficiency (e.g., post-acute infarct)
			❑ cyanotic heart disease
			❑ shunts (intermittent or fixed)
			❑ conduction disturbances
			  • complete AV block
			  • left BBB
			  • Wolff-Parkinson-White syndrome
			❑ dysrhythmias—controlled
			❑ fixed rate pacemakers
				• clinical exercise test may be warranted in selected cases, for specific determination of functional capacity and limitations and precautions (if any).
				• slow progression of exercise to levels based on test performance and individual tolerance.
				• consider individual need for initial conditioning program under medical supervision (indirect or direct).

			❑ intermittent claudication	progressive exercise to tolerance
			❑ hypertension: systolic 160-180; diastolic 105+	progressive exercise; care with medications (serum electrolytes; post-exercise syncope; etc.)
Infections	❑ acute infectious disease (regardless of etiology)	❑ subacute/chronic/recurrent infectious diseases (e.g., malaria, others)	❑ chronic infections ❑ HIV	variable as to condition
Metabolic		❑ uncontrolled metabolic disorders (diabetes mellitus, thyrotoxicosis, myxedema)	❑ renal, hepatic & other metabolic insufficiency	variable as to status
			❑ obesity ❑ single kidney	dietary moderation, and initial light exercises with slow progression (walking, swimming, cycling)
Pregnancy		❑ complicated pregnancy (e.g., toxemia, hemorrhage, incompetent cervix, etc.)	❑ advanced pregnancy (late 3rd trimester)	refer to the "PARmed-X for PREGNANCY"

References:

Arraix, G.A., Wigle, D.T., Mao, Y. (1992). Risk Assessment of Physical Activity and Physical Fitness in the Canada Health Survey Follow-Up Study. **J. Clin. Epidemiol.** 45:4 419-428.

Mottola, M., Wolfe, L.A. (1994). Active Living and Pregnancy, In: A. Quinney, L. Gauvin, T. Wall (eds.), **Toward Active Living: Proceedings of the International Conference on Physical Activity, Fitness and Health.** Champaign, IL: Human Kinetics.

PAR-Q Validation Report, British Columbia Ministry of Health, 1978.

Thomas, S., Reading, J., Shephard, R.J. (1992). Revision of the Physical Activity Readiness Questionnaire (PAR-Q). **Can. J. Spt. Sci.** 17: 4 338-345.

The PAR-Q and PARmed-X were developed by the British Columbia Ministry of Health. They have been revised by an Expert Advisory Committee of the Canadian Society for Exercise Physiology chaired by Dr. N. Gledhill (2002).

No changes permitted. You are encouraged to photocopy the PARmed-X, but only if you use the entire form.

Disponible en français sous le titre
«Évaluation médicale de l'aptitude à l'activité physique (X-AAP)»

Continued on page 3...

	Special Prescriptive Conditions	**ADVICE**
Lung	❑ chronic pulmonary disorders	special relaxation and breathing exercises
	❑ obstructive lung disease	breath control during endurance exercises to tolerance; avoid polluted air
	❑ asthma	
	❑ exercise-induced bronchospasm	avoid hyperventilation during exercise; avoid extremely cold conditions; warm up adequately; utilize appropriate medication.
Musculoskeletal	❑ low back conditions (pathological, functional)	avoid or minimize exercise that precipitates or exasperates e.g., forced extreme flexion, extension, and violent twisting; correct posture, proper back exercises
	❑ arthritis—acute (infective, rheumatoid; gout)	treatment, plus judicious blend of rest, splinting and gentle movement
	❑ arthritis—subacute	progressive increase of active exercise therapy
	❑ arthritis—chronic (osteoarthritis and above conditions)	maintenance of mobility and strength; non-weightbearing exercises to minimize joint trauma (e.g., cycling, aquatic activity, etc.)
	❑ orthopaedic	highly variable and individualized
	❑ hernia	minimize straining and isometrics; stregthen abdominal muscles
	❑ osteoporosis or low bone density	avoid exercise with high risk for fracture such as push-ups, curl-ups, vertical jump and trunk forward flexion; engage in low-impact weight-bearing activities and resistance training
CNS	❑ convulsive disorder not completely controlled by medication	minimize or avoid exercise in hazardous environments and/or exercising alone (e.g., swimming, mountainclimbing, etc.)
	❑ recent concussion	thorough examination if history of two concussions; review for discontinuation of contact sport if three concussions, depending on duration of unconsciousness, retrograde amnesia, persistent headaches, and other objective evidence of cerebral damage
Blood	❑ anemia—severe (< 10 Gm/dl)	control preferred; exercise as tolerated
	❑ electrolyte disturbances	
Medications	❑ antianginal ❑ antiarrhythmic ❑ antihypertensive ❑ anticonvulsant ❑ beta-blockers ❑ digitalis preparations ❑ diuretics ❑ ganglionic blockers ❑ others	NOTE: consider underlying condition. Potential for: exertional syncope, electrolyte imbalance, bradycardia, dysrhythmias, impaired coordination and reaction time, heat intolerance. May alter resting and exercise ECG's and exercise test performance.
Other	❑ post-exercise syncope	moderate program
	❑ heat intolerance	prolong cool-down with light activities; avoid exercise in extreme heat
	❑ temporary minor illness	postpone until recovered
	❑ cancer	if potential metastases, test by cycle ergometry, consider non-weight bearing exercises; exercise at lower end of prescriptive range (40-65% of heart rate reserve), depending on condition and recent treatment (radiation, chemotherapy); monitor hemoglobin and lymphocyte counts; add dynamic lifting exercise to strengthen muscles, using machines rather than weights.

*Refer to special publications for elaboration as required

The following companion forms are available online: http://www.csep.ca/forms.asp

The **Physical Activity Readiness Questionnaire (PAR-Q)** - a questionnaire for people aged 15-69 to complete before becoming much more physically active.

The **Physical Activity Readiness Medical Examination for Pregnancy (PARmed-X for PREGNANCY)** - to be used by physicians with pregnant patients who wish to become more physically active.

For more information, please contact the:

Canadian Society for Exercise Physiology
202 - 185 Somerset St. West
Ottawa, ON K2P 0J2
Tel. 1-877-651-3755 • FAX (613) 234-3565 • Online: www.csep.ca

Note to physical activity professionals...

It is a prudent practice to retain the completed Physical Activity Readiness Conveyance/Referral Form in the participant's file.

 © Canadian Society for Exercise Physiology

Supported by: Health Santé
Canada Canada

Continued on page 4...

3

PARmed-X PHYSICAL ACTIVITY READINESS MEDICAL EXAMINATION

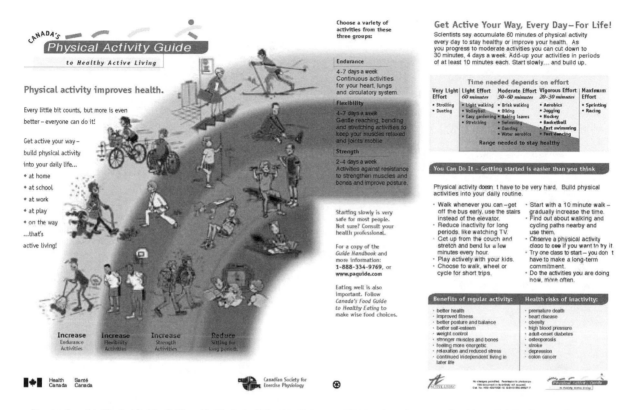

Source: Canada's Physical Activity Guide to Healthy Active Living, Health Canada, 1998 http://www.hc-sc.gc.ca/hppb/paguide/pdf/guideEng.pdf

© Reproduced with permission from the Minister of Public Works and Government Services Canada, 2002.

- - - - - ✂ -

PARmed-X Physical Activity Readiness Conveyance/Referral Form

Based upon a current review of the health status of _____ _____, I recommend:

❏ No physical activity

❏ Only a medically-supervised exercise program until further medical clearance

❏ Progressive physical activity

    ❏ with avoidance of: _____

    ❏ with inclusion of: _____

    ❏ under the supervision of a CSEP-Professional Fitness &

Lifestyle Consultant or CSEP-Exercise Therapist™

❏ Unrestricted physical activity — start slowly and build up gradually

Further Information:
❏ Attached
❏ To be forwarded
❏ Available on request

Physician/clinic stamp:

_____ M.D.

_____ 20_____
(date)

NOTE: This physical activity clearance is valid for a maximum of six months from the date it is completed and becomes invalid if your medical condition becomes worse.

4

Bibliography and References

Introduction

Anderson, R.K., and W.L. Kenney. Effect of age on heat-activated sweat gland density and flow during exercise in dry heat. *Journal of Applied Physiology* 63: 1089-1094, 1987.

Anderton, B.H. Ageing of the brain. *Mechanisms in Ageing and Development* 123: 811-817, 2002.

Balcombe, N.R. and A. Sinclair. Ageing: Definitions, Mechanisms and the Magnitude of the Problem. *Best Practice and Research in Clinical Gastroenterology* 15: 835-840, 2001.

Bassey, E.J. Age, inactivity, and some physiological responses to exercise. *Gerontology* 24: 6-77, 1978.

Blair, S.N., H.W. Kohl, R.S. Paffenbarger, D.G. Clark, K.H. Cooper, and L.W. Gibbons. Health benefits of activity. *Exercise and Sport Science Reviews,* 12: 205-244, 1989.

Brody, H. *Biological Mechanisms of Aging.* Washington, DC: U.S. Department of Health and Human Services, 1980.

Esposito, J.L. Conceptual problems in theoretical gerontology. *Perspectives in Biology and Medicine* 26: 522-546, 1983.

Failla, P.M., and G. Failla. Measurement of the dose in small tissue volumes surrounding "point" sources of radioisotopes. *Radiation Research* 13: 61-91, 1960.

Farmer, M.E. Anthropometric indicators and hip fracture: The HHANES 1 Epidemiological Follow-Up Study. *Journal of the American Geriatric Society.* 37: 9-16, 1989.

Fries, J.F. Aging, natural death and the compression of morbidity. *The New England Journal of Medicine.* 303: 130-135, 1980.

Hayflick, L. The cell biology of human aging. *New England Journal of Medicine* 295: 1302-1308, 1976.

Health Canada. *Canada's Physical Activity Guide for Active Older Adults.* Health Canada, Ottawa, 2001.

Health Canada, Division of Aging and Seniors. *Canada's Aging Population (Report #H39-608/2002E).* Ottawa, Ministry of Public Works and Government Services, 2002a.

Health Canada, Division of Aging and Seniors. *Canada's Aging Population (Report #H39-608/2002E-4E)*. Ottawa, Ministry of Public Works and Government Services, 2002b.

Joseph, J.A., and J.C. Cutler. The role of oxidative stress in signal transduction changes and cell loss in senescence. *Annals of the New York Academy of Science* 738: 37-43, 1994.

Katz, S., L.G. Branch, M.H. Branson, J.A. Papsidero, J.C. Beck, and D.S. Greer. Active life expectancy. *New England Journal of Medicine* 309: 1218-1224, 1983.

Kenney, R.A. Physiology of aging. *Clinical Geriatric Medicine*. 1: 37-59, 1985.

Kunze, P. Magnetic deflection of cosmic corpuscles in the wilson champer. *Ztitschrift fur Physik* 80: 559-572, 1933.

Manton, K. and J. Vaupel. Survival after the age of 80 in the United States, Sweden, France, England, and Japan. *The New England Journal of Medicine* 333. 1232-1235, 1995.

Medawar, P.B. *An unsolved problem in biology*. London: Lewis, 1952.

Munnell, A.H., R.E. Hatch, and J.G. Lee. *Why is life expectancy too low in the United States?* Boston: Center for Retirement Research, www.bc.edu/crr.

Olshansky, S.L, B.A. Carnes, and C. Cassel. In search of Methuselah: Estimating the limits to human longevity. *Science* 250: 634-640, 1990.

Orentreich, N., J.L. Brind, J.H. Vogelman, R. Andres, and H. Baldwin. Long-term longitudinal measurements of plasma dehydroepiandrosterone sulfate in normal men. *Journal of Clinical Endorcrinology and Metabolism* 75: 1002-1004, 1992.

Organization for Economic Cooperation and Development. *OECD Health Date 2003 (3rd ed.)*.

Orgel, L.E. The maintenance of the accuracy of protein synthesis and its relevance to aging. *Proceedings of the National Academy of Science (USA)* 49: 517-521, 1963.

Shock, N.W., Physical activity and the rate of aging. *Canadian Medical Association Journal*. 96: 836-840, 1967.

Skinner, J.S. In: J. Keul (ed.) *Limiting Factors of Human Performance*. Stuttgart: Georg Thieme. Pp. 271-282, 1973.

Spirduso, W.W. *Physical Dimensions of Aging*. 2nd ed. Champaign, Illinois: Human Kinetics, 2005.

Strehler, B.L., D.D. Mark, and A.S. Mildvan. Rate and magnitude of age pigment accumulation in the human myocardium. *Journal of Gerontology* 14: 430-439, 1959.

Taylor, A.W. Ageing, a normal degenerative process—with or without regular exercise. *Canadian Journal of Sport Sciences* 17: 163-167, 1992.

United Nations Department of Economic and Social Affairs, Population Division. *World Population Ageing: 1950-2050 (Report # ST/ESA/SER.A/207)*. New York, 2002.

U.S. Bureau of Census. 2003. www.census.gov/prod/2003pubs/p60-221.pdf.

Taylor, A.W., and E.G. Noble. Overview of exercise and aging. *Biochemistry of Exercise*: 264-271, 1996.

Chapter 1

Anderson, T.J., A. Uehata, M.D. Gerhard, I.T. Meredith, S. Knab, D. Delagrange, E.H. Lieberman, P. Ganz, M.A. Creager, and A.C. Yeung. 1995. Close relation of endothelial function in the human coronary and peripheral circulations. *J Am Coll Cardiol* 26: 1235-1241.

Bassuk, S.S., and J.E. Manson. 2003. Physical activity and cardiovascular disease prevention in women: How much is good enough? *Exerc Sport Sci Rev* 31: 176-181.

Benarroch, E.E. 1993. The central autonomic network: Functional organization, dysfunction, and perspective. *Mayo Clin Proc* 988-1001.

Booth, F.W., S.E. Gordon, C.J. Carlson, and M.T. Hamilton. 2000. Waging war on modern chronic diseases: Primary prevention through exercise biology. *J Appl Physiol* 88: 774-787.

Cechetto, D.F. 1993. Experimental cerebral ischemic lesions and autonomic and cardiac effects in cats and rats. *Stroke* 24(Suppl I): I6-I9.

Celermajer, D.S., K.E. Sorensen, C. Bull, J. Robinson, and J.E. Deanfield. 1994. Endothelium-dependent dilation in the systemic arteries of asymptomatic subjects relates to coronary risk factors and their interaction. *J Am Coll Cardiol* 24: 1468-1474.

Doyle, A.E., and G.A. Donnan. 1990. Stroke as a clinical problem in hypertension. *J Cardiovasc Pharmacol* 15(Suppl 1): S34-S37.

Du, X., H.S. Cox, A.M. Dart, and M.D. Esler. 1999. Sympathetic activation triggers ventricular arrhythmias in rat heart with chronic infarction and failure. *Cardiovasc Res* 43: 919-929.

Grassi, G., G. Seravalle, G. Bertinieri, C. Turri, R. Dell'Oro, M.L. Stella, and G. Mancia. 2000. Sympathetic and reflex alterations in systo-diastolic and systolic hypertension of the elderly. *J Hypertens* 587-593.

Grassi, G., G. Seravalle, B.M. Cattaneo, A. Lanfranchi, S. Vailati, C. Giannattasio, A. Del Bo, C. Sala, G.B. Bolla, M. Pozzi, and G. Mancia. 1995. Sympathetic activation and loss of reflex sympathetic control in mild congestive heart failure. *Circulation* 92: 3206-3211.

Hachinski, V.C., K.E. Smith, M.D. Silver, C.J. Gibson, and J. Ciriello. 1986. Acute myocardial and plasma catecholamine changes in experimental stroke. *Stroke* 17: 387-390.

Hachinski, V.C., J.X. Wilson, L. Tichenoff, K.E. Smith, and D.F. Cechetto. 1992. Effect of age on autonomic and cardiac responses in a rat stroke model. *Arch Neurol* 49: 690-696.

Iwase, S., T. Mano, T. Watanabe, M. Saito, and F. Kobayashi. 1991. Age-related changes of sympathetic outflow to muscle in humans. *J Gerontol* 46: M1-M5.

Izzo, J.L., and A.A. Taylor. 1999. The sympathetic nervous system and baroreflexes in hypertension and hypotension. *Curr Hypertens Rep* 1: 254-263.

Kaye, D.M., J. Lefkovits, G.L. Jennings, P. Bergin, A. Broughton, and M.D. Esler. 1995. Adverse consequences of high sympathetic nervous activity in the failing human heart. *J Am Coll Cardiol* 26: 1257-1263.

Laughlin, M.H. 2004. Wolfe memorial lecture. Physical activity in prevention and treatment of coronary disease: The battle line is in exercise vascular cell biology. *Med Sci Sports Exerc* 36: 352-362.

Matsukawa, T., Y. Sugiyama, T. Watanabe, F. Kobayashi, and T. Mano. 1998. Gender difference in age-related changes in muscle sympathetic nerve activity in healthy subjects. *Am J Physiol* 275: R1600-R1604.

Middlekauff, H.R. 1997. Mechanisms and implications of autonomic nervous system dysfunction in heart failure. *Curr Opin Cardiol* 12: 265-275.

Narkiewicz, K., C.A. Pesek, P. van de Borne, M. Kato, and V. Somers. 1999. Enhanced sympathetic and ventilatory responses to central chemoreflex activation in heart failure. *Circulation* 100: 262-267.

Palmer, G.J., M.G. Ziegler, and C.R. Lake. 1978. Response of norepinephrine and blood pressure to stress increases with age. *J Geront* 33: 482-487.

Pauletto, P., G. Scannapieco, and A.C. Pessina. 1991. Sympathetic drive and vascular damage in hypertension and atherosclerosis. *Hypertension* 17(Suppl): III75-III81.

Proctor, D.N., K.U. Le, and S.J. Ridout. 2005. Age and regional specificity of peak limb vascular conductance in men. *J Appl Physiol* 98. 193-202.

Rowell, L.B. 1993. *Human cardiovascular control.* New York: Oxford University Press.

Seals, D.R., and E.A. Dinenno. 2004. Collateral damage: Cardiovascular consequences of chronic sympathetic activation with human aging. *Am J Physiol Heart Circ Physiol* 287: H1895-H1905.

Seals, D.R., and M.D. Esler. 2000. Human ageing and the sympathoadrenal system. *J Physiol* 528(Pt 3): 407-417.

Sowers, J.R., L.Z. Rubenstein, and N. Stern. 1983. Plasma norepinephrine responses to posture and isometric exercise increase with age in the absence of obesity. *J Geront* 38: 315-317.

Stoney, C., M. Davis, and K. Matthews. 1987. Sex differences in physiological responses to stress and in coronary heart disease: A causal link? *Psychophysiology* 24: 127-131.

Sundlöf, G., and B.G. Wallin. 1978. Human muscle nerve sympathetic activity at rest. Relationship to blood pressure and age. *J Physiol* 274: 637.

Walther, C., S. Gielen, and R. Hambrecht. 2004. The effect of exercise training on endothelial function in cardiovascular disease in humans. *Exerc Sport Sci Rev* 32: 129-134.

Watts, K., P. Beye, A. Siafarikas, E.A. Davis, T.W. Jones, G. O'Driscoll, and D.J. Green. 2004. Exercise training normalizes vascular dysfunction and improves central adiposity in obese adolescents. *J Am Coll Cardiol* 43: 1823-1827.31.

WHO. The World Health Report 2002. ISBN# 9789241562072.

Wilmore, J.M. and D.L. Costill. (2004). Physiology of sport and exercise. Champaign, Illinois: Human Kinetics.

Zhang, H., and J.E. Faber. 2001a. Norepinephrine stimulation of injured aorta ex vivo increases growth of the intima-media via alpha 1A-and the adventitia via alpha 1B-adrenoceptors. *FASEB J* 15: A248.

Zhang, H., and J.E. Faber. 2001b. Trophic effect of norepinephrine on arterial intima-media and adventitia is augmented by injury and mediated by different alpha 1-adrenoceptor subtypes. *Circ Res* 89: 815-822.

Zucker, I.H., W. Wang, R.U. Pliquett, J.L. Liu, and K.P. Patel. 2001. The regulation of sympathetic outflow in heart failure. The roles of angiotensin II, nitric oxide, and exercise training. *Ann NY Acad Sci* 940: 431-443.

Chapter 2

Abernethy, P.J., J. Jurimae, P.A. Logan, A.W. Taylor, R.E. Thayer. 1994. Acute and chronic responses of skeletal muscle to resistance exercise. *Sports Medicine* 17: 22-38.

American College of Sports Medicine. 1998. Position stand on exercise and physical activity for older adults. *Medicine and Science in Sports and Exercise* 30: 992-1008.

Camerlain, M. 2004, August. Aging, arthritis and active living. *ALCOA Research to Action.* pp. 1-6

Chilibeck, P.D., C.R. McCreary, G.D. Marsh, D.H. Paterson, E.G. Noble, A.W. Taylor, and T.T. Thompson. 1998. Evaluation of muscle oxidative potential by 31P-MRS during incremental exercise in old and young humans. *European Journal of Applied Physiology* 78: 460-465.

Chilibeck, P.D., D.H. Paterson, D.A. Cunningham, A.W. Taylor, and E.G. Noble. 1997. Muscle capillarization, O_2 diffusion distance, and VO_2 kinetics in old and young individuals. *Journal of Applied Physiology* 82: 63-69.

Coggan, A.R., A.J. Spina, D.S. King, M.A. Rogers, M. Brown, P.M. Nemeth, J.O. Holloszy. 1992. Skeletal muscle adaptations to endurance training in 60– to 70 yr–old men and women. *Journal of Applied Physiology* 75: 1780-1786.

Cunningham, D.A., P.A. Rechnitzer, J.H. Howard, and A.P. Donner. 1987. Exercise training of men at retirement: A clinical trial. *Journal of Gerontology* 42: 17-23.

Doherty, T.J., and W.E. Brown. 1993. The estimated numbers and relative sizes of thenar motor units as selected by multiple point stimulation in young and older adults. *Muscle and Nerve* 16: 355-366.

Doherty, T.J., A.A. Vandervoort, A.W. Taylor, W.F. Brown. 1993. Effects of motor unit losses on strength in older men and women. *Journal of Applied Physiology* 74: 868-874.

Fiatarone, M.A., E.C. Marts, N.D. Ryan, C.N. Merideth, L.A. Lipsitz, W.J. Evans. 1990. High intensity strength training in nonagenarians. *Journal of the American Medical Association* 263: 3029-3034.

Grimby, G., A. Aniansson, M. Hedberg, G.-B. Henning, U. Grangard, and H. Kvist. 1992. Training can improve muscle strength and endurance. *Journal of Applied Physiology* 73: 2517-2523.

Jones, D.A., and J.M. Round. 1990. *Skeletal muscle in health and disease: A textbook of muscle physiology.* Manchester, England: Manchester University Press.

Keh-Evans, L., C.L. Rice, E.G. Noble, D.H. Paterson, D.A. Cunningham, A.W. Taylor. 1992. Comparison of histochemical, biochemical, and contractile properties of triceps surae of trained aged subjects. *Canadian Journal of Ageing* 11: 412-425.

Klein, C., D.A. Cunningham, D.H. Paterson, and A.W. Taylor. 1988. Fatigue and recovery of contractile properties of young and elderly men. *European Journal of Applied Physiology* 57: 684-690.

Klein, C.S., C.L. Rice, and G.D. Marsh. 2001. Normalized force, activation, and co-activation in the arm muscles of young and old men. *Journal of Applied Physiology* 91: 1341-1349.

Klitgaard, H., M. Mantoni, S. Schiaffino, S. Ausoni, L. Gorza, C. Laurent-Winter, P. Schnohr, and B. Saltin. 1990. Function, morphology and protein expression of ageing skeletal muscle: A cross-sectional study of elderly men with different training backgrounds. *Acta Physiologica Scandinavica* 140: 41-54.

Klitgaard, H., M. Zhou, S. Schiaffino, R. Betto, G. Salviati, and B. Saltin. 1990. Ageing alters the myosin heavy chain composition of single fibres from human skeletal muscle. *Acta Physiologica Scandinavica* 140: 55-62.

Larsson, L., and T. Ansved. 1985. Effects of long-term physical training and detraining on enzyme, histochemical, and functional skeletal muscle characteristics in man. *Muscle and Nerve* 8: 714-722.

Larsson, L., X. Li, and W.R. Frontera. 1997. Effects of aging on shortening velocity and myosin isoform composition in single human skeletal muscle cells. *American Journal of Physiology* 272: C638-C649.

Lexell, J., K. Henriksson-Larsen, and M. Sjostrom. 1983. Distribution of different fiber types in human skeletal muscle. 2. A study of cross-sections of whole m. vastus lateralis. *Acta Physiologica Scandinavica* 117: 115-122.

Lexell, J., M. Sjostrom, A.S. Nordlund, and C.C. Taylor. 1992. Growth and development of human muscle: A quantitative morphological study of whole vastus lateralis from childhood to adult age. *Muscle and Nerve* 15: 404-409.

Lexell, J., C.C. Taylor, and M. Sjostrom. 1988. What is the cause of the ageing atrophy? Total number, size and proportion of different fiber types studied in whole vastus lateralis muscles from 15-83 year old men. *Journal of Neurological Science* 84: 275-294.

MacDougall, J.D., D.G. Sale, S.E. Always, and J.R. Sutton. 1984. Muscle fiber number in biceps brachii in body-builders and control subjects. *Journal of Applied Physiology* 57: 1399-1403.

McDonagh, M.J., and C.T. Davies. 1984. Adaptive response of mammalian skeletal muscle to exercise with high loads. *European Journal of Applied Physiology and Occupational Physiology* 52: 139-155.

Noble, E.G., C.L. Rice, R.E. Thayer, and A.W. Taylor. 2004. Evolving concepts of skeletal muscle. In J.R. Poortmans (Ed.), *Principles of exercise biochemistry: Medicine and sport science series,* 46, pp. 36-61.

O'Neill, D.E., R.E. Thayer, A.W. Taylor, T.M. Dzialoszynski, and E.G. Noble. 2000. Effects of short-term resistance on muscle strength and morphology in the elderly. *Journal of Aging and Physical Activity* 8: 312-324.

Overend, T.J., D.A. Cunningham, D.H. Paterson, and M.S. Lefcoe. 1992. Knee extensor and knee flexor strength: Cross sectional area ratios in young and elderly men. *Journal of Gerontology* 47: M204-M210.

Porter, M.M., A.A. Vandervoort, and J. Lexell. 1995. Aging of human muscle: Structure, function and adaptability. *Scandinavian Journal of Medicine and Science in Sports* 5: 129-142.

Radak, Z., and A.W. Taylor. 2004. Exercise and cancer. In Z. Radak (Ed.), *Exercise and diseases.* Aauchen: Meyer and Meyer, pp. 168-190.

Rice, C.L. 2000. Muscle function at the motor unit level: Consequences of aging. *Topics in Geriatric Rehabilitation* 15: 70-82.

Rice, C.L., D.A. Cunningham, D.H. Paterson, and M.S. Lefcoe. 1989. Arm and leg composition determined by computed tomography in young and elderly men. *Clinical Physiology* 9: 207-220.

Rice, C.L., D.A. Cunningham, D.H. Paterson, and M.S. Lefcoe. 1990. A comparison of anthropometry with computed tomography in limbs of young and aged men. *Journal of Gerontology* 45: M175-M179.

Rice, C.L., D.A. Cunningham, A.W. Taylor, D.H. Paterson. 1988. Comparison of the histochemical and contractile properties of human triceps surae. *European Journal of Applied Physiology and Occupational Physiology* 58: 165-170.

Taylor, A.W. 1975. The effects of exercise and training on the activities of human skeletal muscle glycogen cycle enzymes. In J. Poortmans, H. Howald, J. Keul (Eds.), *Metabolic adaptation to prolonged physical exercise.* Basel: Birkhauer Press, pp. 451-462.

Taylor, A.W., L. Bachman. 1999. The effects of endurance training on muscle fibre types and enzyme activities. *Canadian Journal of Applied Physiology* 21: 41-53.

Taylor, A.W., N.A. Ecclestone, G.R. Jones, and D.H. Paterson (Eds.). 1999. *Activity for older adults: From research to action.* London, Canada: Double Q Press.

Taylor, A.W., G. Jones, N. Ecclestone (Eds.). 2005. *Proceedings of the 6th International Congress on Aging and Physical Activity: From research to practice.* London, Canada: CCAA Press.

Taylor, A.W., S. Lavoie, G. Lemieux, C. Dufresne, J.S. Skinner. 1978. Effects of endurance training on fiber area and enzyme activities of skeletal muscle of French Canadians. In *Third International Symposium in Biochemistry of Exercise.* Miami: Symposium Specialists Inc., pp. 267-278.

Taylor, A.W., E.G. Noble. 1996. Overview of exercise and aging. In J.R. Poortmans (Ed.), *Biochemistry of exercise IX,* chapter 21, pp. 279-286.

Taylor, A.W., E.G. Noble, D.A. Cunningham, D.H. Paterson, and P.A. Rechnitzer. 1992. Ageing, skeletal muscle contractile properties, and enzyme activities with exercise. In Y. Sato, J. Poortmans, I. Hashimoto, Y. Oshida (Eds.), *Integration of medical sports sciences.* Basel: Karger, pp. 109-125.

Thayer, R., J. Collins, E.G. Noble, A.W. Taylor. 2000. A decade of endurance aerobic training: Histological evidence for fibre type transformation. *Journal of Sports Medicine and Physical Fitness* 40: 284-289.

Thayer, R., C.L. Rice, F.P. Pettigrew, E.G. Noble, A.W. Taylor. 1993. The fibre composition of skeletal muscle. In J.R. Poortmans (Ed.), *Principles of exercise biochemistry.* Basel: Karger, pp. 25-50.

Tomlinson, B.E., D. Irving. 1977. The numbers of limb motor neurons in the human lumbosacral cord throughout life. *Journal of Neurological Sciences* 34: 213-219.

Williams, G.N., M.J. Higgins, M.D. Lewek. 2002. Aging skeletal muscle: Physiologic changes and the effects of training. *Physical Therapy* 82: 62-68.

Young, A., M. Stokes, M. Crowe. 1984. Size and strength of the quadriceps muscles of old and young women. *European Journal of Clinical Investigation* 14: 282-287.

Young, A., M. Stokes, M. Crowe. 1985. Size and strength of the quadriceps muscles of old and young men. *Clinical Physiology* 5: 145-154.

Chapter 3

Colcombe, S.J., Erickson, K.I., Raz, N., Webb, A.G., Cohen, N.J., McAuley, E., et al. 2003. Aerobic fitness reduces brain tissue loss in aging humans. *J Gerontol A Biol Sci Med Sci* 58: 176-180.

Colcombe, S.J., Kramer, A.F., Erickson, K.I., Scalf, P., McAuley, E., Cohen, N.J., et al. 2004. Cardiovascular fitness, cortical plasticity, and aging. *Proc Natl Acad Sci USA* 101: 3316-3321.

Doherty, T.J. 2003. Invited review: Aging and sarcopenia. *J Appl Physiol* 95: 1717-1727.

Doherty, T.J., Vandervoort, A.A., Taylor, A.W., Brown, W.F. 1993. Effects of motor unit losses on strength in older men and women. *J Appl Physiol* 74: 868-874.

Fries, J.F., Crapo, L. 1981. *Vitality and aging.* San Francisco: Freeman.

Jernigan, T.L., Archibald, S.L., Fennema-Notestine, C., Gamst, A.C., Stout, J.C., Bonner, J., et al. 2001. Effects of age on tissues and regions of the cerebrum and cerebellum. *Neurobiol Aging* 22: 581-594.

Lexell, J., Vandervoort, A.A. 2002. Age-related changes in the neuromuscular system. In W.F. Brown, C.F. Bolton, and M.J. Aminoff (Eds.), *Clinical neurophysiology and neuromuscular disease.* Philadelphia: Saunders, pp. 591-601.

Macintosh, B.R., Gardner, P., McComas, A.J. 2006. *Skeletal muscle: Form and function* (2nd ed.). Champaign, IL: Human Kinetics.

Magnoni, M.S., Govoni, S., Battaini, F., Trabucchi, M. 1991. The aging brain: Protein phosphorylation as a target of changes in neuronal function. *Life Sciences* 48: 373-385.

National Advisory Council on Aging. 1996. *Aging vignettes.* Ohawa: Government of Canada.

Porter, M.M. 2001. The effects of strength training on sarcopenia. *Can J Appl Physiol* 26: 123-141.

Vandervoort, A.A. 1999. Ankle mobility and postural stability. *Physiother Theory Pract* 15: 91-103.

Vaynman, S., F. Gomez-Pinilla. 2005. License to run: Exercise impacts functional plasticity in the intact and injured central nervous system by using neurotrophins. *Neurorehabil Neural Repair* 19: 283-295.

Chapter 4

Boyce, J.M., Shone, G.R. (2006). Effects of ageing on smell and taste. *Postgraduate medical journal,* 82: 966, 239-241.

Katzman, R., R. Terry. 1983. *The neurology of aging.* Philadelphia: FA Davis.

Leslie, D.K. 1989. *Nature stuff: Physical activity for the older adult.* Reston, VA: American Alliance for Health, Physical Education, Recreation and Dance.

Wallhagen, M.I., Pettengill, E., Whiteside, M. (2006). Sensory impairment in older adults: Part I: Hearing Loss. *The American Journal of Nursing,* 106: 10, 40-48; quiz 48-49.

Whiteside, M.M., Wallhagen, M.I., Pettengill, E. (2006). Sensory impairment in older adults: Part II: Vision loss. *The American Journal of Nursing,* 106: 11, 52-61; quiz 61-62.

Wilmore, J.H., and D.L. Costill. 2004. *Physiology of sport and exercise* (3rd ed.). Champaign, IL: Human Kinetics.

Chapter 5

American Academy of Family Physicians, American Dietetic Association, National Council on Aging. 2000. *Determine your nutritional health.* Washington, DC: Nutrition Screening Initiative.

Bunout D, Barrera G, de la Maza P, Gattas V, Hirsch S. 2003. Seasonal variation in insulin sensitivity in healthy elderly people. *Nutrition* 19: 310-316.

Campbell WW, Trappe TA, Jozsi AC, Kruskall LJ, Wolfe RR, Evans WJ. 2002. Dietary protein adequacy and lower body versus whole body resistive training in older humans. *J Physiol* 542(Pt 2): 631-642.

Canadian Diabetes Association. 2000. *Things you should know about type II diabetes.* Toronto: CDA.

Dela F, Mikines KJ, Larsen JJ, Galbo H. 1999. Glucose clearance in aged trained skeletal muscle during maximal insulin with superimposed exercise. *J Appl Physiol* 87: 2059-2067.

Dela F, Ploug T, Handberg A, Petersen LN, Larsen JJ, Mikines KJ, Galbo H. 1994. Physical training increases muscle GLUT4 protein and mRNA in patients with NIDDM. *Diabetes* 43: 862-865.

Donaldson A. 2000. *Canadian diabetes care guide.* Toronto: Hotspur Communications.

Dorrens J, Rennie MJ. 2003. Effects of ageing and human whole body and muscle protein turnover. *Scand J Med Sci Sports* 13: 26-33.

Drug Trading Co. Ltd. 2000. *Nutrition care guide.* Markham, ON: Drug Trading Co.

Health Canada. 1997. *Canada's food guide to healthy eating.* Ottawa, ON: Minister of Public Works and Government Services Canada.

Health Canada. 1998. *Canada's physical activity guide to healthy active living for older adults.* Ottawa, ON: Minister of Public Works and Government Services Canada.

Health Canada. 2002. *The Canadian diabetes strategy.* Ottawa, ON: Health Canada.

Ivy JL 1997. Role of exercise training in the prevention and treatment of insulin resistance and non-insulin-dependent diabetes mellitus. *Sports Med* 24: 321-336.

Johnson S. 2003. Healthy eating and regular physical activity: A winning combination for older adults. *ALCOA Res Update,* no. 6.

Kesavadev JD, Short KR, Nair KS. 2003. Diabetes in old age: An emerging epidemic. *J Assoc Physicians India* 51: 1083-1094.

McReynolds JL, Rossen EK. 2004. Importance of physical activity, nutrition, and social support for optimal aging. *Clin Nurse Spec* 18: 200-206.

Mitchell D, Haan MN, Steinberg FM, Visser M. 2003. Body composition in the elderly: The influence of nutritional factors and physical activity. *J Nutr Health Aging* 7: 130-139.

Miyasaka K, Ichikawa M, Kawanami T, Kanai S, Ohta M, Sato N, Ebisawa H, Funakoshi A. 2003. Physical activity prevented age-related decline in energy metabolism in genetically obese and diabetic rats, but not in control rats. *Mech Ageing Dev* 124: 183-190.

O'Brien Cousins S, Horne T. 1999. *Active living among older adults: Health benefits and outcomes.* Philadelphia: Taylor & Francis.

Oiknine R, Mooradian AD. 2004. Epidemiology of diabetes. *J Clin Pharmacol* 44: 397-405.

Richter EA, Galbo H. 1986. Diabetes, insulin and exercise. *Sports Med* 3: 275-288.

Ryan AS. 2000. Insulin resistance with aging: Effects of diet and exercise. *Sports Med* 30: 327-346.

Singh I, Marshall MC Jr. 1995. Diabetes mellitus in the elderly. *Endocrinol Metab Clin North Am* 24: 255-272.

Strano-Paul L, Phanumas D. 2000. Diabetes management: Analysis of the American Diabetes Association's clinical practice recommendations. *Geriatrics* 55: 57-62; quiz 65.

Takemura Y, Kikuchi S, Inaba Y, Yasuda H, Nakagawa K. 1999. The protective effect of good physical fitness when young on the risk of impaired glucose tolerance when old. *Prev Med* 28: 14-19.

Tipton KD. 2001. Muscle protein metabolism in the elderly: Influence of exercise and nutrition. *Can J Appl Physiol* 26: 588-606.

Winer N, Sowers JR. 2004. Epidemiology of diabetes. *J Clin Pharmacol* 44: 397-405.

Yarasheski KE. 2003. Exercise, aging, and muscle protein metabolism. *J Gerontol A Biol Sci Med Sci* 58: M918-922.

Chapter 6

Adachi JD, Olszynski WP, Hanley DA, Hodsman AB, Kendler DL, Siminoski KG. 2000. Management of corticosteroid-induced osteoporosis. *Semin Arthritis Rheum* 29: 228-215.

Adams, M.A., Pollintine, P., Tobias, J.P., Wakley, G.K., Dolan, P. (2006). Intervertebral disc degeneration can predispose to anterior vertebral fractures in the thoracolumbar spine. *J Bone Miner Res.* 21: 1405-1416.

Bailey DA, Faulkner RA, McKay HA. 1996. Growth, physical activity and bone mineral acquisition. In Holloszy JO (Ed.), *Exercise and sports sciences reviews.* Baltimore: Williams & Wilkins, 24, pp. 233-266.

Bass S, Pearce G, Bradney M, Hendrich E, Delmas PD, Harding A, Seeman E. 1998. Exercise before puberty may confer residual benefits in bone density in adulthood: Studies in active prepubertal and retired female gymnasts. *J Bone Miner Res* 13: 500-507.

Bilanin JE, Blanchard MS, Russek-Cohen E. 1989. Lower vertebral bone density in male long distance runners. *Med Sci Sports Exerc* 21: 66-70.

Bischoff HA, Stahelin HN, Dick W, Akos R, Knecht M, Salis C, Nebiker M, Theiler R, Pfeifer M, et al. 2003. Effects of vitamin D and calcium supplementation on falls: A randomized controlled trial. *J Bone Min Res* 18: 343-351.

Bischoff-Ferrari HA, Borchers M, Gudat F, Durmuller U, Stahelin HB, Dick W. 2004a. Vitamin D receptor expression in human muscle tissue decreases with age *J Bone Miner Res* 19: 265-269.

Bischoff-Ferrari HA, Dietrich T, Orav J, Dawson-Hughes B. 2004b. Positive association between 25-hydroxyvitamin D levels and bone mineral density: A population-based study of younger and older adults. *JAMA* 116: 634-639.

Bouxsein ML, Melton III LJ, Riggs BL, Muller J, Atkinson EJ, Oberg AL, Robb RA, Camp JJ, Rouleau PA, McCollough CH, Khosla S. (2006). Age- and sex-specific differences in the factor of risk for vertabral fracture: A population-based study using QCT. *J Bone Miner Res.* 21: 1475-1482.

Brooke-Wavell K, Jones PRM, Hardman AE. 1997. Brisk walking reduces calcaneal bone loss in post-menopausal women. *Clin Sci (Lond)* 92: 75-80.

Brown J, Josse RG for the Scientific Advisory Council of the Osteoporosis Society of Canada. 2002. Clinical practice guidelines for the diagnosis and management of osteoporosis in Canada. *CMAJ* 167(10 Suppl).

Campbell AJ, Robertson MC, Gardner MM, et al. 1997. Randomised controlled trial of a general practice programme of home based exercise to prevent falls in elderly women *Brit Med J* 315: 1065-1069.

Chow R, Harrison J, Dornan J. 1989. Prevention and rehabilitation of osteoporosis program: Exercise and osteoporosis. *Int J Rehab Res* 12: 49-56.

Chow R, Harrison JE, Notarius C. 1987. Effect of two randomised exercise programs on bone mass of healthy post-menopausal women. *Br Med J* 295: 1441-1444.

Coupland C, Wood D, Cooper C. 1988. Physical inactivity is an independent risk fracture for hip fracture in the elderly. *J Epidemiol Comm Health* 47: 441-443.

Cranney A, Papaioannou A, Zytaruk N, Hanley D, Adachi J, Goltzman D, Murray T, Hodsman A for the Clinical Guidelines Committee of Osteoporosis Canada. 2006, July 4. Parathyroid hormone for the treatment of osteoporosis: A systematic review *CMAJ* 175(1): 52-59.

Dalsky GP, Stocke KS, Ehsani AI, Slatopolsky E, Lee W, Birge SJ. 1988. Weight-bearing exercise training and lumbar bone mineral content in post-menopausal women. *Ann Intern Med* 108: 824-828.

Davison KS, Siminoski K, Adachi JD, Hanley DA, Goltzman D, Hodsman AB, Josse R, Kaiser S, Olszynski WP, Papaioannou A, Ste-Marie LG, Kendler DL, Tenenhouse A, Brown JP. 2006. Bone strength: The whole is greater than the sum of its parts. *Semin Arthritis Rheum,* August 1; 36(1): 22-31.

Dilsen G, Berker C, Oral A, Varan G. 1989. The role of physical exercise in prevention and management of osteoporosis. *Clin Rheumatol* 8(Suppl 2): 70-75.

Ebrahim S, Thompson PW, Baskaran V, Evans K. 1997. Randomised placebo controlled trial of brisk walking in the prevention of postmenopausal osteoporosis. *Age Ageing* 26: 253-260.

Ecclestone NA, Tudor-Locke C, Lazowski D, Myers AM. 1995. Programming and evaluation insights into physical activity for special older populations. Proceedings of the International Conference on Aging and Physical Activity. *J Aging Phys Act* 3: 424-425.

Embry AF, Snowdon LR, Vieth R. 2000. Vitamin D and seasonal fluctuations of gadolinium-enhancing magnetic resonance imaging lesions in multiple sclerosis. *Ann Neurol* 48: 271-272.

Forwood MR, Burr DB. 1993. Physical activity and bone mass: Exercises in futility? *Bone and Miner* 21: 89-112.

Francis RM, Baillie SP, Chuck AJ, Crook PR, Dunn N, Fordham JN, Kelly C, Rodgers A. 2004. Acute and long-term management of patients with vertebral fractures. *QJM* 97: 63-74.

Giangregorio L, Papaioannou A, Cranney A, Zytaruk N, Adachi JD. (2006). Fragility fractures and the osteoporosis care gap: An international phenomenon. *Semin Arthritis Rheum* 35: 293-305.

Gillespie LD, Gillespie WJ, Cumming R, Lamb SE, Rowe BH. 2003. Interventions to reduce the incidence of falling in the elderly (Cochrane Review). Cochrane Database Syst Rev. 2003 (4): CD000340.

Grant WB. 2002. An estimate of premature cancer mortality in the U.S. due to inadequate doses of solar ultraviolet-B radiation. *Cancer* 94: 1867-1875.

Hartard M, Haber P, Ilieva D, Preisinger E, Seidl G, Huber J. 1996. Systematic strength training as a model of therapeutic intervention: A controlled trial in postmenopausal women with osteopenia. *Am J Phys Med Rehab* 75: 21-28.

Heinonen A, Oja P, Sievanen H, Pasanen M, Vuori I. 1998. Effect of two training regimens on bone mineral density in healthy perimenopausal women: A randomised controlled trial. *J Bone Miner Res* 13: 483-490.

Helmes E, Hodsman AB, Lazowski DA, Bhardwaj A, Crilly R, Nichol P, Drost D, Vanderburgh L, Peterson L. 1995. A questionnaire to evaluate disability in osteoporotic patients with vertebral compression fractures. *J Gerontol Med Sci 50:* M91-M98.

Henderson NK, White CP, Eisman JA. 1998. The roles of exercise and fall risk reduction in the prevention of osteoporosis. *Endocrinol Metab Clin N Am* 27: 369-387.

Hernandez-Avila M, Colditz GA, Stampfer MJ, Rosner B, Speizer FE, Willett WC. 1991. Caffeine, moderate alcohol intake and risk of fractures of the hip and forearm in middle-aged women. *Am J Clin Nutr* 54: 157-163.

Hetland ML, Haarbo J, Christiansen C. 1993. Low bone mass and high bone turnover in male long distance runners. *J Clin Endocrinol Metab* 77: 770-775.

Holick MF. 2005. The vitamin D epidemic and its health consequences. *J Nutr* 135: 2739S-2748S.

Hypponen E, Laara E, Jarvelin M-R, Virtanen SM. 2001. Intake of vitamin D and risk of type 1 diabetes: A birth-cohort study. *Lancet* 358: 1500-1503.

Ismail AA, Cooper C, Felsenberg D, Varlow J, Kanis JA, Silman AJ, O'Neill TW. 1999. Number and type of vertebral deformities: Epidemiological characteristics and relation to back pain and height loss. European Vertebral Osteoporosis Study Group. *Osteoporos Int* 9: 206-213.

Jackson SA, Tenenhouse A, Robertson L. 2000. Vertebral fracture definition from population-based data: Preliminary results from the Canadian Multicenter Osteoporosis Study (CaMos). *Osteoporos Int* 11(8): 680-687.

Jilka RL. 2003. Biology of the basic multicellular unit and pathophysiology of osteoporosis. *Med Pediatr Oncol* 41: 182-185.

Johnell O, Oden A, Caulin F, Kanis JA. 2001. Acute and long-term increase in fracture risk after hospitalization for vertebral fracture. *Osteoporos Int* 12: 207-214.

Jonsson B, Ringsberg K, Josefson PO, Johnell O, Birch-Jebsen M. 1992. Effects of physical activity on bone mineral content and muscle strength in women: A cross-sectional study. *Bone* 13: 191-195.

Kanis JA, Melton LJ III, Christiansen C, Johnston CC, Khaltaev N. 1994. The diagnosis of osteoporosis. *J Bone Miner Res* 9: 1137-1141.

Kannus P, Haapasalo H, Sankelo M, Siavanen H, Pasanen M, Heinonen A, et al. 1995. Effect of starting age of physical activity on bone mass in the dominant arm of tennis and squash players. *Ann Intern Med* 123: 27-31.

Kerr D, Morton A, Dick I, Prince R. 1996. Exercise effects on bone mass in post-menopausal women are site-specific and load-dependent. *J Bone Miner Res* 11: 218-225.

Khan AA, Hodsman AB, Papaioannou A, Kendler D, Brown JP, Olszynski WP. 2007. Management of osteoporosis in men: An update and case example. *Canadian Medical Association Journal* January 30; 176.

Kohrt WM, Snead DB, Slatopolsky E, Birge SJ Jr. 1995. Additive effects of weight-bearing exercise and estrogen on bone mineral density in older women. *J Bone Miner Res* 10: 1303-1311.

Krause R, Buhring M, Hopfenmuller W, Holick MF, Sharma AM. 1998. Ultraviolet B and blood pressure. *Lancet* 352: 709-710.

Lazowski DA, Ecclestone NA, Myers AM, Paterson DH, Tudor-Locke C, Fitzgerald C, Jones G, Shima N, Cunningham DA. 1999. A randomized outcome evaluation of group exercise programs in long-term care institutions. *J Gerontol A Biol Sci Med Sci* 54: M621-628.

Lazowski DA, Hodsman AB, Helmes E. 1994. The use of postural feedback to treat thoracic kyphosis in osteoporotic women. *Phys Ther* 74: S101.

Lazowski DA, Hodsman AB, Helmes E, Howe D, Carscadden J. 1995. Thoracic kyphosis and back extensor strength in elderly osteoporotic women. *Proceedings of the 24th annual scientific and educational meeting of the Canadian Association on Gerontology,* October 26-29, Vancouver, BC, p. 101.

Lentle, BC, Brown JP, Khan A, Leslie WD, Levesque J, Lyons DJ, Siminoski K, Tarulli G, Josse RG, Hodsman AB. (2007). Recognizing and reporting vertebral fractures: Reducing the risk of future osteoporotic fractures. *Canadian Association of Radiologists Journal,* 27.

Lofman O, Berglund K, Larsson L, Toss G. 2002. Changes in hip fracture epidemiology: Redistribution between ages, genders and fracture types. *Osteoporos Int* 13: 18-25.

Lohman T, Going S, Pamenter R, Hall M, Boyden T, Houtkooper L, et al. 1995. Effect of resistance training on regional and total BMD in premenopausal women: A randomised prospective study. *J Bone Miner Res* 10: 1015-1024.

MacDougall JD, Webber CE, Martin J, Ormerod S, Chesley A, Younglai EV. 1992. Relationship among running mileage, bone density, and serum testosterone in male runners. *J Appl Physiol* 73: 1165-1170.

Melton LJ III, Atkinson EJ, Cooper C, O'Fallon WM, Riggs BL. 1999. Vertebral fractures predict subsequent fractures. *Osteoporos Int* 10: 214-221.

Merlino LA, Curtis J, Mikuls TR, Cerhan JR, Criswell LA, Saag KG. 2004. Vitamin D intake is inversely associated with rheumatoid arthritis. *Arthritis Rheum* 50: 72-77.

Nelson ME, Fiatarone MA, Morganti CM, Trice I, Greenberg RA, Evans WJ. 1994. Effects of high intensity strength training on multiple risk factors for osteoporotic fractures: A randomised controlled trial. *JAMA* 272: 1909-1913.

Nelson ME, Fisher EC, Dilmanian FA, Dallal GE, Evans WJ. 1991. A 1-year walking program and increased dietary calcium in post-menopausal women: Effects on bone. *Am J Clin Nutr* 53: 1305-1311.

Nguyen T, Sambrook P, Kelly P, Lord S, Freund J, Eisman J. 1993. Prediction of osteoporotic fractures by postural instability and BMD. *Brit Med J* 307: 1111-1115.

Parfitt AM. 1996. Skeletal heterogeneity and the purposes of bone remodeling. In *Osteoporosis.* New York: Academic Press, pp. 315-329.

Prince RL, Smith M, Dick IM, Price RI, Webb PG, Henderson NK, et al. 1991. Prevention of post-menopausal osteoporosis. A comparative study of exercise, calcium supplementation, and hormone-replacement therapy. *N Engl J Med* 32517: 1189-1195.

Rikli R, Busch S. 1986. Motor performance of women as a function of age and physical activity level. *J Gerontol* 41: 645-649.

Rikli R, McManus BG. 1990. Effects of exercise on bone mineral content in post-menopausal women. *Res Quart Exerc Sport* 61: 243-249.

Rosen CJ, Glowacki J, Bilezikian JP (Eds.). 1999. *The aging skeleton.* New York: Academic Press.

Rostand SG. 1979. Ultraviolet light may contribute to geographic and racial blood pressure differences. *Hypertension* 30: 150-156.

Seeman E. 2002. Pathogenesis of bone fragility in women and men. *Lancet* 25(359) 1841-1850.

Simmons V, Hansen PD. 1996. Effectiveness of water exercise on postural mobility in the well elderly: An experimental study on balance enhancement. *J Gerontol* 51A: M233-M238.

Sinaki M, Wahner HW, Offord KP, Hodgson SF. 1989. Efficacy of non-loading exercises in prevention of vertebral bone loss in postmenopausal women: A controlled trial. *Mayo Clin Proc* 64: 762-769.

Smith EL, Gilligan C, Shea MM, Ensign CP, Smith PE. 1989. Exercise reduces bone involution in middle aged women. *Calcif Tissue Int* 44: 312-321.

Snow-Harter C, Bouxsein ML, Lewis BT, Carter DR, Marcus R. 1992. Effects of resistance training and endurance exercise on bone mineral status of young women: A randomised exercise intervention trial. *J Bone Miner Res* 7: 761-769.

Specker BL. 1996. Evidence for an interaction between calcium intake and physical activity on changes in bone mineral density. *J Bone Miner Res* 11: 1539-1544.

Tangpricha V, Turner A, Spina C, Decastro S, Chen T, Holick MF. 2004. Tanning is associated with optimal vitamin D status (serum 25-hydroxyvitamin D concentration) and higher bone mineral density. *Am J Clin Nutr* 80: 1645-1649.

Webb K, Lazowski DA. 2006. *Body basics for bones: Beat osteoporosis, build better bones!* (2nd ed.). Thornburg, ON, Canada: Birchcliff.

Welten DC, Kemper HC, Post GB, Van Mechelen W, Twisk J, Lips P, Teule GJ. 1994. Weight-bearing activity during youth is a more important factor for peak bone mass than calcium intake. *J Bone Miner Res* 9: 1089-1096.

World Health Organization. 1994. Assessment of fracture risk and its application to screening for postmenopausal osteoporosis: Report of a WHO Study Group. *WHO Tech Rep Series.* Geneva: WHO.

World Health Organization. 1998. *Guidelines for preclinical evaluation and clinical trials in osteoporosis.* Geneva: WHO, p. 59.

Zittermann A, Schleithoff SS, Tenderich G, Berthold HK, Korfer R, Stehle P. 2003. Low vitamin D status: A contributing factor in the pathogenesis of congestive heart failure? *J Am Coll Cardiol* 41: 105-112.

Chapter 7

Ainsworh BE, Haskell WL, Leon AS, Jacobs DR, Montoye HJ, Sallis JF, Paffenbarger RS. 1993. Compendium of physical activities: Classification of energy costs of human physical activities. *Med Sci Sports Exerc.* 25 (1): 71-80.

American College of Sports Medicine. 2005. *ACSM's guidelines for exercise testing and prescription* (7th ed.). Philadelphia: Lippincott, Williams & Wilkins.

American College of Sports Medicine. 2001. *ACSM's resource manual for guidelines for exercise testing and prescription* (4th ed.). Philadelphia: Lippincott, Williams & Wilkins.

American Thoracic Society. 2002. ATS statement: Guidelines for the six-minute walk test. *American Journal of Respiratory and Critical Care Medicine* 166: 111-117.

Baker MK, Kennedy DL, Bohle PL, Campbell DS, Knapman L, Grady J, Wiltshire J, McNamara M, Evans WJ, Atlantis E, Fiatarone Singh MA. 2007. *Journal of the American Geriatricts Society* 55 (1): 1-10.

Berg KO, Wood-Dauphinee SL, Williams JI, Maki B. 1992. Measuring balance in the elderly: Validation of an instrument. *Canadian Journal of Public Health* 83(Suppl 2): S7-S11.

Berg KO, Wood-Dauphinee SL, Williams JI, Gayton D. 1989. Measuring balance in the elderly: Preliminary development of an instrument. *Physiotherapy Canada* 41 (6): 304-311.

Borg G. 1998. *Borg's rating of perceived exertion and pain scales.* Champaign, IL: Human Kinetics.

Brandon LJ, Boyette LW, Lloyd A, Gaasch DA. 2004. Resistive training and long-term function in older adults. *Journal of Aging and Physical Activity* 12: 10-28.

Bruce DG, Devine A, Prince RL. 2002. Recreational physical activity levels in healthy older women: The importance of fear of falling. *Journal of the American Geriatrics Society* 50 (1): 84-89.

Bryant CX, Peterson JA, Graves JE. 2001. Muscular strength and endurance. In Darcy P (Ed.), *ACSM's resource manual for guidelines for exercise testing and prescription* (4th ed.). Champaign, IL: Human Kinetics, chapter 53, pp. 460-467.

Butland RJA, Pang J, Gross ER, Woodcock AA, Geddes DM. 1982. Two-, six-, and 12-minute walking tests in respiratory disease. *British Medical Journal* 284: 1607-1608.

Canadian Centre for Activity and Aging. www.ccaa-outreach.com/show_course. php?coursetypeid=1.

Canadian Society for Exercise Physiology. www.csep.ca/forms.asp.

Carriere Y, Jenkins E, Gupta N, Legare J. 1996. The needs for home care services for the elderly in a context of population aging. *Facts and Research in Gerontology Home Care*, 31-52.

Chang M, Cohen-Mansfield J, Ferrucci L, Leveille S, Volpato S, de Rekeneire N, Guralnik JM. 2004. Incidence of loss of ability to walk 400 meters in a functionally limited older population. *Journal of the American Geriatrics Society* 52: 2094-2098.

College of Physiotherapists of Ontario. 2004. *Professional Portfolio Guide*, p. 14.

Collette M, Godin G, Bradet R, Gionet NJ. 1994. Active living in communities: Understanding the intention to take up physical activity as an everyday way of life. *Canadian Journal of Public Health* 85 (6): 418-421.

Connelly DM. 2000. Resisted exercise training of institutionalized older adults for improved strength and functional mobility: A review. *Topics in Geriatric Rehabilitation* 15 (3): 6-28.

Connelly DM, Stevenson TJ, Vandervoort AA. 1996. Between- and within-rater reliability of walking tests in a frail elderly population. *Physiotherapy Canada* 48: 47-51.

Connelly DM, Vandervoort AA. 1995. Improvement in knee extensor strength of institutionalized elderly women after exercise with ankle weights. *Physiotherapy Canada* 47 (1): 15-23.

Dipietro L, Caspersen CJ, Ostfeld AM, Nadel ER. 1993. A survey for assessing physical activity among older adults. *Medicine and Science in Sports and Exercise* 25: 628-642.

Durstine JL, Moore GE. 2003. *ACSM's exercise management for persons with chronic disease and disabilities* (2nd ed.). Champaign, IL: Human Kinetics.

Federici A, Bellaqamba S, Rocchi MB. 2005. Does dance-based training improve balance in adult and young old subjects? A pilot randomized controlled trial. *Aging Clinical and Experimental Research* 17 (5): 385-389.

Folstein M, Folstein SE, McHugh PR. 1975. Mini-Mental State: A practical method for grading the cognitive state of patients for the clinician. *Journal of Psychiatric Research* 12: 189-198.

Gillespie LD, Gillespie WJ, Cumming R, Lam SE, Rowe BH, 1998. Interventions to reduce the incidence of falling in the elderly (Cochrane review). In: The Cochrane Library, Issue 4, Oxford: Update Software.

Gowland C, Gambarotto C. 1994. Assessment and treatment of physical impairment leading to physical disability after brain injury. In Finlayson MAJ and Garner SH (Eds.), *Brain injury rehabilitation: Clinical considerations*. Baltimore: Williams & Wilkins, pp. 103-108.

Hardman AE. 2001. Issues of fractionization of exercise (short vs long bouts). *Medicine and Science in Sports and Exercise* 33(6 Suppl): S421-427; discussion S452-453.

Hippocrates. 400 BCE. *Of the epidemics*. Book I. Translated by F. Adams. http://etext.library.adelaide.edu.au/mirror/classics.mit.edu/Hippocrates/epidemics.html.

http://walking.about.com/cs/fitnesswalking/a/hearttrainig_2.htm.

International Curriculum Guidelines for Preparing Instructors of Older Adults. www.seniorfitness.net/international_curriculum_guidelines_for_preparing_physical_activity_instructors_of_older_adults.htm.

Jones GJ, Rose DJ (Eds.). 2005. *Physical activity instruction of older adults.* Champaign, IL: Human Kinetics.

Karvonen J, Vuorimaa T. 1988. Heart rate and exercise intensity during sports activities. Practical application. *Sports Medicine* 5: 303-311.

Lachenmayr S, Mackenzie G. 2004. Building a foundation for systems change: Increasing access to physical activity programs for older adults. *Health Promotion Practice* 5: 451-458.

Lawlor DA, Taylor M, Bedford C, Ebrahim S. 2002. Is housework good for health? Levels of physical activity and factors associated with activity in elderly women. Results from the British Women's Heart and Health Study. *Journal of Epidemiology and Community Healthy* 56 (6): 473-478.

Lawton MP, Brody EM. 1969. Assessment of older people: Self-maintaining and instrumental activities of daily living. *Gerontologist* 9: 179-186.

Lees FD, Clark PG, Nigg CR, Newman P. 2005. Barriers to exercise behavior among older adults: A focus-group study. *Journal of Aging and Physical Activity* 13 (1): 23-33.

Li F, Fisher, KJ, Harmer P, McAuley E, Wilson, NL. 2003. Fear of falling in elderly persons: Association with falls, functional ability, and quality of life. *Journal of Gerontology: Psychological Sciences* 58B (5): 283-290.

Li F, Harmer P, Fisher KJ, McAuley E. 2004. Tai Chi: Improving functional balance and predicting subsequent falls in older persons. *Medicine in Science and Sports and Exercise* 36 (12): 2046-2052.

Mahoney FI, Barthel D. 1965. Functional evaluation: The Barthel index. *Maryland State Medical Journal* 14: 56-61.

Mazzeo RS, Cavanagh P, Evans WJ, Fiatarone M, Hagberg J, McAuley E, Startzell J. 1998. American College of Sports Medicine position stand. Exercise and physical activity for older adults. *Medicine and Science in Sports and Exercise* 30: 992-1008.

Meyer P. http://www.topachievement.com/smart.html.

Persinger R, Foster C, Gibson M, Fater DCW, Porcari JP. 2004. Consistency of the talk test for exercise prescription. *Medicine and Science in Sports and Exercise* 36 (9): 1632-1636.

Pescatello LS, Murphy D, Costanzo D. 2000. Low-intensity physical activity benefits blood lipids and lipoproteins in older adults living at home. *Age and Ageing* 29: 433-439.

Podsiadlo D, Richardson S. 1991. The timed "up & go": A test of basic functional mobility for frail elderly persons. *Journal of the American Geriatrics Society* 39: 142-148.

Prochaska JO, DiClemente CC. 1982. Transtheoretical therapy toward a more integrative model of change. *Psychotherapy: Theory, Research and Practice* 19 (3): 276-287.

Rikli RE, Jones CJ. 1997. Assessing physical performance in independent older adults: Issues and guidelines. *Journal of Aging and Physical Activity* 5: 244-261.

Rikli RE, Jones CJ. 1999. Functional fitness normative scores for community-residing older adults, ages 60-94. *Journal of Aging and Physical Activity* 7: 162-181.

Rikli RE, Jones CJ. 2001. *Senior fitness test manual.* Champaign, IL: Human Kinetics.

Rose DJ. 2003. *Fallproof: A comprehensive balance and mobility program.* Champaign, IL: Human Kinetics.

Sayers SP, Jette AM, Haley SM, Heeren TC, Guralnik JM, Fielding RA. 2004. Validation of the late-life function and disability instrument. *Journal of the American Geriatrics Society* 52: 1554-1559.

Shephard RJ. 1997. What is the optimal type of physical activity to enhance health? *British Journal of Sports Medicine* 31: 277-284.

Shigematsu R, Okura T. 2006. A novel exercise for improving lower-extremity functional fitness in the elderly. *Aging Clinical and Experimental Research* 18 (3). 242-248.

Shigematsu R, Ueno LM, Nakagaichi M, Nho H, Tanaka K. 2004. Rate of perceived exertion as a tool to monitor cycling exercise intensity in older adults. *Journal of Aging and Physical Activity* 12: 3-9.

Skinner JS. (Ed.). 1993. *Exercise testing and exercise prescription for special cases: Theoretical basis and clinical application.* Philadelphia: Lippincott, Williams & Wilkins.

Steffen TM, Hacker TA, Mollinger L. 2002. Age- and gender-related test performance in community-dwelling elderly people: Six-minute walk test, Berg balance scale, timed up & go test and gait speeds. *Physical Therapy* 82: 128-137.

Tanaka H, Monahan KD, Seals DR. 2001. Age-predicted maximal heart rate revisited. *Journal of the American College of Cardiology* 37: 153-156.

Thomas SG. 1995. Exercise and activity programmes. In Pickles B, Compton A, Cott C, Simpson J, Vandervoort A (Eds.), *Physiotherapy with older people.* London, UK: Saunders, chapter 12, pp. 148-170.

Washburn RA, Smith KW, Jette AM, Janney CA. 1993. The Physical Activity Scale for the Elderly (PASE): Development and evaluation. *Journal of Clinical Epidemiology* 46: 153-162.

Webb K, Laxowski D. 1998. Body basics for bones. Thornbury, ON: Birchcliff Publishing.

Webb K, Lazowski DA, 2001. Body Basics for Bones: Beat Osteoporosis, Build Better Bones! (1st ed.) Thonrburg, ON, Canada: Birchcliff.

www.hc-sc.gc.ca/hc-cs/media/nr-cp_e.html.

Chapter 8

American College of Sports Medicine. 2000. *Guidelines for exercise testing and prescription* (6th ed.). Baltimore: Lippincott, Williams & Wilkins.

American College of Sports Medicine. 1998a. ACSM position stand on the recommended quantity and quality of exercise for developing and maintaining cardiorespiratory and muscular fitness, and flexibility in healthy adults. *Medicine and Science in Sports and Exercise* 30: 975-991.

American College of Sports Medicine. 1998b. Position stand on exercise and physical activity in older adults. *Medicine and Science in Sports and Exercise* 30: 992-1008.

Benyo R. 1998. *Running past 50.* Champaign, IL: Human Kinetics.

Billat LV. 2001a. Interval training for performance: A scientific and empirical practice. Special recommendations for middle and long-distance running. Part I: Aerobic interval training. *Sports Medicine* 31: 13-31.

Billat LV. 2001b. Interval training for performance: A scientific and empirical practice. Special recommendations for middle and long-distance running. Part II: Anaerobic interval training. *Sports Medicine* 31: 75-90.

Binder EF, Birge SJ, Spina R, Ehsani AA, Brown M, Sinacore DR, Kohrt WM. 1999. Peak aerobic power is an important component of physical performance in older women. *Journals of Gerontology* 54A: M353-356.

Bonnefoy M, Kostka T, Arsac LM, Berthouze SE, Lacour JR. 1998. Peak anaerobic power in elderly men. *European Journal of Applied Physiology* 77: 182-188.

Borg GV. 1998. *Borg's perceived exertion and pain scales.* Champaign, IL: Human Kinetics.

Cahill BR, Misner JE, Boileau RA. 1997. The clinical importance of the anaerobic energy system and its assessment in human performance. *American Journal of Sports Medicine* 25: 863-872.

Charmari K, Ahmaidi S, Fabre C, Massé-Biron J, Préfaut Ch. 1995. Anaerobic and aerobic peak power output and the force-velocity relationship in endurance-trained athletes: Effects of aging. *European Journal of Applied Physiology* 71: 230-234.

Doherty TJ. 2003. Invited review: Aging and sarcopenia. *Journal of Applied Physiology* 95: 1717-1727.

Evans WJ. 1999. Exercise training guidelines for the elderly. *Medicine and Science in Sports and Exercise* 31: 12-17.

Fox EL, Mathews DK, Bairstow JN. 1980. *I.T.: Interval training for lifetime fitness.* New York: Dial Press.

Friel, J. 1998. *Cycling past 50.* Champaign, IL: Human Kinetics.

Frontera WR, Hughes VA, Fielding RA, Fiatarone MA, Evans WJ, Roubenoff R. 2000. Aging of skeletal muscle: A 12-yr longitudinal study. *Journal of Applied Physiology* 88: 1321-1336.

Goldstein M, Tanner D. 1999. *Swimming past 50.* Champaign, IL: Human Kinetics.

Hawkins SA, Wiswell RA. 2003. Rate and mechanism of maximal oxygen consumption decline with aging. *Sports Medicine* 33: 877-888.

Katzel LI, Sorkin JD, Fleg JL. 2001. A comparison of longitudinal changes in aerobic fitness in older endurance athletes and sedentary men. *Journal of the American Geriatrics Society* 49: 1657-1664.

Kostka T, Bonnefoy M, Arsac LM, Berthouze SE, Belli A, Lacour JR. 1997. Habitual physical activity and peak anaerobic power in elderly women. *European Journal of Applied Physiology* 76: 81-87.

Lauretani F, Russo CR, Bandinelli S, Bartali B, Cavazzini C, Di Iorio A, Corsi AM, Rantanen T, Guralnik JM, Ferrucci L. 2003. Age-associated changes in skeletal muscles and their effect on mobility: An operational diagnosis of sarcopenia. *Journal of Applied Physiology* 95: 1851-1860.

Lemura LM, Von Duvillard SP, Mookerjee S. 2000. The effects of physical training of functional capacity in adults ages 46-90: A meta-analysis. *Journal of Sports Medicine and Physical Fitness* 40: 1-10.

Lexell J, Taylor CC, Sjostrom M. 1988. What is the cause of the aging atrophy? Total number, size and proportion of different fiber types studied in whole vastus lateralis muscle from 15- to 83-year-old men. *Journal of Neurological Sciences* 84: 275-294.

Malbut KE, Dinan S, Young A. 2002. Aerobic training in the "oldest old": The effect of 24 weeks of training. *Age and Ageing* 31: 255-260.

Metter EJ, Conwit R, Tobin J, Fozard JL. 1997. Age-associated loss of power and strength in the upper extremities in women and men. *Journals of Gerontology: Biological Sciences* 2: B267-276.

Mitchell TL, Gibbons LW, Devers SM, Earnest CP. 2004. Effects of cardiorespiratory fitness on healthcare utilization. *Medicine and Science in Sports and Exercise* 36(12): 2088-2092.

Moreland JD, Richardson JA, Goldsmith CH, Clase CM. 2004. Muscle weakness and falls in older adults: A systematic review and meta-analysis. *Journal of the American Geriatrics Society* 52: 1121-1129.

Pate RR, Pratt M, Blair SN, Haskell WL, Macera CA, Bouchard C, Buchner D, Ettinger W, Heath GW, King AC, et al. 1995. Physical activity and public health. A recommendation from the Centers for Disease Control and Prevention and the American College of Sports Medicine. *Journal of the American Medical Association* 273: 402-407.

Paterson DH, Govindasamy D, Vidmar M, Cunningham DA, Koval JJ. 2004. Longitudinal study of determinants of dependence in an elderly population. *Journal of the American Geriatrics Society* 52: 632-638.

Pollock ML, Mengelkoch LJ, Graves JE, Lowenthal DT, Limacher MC, Foster C, Wilmore JH. 1997. Twenty-year follow-up of aerobic power and body composition of older track athletes. *Journal of Applied Physiology* 82: 1508-1516.

Posner JD, McCully KK, Landsberg LA, Sands LP, Tycenski P, Hofmann MT, Wetterholt KL, Shaw CE. 1995. Physical determinants of independence in mature women. *Archives of Physical Medicine and Rehabilitation* 76: 373-380.

Ramsbottom R, Ambler A, Potter J, Jordan B, Nevill A, Williams C. 2004. The effect of 6 months training on leg power, balance, and functional mobility of independently living adults over 70 years old. *Journal of Aging and Physical Activity* 12: 497-510.

Rogers MA, Wernicki PG, Shamoo AE. 2000. *Sports medicine for coaches and athletes: Older individuals and athletes over 50.* Malaysia: Harwood Academic.

Shephard RJ. 1987. *Physical activity and aging.* Rockville, MD: Aspen.

Shephard RJ. 1993. Exercise and aging: Extending independence in older adults. *Geriatrics* 48: 61-64.

Swain DP, Leutholtz BC. 2002. *Exercise prescription.* Champaign, IL: Human Kinetics.

Tanaka H, Monahan KD, Seals DR. 2001. Age-predicted maximal heart rate revisited. *Journal of the American College of Cardiology* 37: 153-156.

Weiss JP, Froelicher VF, Myers JN, Heidenreich PA. 2004. Health-care costs and exercise capacity. *Chest* 126: 608-613.

Williams GN, Higgins MJ, Lewek MD. 2002. Aging skeletal muscle: Physiologic changes and the effects of training. *Physical Therapy* 82: 62-68.

Chapter 9

Abernethy, P.J., and B.M. Quigley. 1993. Concurrent strength and endurance training of the elbow extensors. *J Strength Cond Res* 7: 234-240.

Adams, R., C. Craig, J. Gordon, B. Harwood, B. Hearst, A.W. Taylor, B. Taylor, A. Nikolai, and M. Wilson. 1999. *Canada's physical activity guide to healthy active living for older adults handbook.* Ottawa: Health Canada, 1999.

Bell, G.J., G.D. Snydmiller, J.P. Neary, and H.A. Quinney. 1989. The effect of high and low velocity resistance training on anaerobic power output in cyclists. *J Hum Mov Std* 16: 173-181.

Centers for Disease Control and Prevention. 2004. Strength training among adults aged ≥ 65 years—United States, 2001. *Morb Mortal Wkly Rep* 53(2): 25-28.

Connelly, D.M., and A.A. Vandervoort. 1997. Effects of detraining on knee extensor strength and functional mobility in a group of elderly women. *J Orthop Sports Phys Ther* 25: 340-346.

Doherty, T.J. 2003. Invited review: Aging and sarcopenia. *J Appl Physiol* 95: 1717-1727.

Dudley, G.A., and S.J. Fleck. 1987. Strength and endurance training. Are they mutually exclusive? *Sports Med* 4: 79-85.

Fiatarone, M.A., E.C. Marks, N.D. Ryan, C.N. Meredith, L.A. Lipsitz, and W.J. Evans. 1990. High-intensity strength training in nonagenarians: Effects on skeletal muscle. *JAMA* 263: 3029-3034.

Frontera W.R., C.N. Meredith, K.P. O'Reilly, H.G. Knuttgen, and W.J. Evans. 1988. Strength conditioning in older men: Skeletal muscle hypertrophy and improved function. *J Appl Physiol* 68: 1038-1044.

Hickson, R.C. 1980. Interference of strength development by simultaneously training for strength and endurance. *Eur J Appl Physiol* 45: 255-263.

Hunter, G., R. Demment, and D. Miller. 1987. Development of strength and maximum oxygen uptake during simultaneous training for strength and endurance. *J Sports Med Phys Fitness* 27: 269-275.

Izquierdo, M., J. Ibanez, K. Hakkinen, W.J. Kraemer, J.L. Larrion, and E.M. Gorostiaga. 2004. Once weekly combined resistance and cardiovascular training in healthy older men. *Med Sci Sports Exerc* 36: 435-443.

Kraemer, W.J., K. Adams, E. Cafarelli, G.A. Dudley, C. Dooly, M.S. Feigenbaum, S.J. Fleck, B. Franklin, A.C. Fry, J.R. Hoffman, R.U. Newton, J. Potteiger, M.H. Stone, N.A. Ratamess, and T. Triplett-McBride. 2002. American College of Sports Medicine position stand. Progression models in resistance training for healthy adults. *Med Sci Sports Exerc* 34: 364-380.

Latham, N.K., D.A. Bennett, C.M. Stretton, and C.S. Anderson. 2004. Systematic review of progressive resistance strength training in older adults. *J Gerontol: Med Sci* 59: 48-61.

Lexell, J., and A.A. Vandervoort. 2002. Age-related changes in the neuromuscular system. In W.F. Brown, C.F. Bolton, and M.J. Aminoff (Eds.), *Clinical neurophysiology and neuromuscular disease.* Philadelphia: Saunders.

Marcinik, E.J., J. Potts, G. Schlabach, S. Will, P. Dawson, and B.F. Hurley. 1991. Effects of strength training on lactate threshold and endurance performance. *Med Sci Sports Exerc* 23: 739-743.

Mazzeo, R.S., P. Cavanagh, W.J. Evans, M. Fiatarone, J. Hagberg, E. McAuley, and J. Startzell. 1998. American College of Sports Medicine position stand. Exercise and physical activity for older adults. *Med Sci Sports Exerc* 30: 992-1008.

Mazzeo, R.S., and H. Tanaka. 2001. Exercise prescription for the elderly: Current recommendations. *Sports Med* 31: 809-818.

McCartney, N., A.L. Hicks, J. Martin, and C.E. Webber. 1996. A longitudinal trial of weight training in the elderly: Continued improvements in year 2. *J Gerontol A Biol Sci Med Sci* 51: B425-B433.

McCarthy, J.P., M.A. Pozniak, and J.C. Agre. 2002. Neuromuscular adaptations to concurrent strength and endurance training. *Med Sci Sports Exerc* 34: 511-519.

Porter, M.M., A.A. Vandervoort, and J.F. Kramer. 1997. Eccentric peak torque of plantar and dorsiflexors is maintained in older women. *J Gerontol A Biol Sci Med Sci* 52: 125-131.

Sale, D.G., J.D. MacDougall, I. Jacobs, and S. Garner. 1990. Interaction between concurrent strength and endurance training. *J Appl Physiol* 68: 260-270.

Sale, D.G., and L.L. Spriet. 1996. Skeletal muscle metabolism and energy. In O. Bar-Or, D.R. Lamb, and P.M. Clarkson (Eds.), *Perspectives in exercise science and sports medicine.* Volume 9: *Exercise and the female—a lifespan approach.* Carmel, IN: Cooper, pp. 289-359.

Seynnes, O., M. Fiatarone, M.A. Singh, O. Hue, P. Pras, P. Legros, and P.L. Bernard. 2004. Physiological and functional responses to low-moderate versus high-intensity progressive resistance training in frail elders. *J Gerontol: Med Sci* 59: 503-509.

Tracy, B.L., F.M. Ivey, D. Hurlbut, G.F. Martel, J.T. Lemmer, E.L. Siegel, E.J. Metter, J.L. Fozard, J.L. Fleg, and B.F. Hurley. 1999. Muscle quality. II. Effects of strength training in 65- to 75-yr-old men and women. *J Appl Physiol* 86: 195-201.

Vandervoort, A.A., and A.J. McComas. 1986. Contractile changes in opposing muscles of the human ankle joint with aging. *J Appl Physiol* 61: 361-367.

Wood, R.H., R. Reyes, M.A. Welsch, J. Favaloro-Sabatier, M. Sabatier, L.C. Matthew, L.G. Johnson, and P.F. Hooper. 2001. Concurrent cardiovascular and resistance training in healthy older adults. *Med Sci Sports Exerc* 33: 1751-1758.

Chapter 10

Canadian Centre for Activity and Aging. 1994. *Senior fitness instructor's course.* London, Canada: CCAA Press.

Courneya, K.S., J.K. Vallance, M.L. McNeely, K.H. Karvinen, C.J. Peddle, and J.R. Mackey. 2004. Exercise issues in older cancer survivors. *Critical Reviews in Oncological Hematology* 51: 249-261.

Dean, E. 1994. Cardiopulmonary development. In B.R. Bonder and M.B. Wagner (Eds.), *Functional performance in older adults.* Philadelphia: Davis.

Kallinen, M., and A. Markku. 1995. Aging, physical, and sports injuries. An overview of common sports injuries in the elderly. *Sports Medicine* 20: 41-52.

Mazzeo, R.S., P. Cavanaugh, W.J. Evans, M. Fiatarone, J. Hagberg, E. McAuley, and J. Startzell. 1998. American College of Sports Medicine position stand: Exercise and physical activity for older adults. *Medicine and Science in Sports and Exercise* 30: 992-1008.

Mazzeo, R.S., and H. Tanaka. 2001. Exercise prescription for the elderly: Current recommendations. *Sports Medicine* 31: 809-818.

McAuley, E., G.J. Jerome, S. Elavsky, D.X. Marquez, and S.N. Ramsey. 2003. Predicting long-term maintenance of physical activity in older adults. *Preventive Medicine* 27: 110-118.

National Advisory Council on Aging. 2001. *Seniors in Canada: A report card.* Ottawa, ON: Government of Canada.

O'Grady, M., J. Fletcher, and S. Ortiz. 2000. Therapeutic and physical fitness exercise prescription for older adults with joint disease: An evidence-based approach. *Rheumatic Diseases Clinics of North America* 26: 617-646.

Oka, R.K., A.C. King, and D.R. Young. 1995. Sources of social support as predictors of exercise adherence in women and men ages 50 to 65 years. *Women's Health* 1: 161-175.

Rhodes, R.E., A.D. Martin, and J.E. Taunton. 2001. Temporal relationships of self-efficacy and social support as predictors of adherence in a six-month strength-training program for older women. *Perceptual and Motor Skills* 93: 693-703.

Watson, D.L., and R.G. Tharpe. 1997. *Self-directed behavior: Self-modification for personal adjustment* (7th ed.). Pacific Grove, CA: Brooks/Cole.

Williams, P., and S.R. Lord. 1995. Predictors of adherence to a structured exercise program for older women. *Psychological Aging* 10: 617-624.

Young, A. 1997. Ageing and physiological functions. *Philosophical Transactions of the Royal Society of London, B, Biological Sciences* 352: 1837-1843.

Chapter 11

Ballantyne, C.S., S.M. Phillips, J.R. MacDonald, M.A. Tarnopolsky, and J.D. MacDougall. 2000. The acute effects of androstenedione supplementation in healthy young males. *Canadian Journal of Applied Physiology* 25: 68-78.

Balsom, P.D., S.D. Harridge, and K. Soderlund. 1993. Creatine supplementation per se does not enhance endurance exercise performance. *Acta Physiologica Scandinavica* 149: 521-523.

Bermon, S., P. Venembre, C. Sachet, S. Valour, and C. Dolisi. 1998. Effects of creatine monohydrate ingestion in sedentary and weight-trained older adults. *Acta Physiologica Scandinavica* 164: 147-155.

Bhasin, S., T.W. Storer, N. Berman, C. Callegari, B. Clevenger, J. Phillips, T.J. Bunnell, R. Tricker, A. Shirazi, and R. Casaburi. 1996. The effects of supraphysiologic doses of testosterone on muscle size and strength in normal men. *New England Journal of Medicine* 335: 1-7.

Blackman, M.R., J.D. Sorkin, T. Munzer, M.F. Bellatoni, J. Busby-Whitehead, T.E. Stevens, J. Jayme, K.G. O'Connor, C. Christmas, J.D. Tobin, K.J. Srewart, E. Cottrell, C. St. Clair, K.M. Pabst, and S.M. Harman. 2002. Growth hormone and sex hormone administration in healthy aged women and men: A randomized controlled trial. *Journal of the American Medical Association* 288: 2282-2292.

Brown, G.A., M.D. Vukovich, E.R. Martini, M.L. Kohut, W.D. Franke, D.A. Jackson, and D.S. King. 2000. Endocrine response to chronic androstenedione intake in 30-to-56-year-old men. *Journal of Clinical Endocrinology and Metabolism* 85: 4074-4080.

Catlin, D.H., and T.H. Murray. 1996. Performance-enhancing drugs, fair competition, and Olympic sport. *Journal of the American Medical Association* 276: 231-237.

Catlin, D., J. Wright, and H. Pope, Jr, 1993. Assessing the threat of anabolic steroids. *Physician and Sportsmedicine* 21: 37-44.

Chick, T.W., A.K. Halperin, and E.M. Gacek. 1988. The effect of antihypertensive medications on exercise performance: A review. *Medicine and Science in Sports and Exercise* 20: 447-454.

Cohen, J.C., and R. Hickman. 1987. Insulin resistance and diminished glucose tolerance in power lifters ingesting anabolic steroids. *Journal of Clinical and Endocrinological Metabolism* 64: 960-963.

Dziepak, T. 1999, November (revised February 2002). Future doping protocol. www.geocities.com/Colosseum/8682/doping.htm.

Eichner, R.E. 1997. Ergogenic aids: What athletes are using—and why. *Physician and Sportsmedicine* 25: 70.

Gifford, R.W. 1997. Antihypertensive therapy. Angiotensin-converting enzyme inhibitors, angiotensin II receptor antagonists, and calcium antagonists. *Medical Clinics of North America* 81: 1319-1333.

Gifford, R.W., Jr., W. Kirkendall, D.T. O'Connor, and W. Weidman. 1989. Office evaluation of hypertension. A statement for health professionals by a writing group of the Council for High Blood Pressure Research, American Heart Association. *Circulation* 79: 721-731.

Fuentes, R.J., and J.M. Rosenberg. 1999. *Athletic drug reference '99: Complies with NCAA and USCO rules.* Durham, NC: Glaxco Wellcome, pp. 28-36, 52-54, 317-408.

Gaie, M. 1996. Olympic athletes face heat, other health hurdles. *Journal of the American Medical Association* 276: 178-180.

Graham, T.E. 2001. Caffeine and exercise: Metabolism, endurance and performance. *Sports Medicine* 31: 785-807.

Graham, T.E., and L.L. Spriet. 1996. Caffeine and exercise performance. *Sports Science Exchange* 9: 1-6.

Gray, A., H.A. Feldman, J.B. McKinley, and C. Loncope. 1991. Age, disease, changing sex hormone levels in middle-aged men: Results of the Massachusetts Male Aging Study. *Journal of Clinical Endocrinological Metabolism* 73: 1016-1025.

Green, A.L., E.J. Simpson, and J.J. Littlewood. 1996. Carbohydrate ingestion augments retention during creatine feeding in humans. *Acta Physiologica Scandinavica* 158: 195-202.

Greenhaff, P.L. 1997. The nutritional biochemistry of creatine. *Journal of Nutrition and Biochemistry* 8: 610-618.

Greenhaff, P.L., A. Casey, and A.H. Short. 1993. Influence of oral creatine supplementation on muscle torque during repeated bouts of maximal voluntary exercise in men. *Clinical Science* 84: 565-571.

Hartgens, K., and H. Kuipers. 2004. Effects of androgenic-anabolic steroids in athletes. *Sports Medicine* 34: 513-554.

Heath, G.W., J.M. Hagberg, A.A. Ehsani, and J.O. Holloszy. 1981. A physiological comparison of young and older endurance athletes. *Journal of Applied Physiology* 51: 634-640.

Hernelahti, M., U.M. Kujala, J. Kaprio, J. Karjalainen, and S. Sarna. 1998. Hypertension in master endurance athletes. *Journal of Hypertension* 16: 1573-1577.

Hultman, E., K. Soderlund, J.A. Timmons, G. Cederblad, and P.L. Greenhaff. 1996. Muscle creatine loading in man. *Journal of Applied Physiology* 81: 232-237.

Jin, B., L. Turner, W.A.W. Walters, and D.J. Handelsman. 1996. Androgen or estrogen effects on human prostate. *Journal of Clinical and Endocrinological Metabolism* 81: 4290-4295.

Johnson, K.A., M.A. Bernard, and K. Funderburg. 2002. Vitamin nutrition in older adults. *Clinical Geriatric Medicine* 18: 773-799.

Joint National Committee on Prevention, Detection, Evaluation, and Treatment of High Blood Pressure. 1997. The sixth report of the Joint National Committee on Prevention, Detection, Evaluation, and Treatment of High Blood Pressure. *Archives of Internal Medicine* 157: 2413-2446.

Julius, S., and S. Nesbitt. 1996. Sympathetic overactivity in hypertension: A moving target. *American Journal of Hypertension* 9: S113-S120.

Kelly, G.S. 1998. The role of glucosamine sulfate and chondroitin sulfates in the treatment of degenerative joint disease. *Alternative Medicine Reviews* 3: 27-39.

Leffler, C.T., A.F. Philippi, S.G. Leffler, J.C. Mosure, and P.D. Kim. 1999. Glucosamine, chondroitin, and manganese ascorbate for degenerative joint disease of the knee or low back: A randomized, double-blind, placebo-controlled pilot study. *Military Medicine* 164: 85-91.

Maharam, L.G., P.A. Bauman, D. Kalman, H. Skolnik, and S.M. Perle. 1999. Masters athletes: Factors affecting performance. *Sports Medicine* 28: 273-285.

Martineau, L., M.A. Horan, N.J. Rothwell, and R.A. Little. 1992. Salbutamol, a beta-2-adrenoceptor agonist, increases skeletal muscle strength in young men. *Clinical Science* 83: 615-621.

Morreale, P., R. Manopulo, M. Galati, L. Boccanera, G. Saponati, and L. Bocchi. 1996. Comparison of the antiinflammatory efficacy of chondroitin sulfate and diclofenac sodium in patients with knee osteoarthritis. *Journal of Rheumatology* 23: 1385-1391.

Morton, A.R., K. Joyce, S.M. Papalia, N.G. Carroll, and K.D. Fitch. 1996. Is salmeterol ergogenic? *Clinical Journal of Sports Medicine* 6: 220-225.

Muller-Fassbender, H., G.L. Bach, W. Haase, L.C. Rovati, and I. Setnikar. 1994. Glucosamine sulfate compared to ibuprofen in osteoarthritis of the knee. *Osteoarthritis Cartilage* 2: 61-69.

Nativ, A., and J. Puffer. 1991. Lifestyles and health risks in collegiate athletes. *Journal of Family Practice* 33: 585-590.

Nieldfieldt, M.W. 2002. Managing hypertension in athletes and physically active patients. *American Family Physician* 66: 445-452.

Ogawa, T., R.J. Spina, W.H. Martin, V.M. Kohrt, K.B. Schechtman, J.O. Holloszy, and A.A. Ahsani. 1992. Effects of aging, sex, and physical training on cardiovascular responses to exercise. *Circulation* 86: 494-503.

Paluska, S.A. 2003. Caffeine and exercise. *Current Sports Medicine Reports* 2: 213-219.

Papadakis, M.A., D. Grady, D. Black, M.J. Tierney, G.A. Gooding, M. Schambelan, and C. Grunfeld. 1996. Growth hormone replacement in healthy older men improves body composition but not functional ability. *Annals of Internal Medicine* 126(7): 583-584.

Poortmans, J.R., and M. Francaux. 2000. Adverse effects of creatine supplementation: Fact or fiction? *Sports Medicine* 30: 155-170.

Rasmussen, B.B., E. Volpi, D.C. Gore, and R.R. Wolfe. 2000. Androstenedione does not stimulate muscle protein anabolism in young healthy men. *Journal of Clinical Endocrinological Metabolism* 85: 55-59.

Rawson, E.S., M.L. Wehnert, and P.M. Clarkson. 1999. Effects of 30 days of creatine ingestion on body mass. *European Journal of Applied Physiology* 80: 139-144.

Rennic, M.J. 2003. Claims for the anabolic effects of growth hormone: A case of the emperor's new clothes. *British Journal of Sports Medicine* 37: 100-105.

Robertson, W., J. Simkins, S.P. O'Hickey, S. Freeman, and R.M. Cayton. 1994. Does single dose salmeterol affect exercise capacity in asthmatic men. *European Respiration Journal* 7: 1978-1984.

Rock, C.L. 1991. Nutrition of the older athlete. *Clinical Sports Medicine* 10: 445-457.

Ruscin, M., and R.L. Page. 2002, May. The pros and cons of mixing medications with endurance sports. *DOPP Newsletter* 7.

Sacheck, J.M., and R. Roubenoff. 1999. Nutrition in the exercising elderly. *Clinical Sports Medicine* 18: 565-584.

Schwenk, T.L., and C.D. Costley. 2002. When food becomes a drug: Nonanabolic nutritional supplement use in athletes. *American Journal of Sports Medicine* 30: 907-916.

Smith, S.A., S.J. Mountain, R.P. Matott, G.P. Zientara, F.A. Jolesz, and R.A. Fielding. 1998. Creatine supplementation and age influence muscle metabolism during exercise. *Journal of Applied Physiology* 85: 1349-1356.

Spriet, L.L., D.A. MacLean, D.J. Dyck, E. Hultman, G. Cederblad, and T.E. Graham. 1992. Caffeine ingestion and muscle metabolism during prolonged exercise in humans. *American Journal of Physiology* 262: E891-E898.

Tarnopolsky, M.A. 2000. Potential benefits of creatine monohydrate supplementation in the elderly. *Current Opinions in Clinical and Nutritional Metabolic Care* 3: 497-502.

Terjung, R.L., P. Clarkson, E.R. Eichner, P.L. Greenhaff, P.J. Hespel, R.G. Israel, W.J. Kraemer, R.A. Meyer, L.L. Spriet, M.A. Tarnopolsky, A.J. Wagenmakers, and M.H. Williams. 2000. American College of Sports Medicine roundtable. The physiological and health effects of oral creatine supplementation. *Medicine and Science in Sports and Exercise* 32: 706-717.

Toler, S.M. 1997. Creatine is an ergogen for anaerobic exercise. *Nutrition Reviews* 55: 21-25.

Vance, M.L. 2003. Can growth hormone prevent aging? *New England Journal of Medicine* 348: 779-780.

Vandenberghe, K., N. Gillis, M. Van Leemputte, P. Van Hecke, F. Vanstapel, and P. Hespel. 1996. Caffeine counteracts the ergogenic action of muscle creatine loading. *Journal of Applied Physiology* 80: 452-457.

Vandenberghe, K., M. Goris, P. Van Hecke, M. Van Leemputte, L. Vangerven, and P. Hespel. 1997. Long-term creatine intake is beneficial to muscle performance during resistance training. *Journal of Applied Physiology* 83: 2055-2063.

Vander, A.J., J.H. Sherman, and D.S. Luciano. 1998. *Human physiology: Mechanisms of body function* (7th ed.). New York: McGraw-Hill.

Vermeulen, A., and J.M. Kaufman. 1995. Ageing of the hypothalmo-pituitary–testicular axis in men. *Hormone Research* 43: 25-28.

Voy, R., and K.D. Deeter. 1991. *Drugs, sport, and politics*. Champaign, IL: Leisure Press.

Wemyss-Holden, S.A., F.C. Hamdy, and K.J. Hastie. 1994. Steroid abuse in athletes, prostatic enlargement, and bladder outflow obstruction—is there a relationship? *British Journal of Urology* 74: 476-478.

Yarasheski, K.E., J.A. Campbell, K. Smith, M.J. Rennie, J.O. Holloszy, and D.M. Bier. 1992. Effect of growth hormone and resistance exercise on muscle growth in young men. *American Journal of Physiology* 262: E261-E267.

Yarasheski, K.E., J.J. Zachwieja, T.J. Angelopoulos, and D.M. Bier. 1993. Short-term growth hormone treatment does not increase muscle protein synthesis in experienced weight lifters. *Journal of Applied Physiology* 74: 3073-3076.

Index

Note: The letters *f* and *t* after page numbers indicate figures and tables, respectively.

About the Authors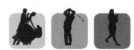

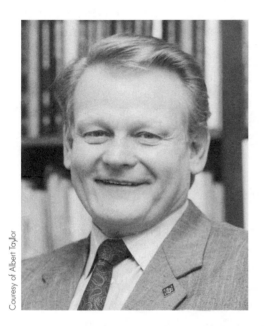

Albert W. Taylor, PhD, DSc, is a professor in the faculties of health sciences and medicine and dentistry at the University of Western Ontario in London, Ontario, Canada, where he teaches courses on healthy aging and the physiology of aging. He also researches the effects of exercise on the aging process—in particular, cancer precursors and metabolic enzyme activities. Professor Taylor has honorary appointments at the University of Toronto, Universite de Moncton, the Ukrainian State University of Physical Education and Sport and Semmelweis University of Budapest Medical University.

During his career, Taylor has published more than 300 research and professional articles, including 54 books and manuals, and made over 500 presentations to scientific and academic groups in more than 50 countries. He has served as a peer reviewer for some 30 journals and 15 granting agencies and has supervised the research of more than 165 students, many of whom now hold leadership roles as research chairs, senior university administrators, and senior scientists with world-renowned status.

In recognition of his research, Taylor has received honorary doctorates from Universite de Sherbrooke (Canada), London Institute for Applied Research (England), Semmelweis University (Hungary), and the Ukrainian State University of Physical Education and Sport (Ukraine). He also has been inducted into five halls of fame and received recognition for his contributions to sport and science. Taylor is a fellow of the American College of Sports Medicine and honorary life member of the Canadian Olympic Association. He has served as president of both the Sports Medicine and Science Council of Canada and Canadian Society of Exercise Physiology. Taylor has received the Honor Award from the Canadian Society of Exercise Physiology, a Certificate of Recognition for Contribution to Sport by the government of Ontario, and the International Wrestling Federation Pin of Merit.

Taylor received his PhD from Washington State University in 1967. Previously he was a member of the board of directors and the chair of the Canadian Centre for Activity and Aging, which is affiliated with the University of Western Ontario. He has also served as the director of the Research Institute for Aging at the University of Waterloo in Ontario, Canada.

In his free time, Taylor enjoys moose hunting, fishing, and playing duplicate bridge. He and his wife, Catherine, live in Mississauga, Ontario, Canada.

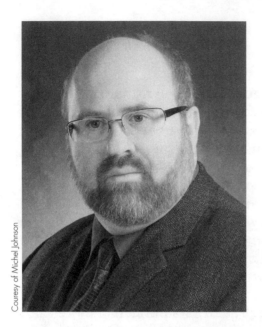

Courtesy of Michel Johnson

Michel J. Johnson, PhD, obtained his PhD from the University of Western Ontario in London, Ontario, Canada, in the area of neurovascular physiology. His current research interests include strength training, skeletal muscle metabolism, and autonomic nervous system regulation in young and older subjects. He is currently an assistant professor of kinesiology and a research member with the Interdisciplinary Research Program on Safe Driving at Lakehead University in Thunder Bay, Ontario, Canada.

Johnson is a certified weightlifting coach and personal trainer. He is a member of both the National Strength and Conditioning Association and the Canadian Society for Exercise Physiology.

In addition to teaching and developing exercise prescription and physiology of aging courses at the university level, Johnson has been a course developer in interprofessional education and health. His experience in these areas combined with more than 15 years as a strength-training consultant for national teams and coaching associations has afforded him extensive practical experience in exercise prescription with athletes and nonathletes of all ages.

Johnson lives in Thunder Bay, Ontario, with his wife, Nicole, and his son, Patrick, where he spends his free time reading, resistance training, and walking.

About the Contributors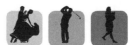

The individuals who have contributed to the writing of this book are all internationally recognized kinesiologists, physiologists, therapists, or medical practitioners who have carried out research on aging and physical activity. Among them, the authors account for more than 500 scientific publications, including more than 50 books and manuals.

Dr. Denise Connelly completed the BSc in biology, the BSc and MSc in physical therapy, and the PhD in kinesiology at the University of Western Ontario (UWO). Her doctorate was completed at the Canadian Centre for Activity and Aging, where she studied the effects of aging and exercise on community-dwelling older adults. Dr. Connelly wrote chapter 7, "A Functional Approach to Exercise." She currently is a member of the professoriate in the School of Physical Therapy at UWO.

Chapter 6, "Bone Health Osteoporosis," was contributed by Dr. Darien Lazowski-Fraher. She completed the BSc in microbiology at the University of British Columbia (UBC), the MSc in pathology (cancer research) at UBC, the PhD in pathology with a special emphasis in bone pathology and osteoporosis at the University of Western Ontario, and her BScPT—clinical degree in physiotherapy—at UWO. She currently leads the Osteoporosis Program at the Downtown Clinic in London, Ontario, Canada, and serves on the Scientific Advisory Council of the Osteoporosis Society of Canada.

Dr. Tom Overend wrote chapter 8, "Training for Aerobic and Anaerobic Fitness." He completed his BPE in physical education at the University of Alberta, the MA in physical education at the University of Western Ontario, and the PhD in kinesiology at the Canadian Centre for Activity and Aging. His PhD studies dealt with aging and aerobic capacity and power. He subsequently completed the BSc in physical therapy at UWO and is currently an associate professor at that school, with research interests in hip fracture rehabilitation and cardiorespiratory physical therapy.

Chapter 1, "Cardiopulmonary System," was written by Dr. Kevin Shoemaker. Dr. Shoemaker completed his undergraduate degree at Wilfrid Laurier University and his MSc and PhD degrees at the University of Waterloo. His dissertation research was on the dynamic control of limb blood flow at the onset of exercise in humans. Subsequently, he examined autonomic control of the circulation at the Pennsylvania State College of Medicine before accepting a position at the University of Western Ontario in the School of Kinesiology. His research interests focus on understanding the manner in which the autonomic nervous system communicates with vascular tissue to regulate blood pressure and the distribution of blood flow.

Dr. Taryn-Lise Taylor completed the BA in kinesiology and the MSc in sports medicine from the University of Western Ontario, and the MD from the University of Ottawa. She has completed her residency in family medicine and a fellowship in sports medicine and is licensed to practice in Canada and the United States. Chapter 11, "Older Athletes and Substance Abuse," is her contribution to this book.

Dr. Anthony Vandervoort coauthored with Dr. Michel Johnson chapters 3, 4, and 9 on the nervous system, sensory systems, and training for muscular fitness, respectively. He received the BSc in kinesiology from the University of Waterloo and the MSc and PhD from McMaster University in kinesiology and neuroscience, respectively. His doctoral and research work has primarily concentrated on falls and strength training in the frail elderly.